Strong Medicine

for

Step 3

Strong Medicine
for
Step 3

Joseph R. DiCostanzo, Jr., M.D.

Resident, Department of Physical Medicine and Rehabilitation
University of Kansas School of Medicine
Kansas City, Kansas

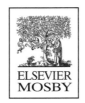

ELSEVIER
MOSBY

ELSEVIER
MOSBY

The Curtis Center
170 S Independence Mall W 300E
Philadelphia, PA 19106

Strong Medicine for Step 3   ISBN 1-56053-631-4
Copyright ©2005, Elsevier Inc. All rights reserved

Note to the reader: Although the information in this book has been carefully reviewed for correctness of dosage and indications, neither the author nor the editor nor the publisher can accept any legal responsibility for any errors or omissions that may be made. Neither the publisher nor the editor makes any warranty, expressed or implied, with respect to the material contained herein. Before prescribing any drug, the reader must review the manufacturer's current product information (package inserts) for accepted indications, absolute dosage recommendations, and other information pertinent to the safe and effective use of the product described. This is especially important when drugs are given in combination or as an adjunct to other forms of therapy.

Library of Congress Control Number: 2004112571

Acquisitions Editor: Linda Belfus
Developmental Editor: Stan Ward

Printed in the United States of America

Last digit is the print number: 9 8 7 6 5 4 3 2 1

Step 3

Contents

Chapter	Subject	Page
	About this book	vii
	Computer-based Case Simulations (CCS)	xi
1	Cardiovascular System	1
2	Dermatology	19
3	Emergency Medicine and Trauma	27
4	Endocrine and Related Issues	43
5	Gastrointestinal System	57
6	Gynecology	73
7	Health Maintenance	87
8	Hematology	97
9	Infectious Disease	109
10	Medical Law and Ethics	133
11	Men's Health	137
12	Musculoskeletal System	141
13	Neurology	157
14	Nonspecific Symptoms	173
15	Obstetrics	179
16	Ophthalmology	193
17	Otolaryngology	199
18	Psychiatry	207
19	Renal System and Urology	217
20	Respiratory System	225
21	Statistics	237
	Index	245

Reviewers

John Alley, MD
General Surgery Resident
Kansas University Medical Center
Kansas City, Kansas

Joseph R DiCostanzo Sr, ME
Dean of Mathematics
Johnson County Community College
Merriam, Kansas

Carlos Fierro, MD
Private Practice, Medicine–Pediatrics
Kansas City, Kansas

Cathy Gordon, ARNP, Certified Nurse Midwife
Private Practice, Family Practice/Women's
Health
Shawnee, Kansas

Christopher M Milford, MD
Critical Care Neurologist
Johns Hopkins University School of Medicine
Baltimore, Maryland

Cynthia Moore, ARNP
Private Practice, Family Practice/
Women's Health
Shawnee, Kansas

Pamela Ramsey, MD
Attending Physician, Emergency Medicine
Kansas University Medical Center
Kansas City, Kansas

About This Book

While preparing for the Step 3 exam, I came to the realization that very little exam preparation material was available for Step 3—unlike the vast array of review guides for Steps 1 and 2. I purchased every Step 3 review book available at the time, yet I found no single review source that covered more than 50% of the subjects tested on the exam. Even the reviews that mentioned the relevant topics did not cover their practical management, which is prominently tested on Step 3.

Thus this book was created out of necessity for my personal use in preparing for the exam. The topics on which this book is based are found in the Problem/Disease List provided by the National Board of Medical Examiners/Federation of State Medical Boards (NBME/FSMB), which can be viewed on their website. When these stated objectives were too narrow, I exercised judgment and expanded them somewhat. These topics appear to change by about 15-20% from year to year, and much of the change is in the "Ill-defined" section. Other important objectives related to statistics, law, and ethics are derived from the Step 1 and Step 2 objectives. This material is repeated throughout all three Steps of the USMLE.

From my experience taking the Step 3 exam, there were no surprises in terms of content. I thought that the test was faithful to the problem/disease list. This book focuses on these key topics and on the practical physician tasks of diagnosis and management, which are the heart of Step 3. The approach I have taken strips away all but essential information, leaves out extraneous detail, and emphasizes high-yield facts.

AUTHORS OF THE STEP 3 EXAMINATION

The Step 3 committee is made up of members who are nominated for 2- to 4-year terms. This is a prestigious appointment that pays a small honorarium. Not surprisingly, over 80% of members are MDs in academic medicine; the remaining 20% are in private practice. Members are divided into organizational groups to author the test: This may give you some idea of the emphasis in each area. Although the computer-based case simulations (CCS) are weighted currently at 25% of the score, the large group assigned to this area may be an indication of future expansion.

Committee	Contributors
Acute Care	10
Ambulatory Care	12
Chronic Illness and Ongoing Conditions	11

continued

Committee	Contributors
Community-based Care	11
Computer-based Case Simulations	38
Family in Community	10
Utilization of Resources	10

REGISTERING FOR STEP 3 USMLE

At minimum to take Step 3 you must:

1. Have officially graduated from medical school
2. Possess a medical diploma (MD or DO)
3. Have passed Steps 1 and 2

Go to the FSMB website to register online at http://www.fsmb.org

You do not have to be a resident of a state in order to be sponsored by it. This is important because many states require completion of residency training and simultaneous application for a permanent medical license. This process can be very expensive. If you were to fail the Step 3, you would lose the Step 3 fee as well as at least a portion of the permanent license application. You would also be at least 12 months into your residency.

After the processing is completed, in about 4 weeks, you will receive a scheduling permit valid for a 105-day period at Sylvan Learning Centers. You can then call and set up 2 days for the test. These days must be consecutive (e.g., Thursday and Friday); you cannot schedule a day off (e.g., Wednesday and Friday). You should expect to receive your scores in about 4 weeks.

SPECIAL PURPOSE EXAMINATON (SPEX)

The SPEX examination is given to practicing physicians who currently hold or have held unrestricted medical licenses to practice in the U.S. or Canada. A Medical Board gives this test to candidates seeking licensure reinstatement/ reactivation after a period of professional inactivity or who are undergoing disciplinary proceedings. SPEX is also given to physicians applying for licensure by endorsement who have not taken a standardized exam or specialty boards for 2-5 years.

While this book is written primary for the Step 3, you might find it helpful in preparing for the SPEX. Out of curiosity, while going through the sample questions for the SPEX, I noticed they were identical to the Step 3 sample questions. This makes sense because the SPEX is an examination of "current knowledge requisite for the general, undifferentiated practice of medicine."

SPEX focuses on clinical encounters:
- Well-care/preventive medicine
- Acute, circumscribed problems
- Ill-defined presentations or problems
- Chronic or progressive illness

- Emergency conditions and critical care
- Behavioral/emotional problems

SPEX also focuses on physician tasks:
- Data gathering
- Diagnostic assessment
- Managing therapy
- Applying scientific concepts

All of these topics are covered in the Step 3 Objectives.

RESPECT THE TEST

There is a common expression regarding preparation for USMLE: "two months, two weeks, number two pencil." This expression indicates the amount of effort that you should put into exams 1–3, respectively. I consider this approach somewhat naïve and believe that you should prepare diligently for Step 3. Many agree that Step 3 has become more difficult in recent years, including one of my attendings, who failed it on the first attempt.

You have invested a great deal of time, money, and energy into your medical education. Generally, medical boards will not allow you to receive a medical license if you have failed Step 3 more than three times. At one extreme, Alaska allows only a single attempt, while at the other extreme some states allow unlimited attempts.

If you are a foreign medical graduate you will find that successful completion of Step 3 can open up preferable Visa status and allow you to stay in the United States since you can then be fully licensed and, in some cases, sponsored for an H1B work Visa.

If you are an American or Canadian medical graduate, early completion of Step 3 can pave the way to an unrestricted medical license and allow moonlighting opportunities as an R2 or R3 that can double your income as a resident. All states require at least completion of one postgraduate year of residency and passing Step 3 to receive a full medical license. States that require at least two years include New Mexico, Illinois, Rhode Island, New Hampshire, Michigan, Washington, Massachusetts, Alaska, Kentucky, South Dakota, Connecticut, New Jersey, Pennsylvania, and the District of Columbia. Utah requires two postgraduate years but will issue a full license after one year to those who are currently in residency programs in Utah. Nevada requires three full years of residency but will issue limited rural licenses for underserved areas with completion of a postgraduate year 1. In most states foreign medical graduates are required to have completed at least two years of residency and sometime three. Some state medical boards require additional postgraduate training if you fail Step 3 even once, thus delaying the license at least another year.

Current guidelines require all three USMLE Step exams to be completed within a seven-year period. If you are an MD/PhD candidate, I suggest taking Step 3 early in your internship, since you will already be nearing the seven-year limit for completion of all three steps. Only a few states make exceptions for the medical scientist or MD/PhD.

Computer-based Case Simulations

GENERAL GUIDELINES

The computer-based case simulation (CCS) format is unique to Step 3. This section of the exam is currently worth 25% of the total score, but it is rumored that eventually it will increase to 75%, although I could not confirm this rumor.

The clinical scenarios (as well as multiple choice questions [MCQs]) that you will encounter are topics from the Problem Disease List; therefore, it is important to study the basic principles of management. You need to practice with the sample CCS cases on the CD provided by the board to become familiar with the computerized order entry. At first try to diagnose the patient's problem quickly and then efficiently manage it. If you can nail the diagnosis and the basic steps of management, passing the CCS section should not be a problem. If the CCS grows to be worth more than the current 25%, however, hammering out the exact standard of care treatment will become ever more important. *I have included sample order entries for some CCS cases with commands that CCS will recognize.*

It is fun to play around with different commands, even wildly inappropriate ones, to see what happens. You will be amazed by what commands the program will recognize and the results that will come back that are appropriate to the diagnosis. For example, I moved a completely stable patient who came to the clinic for a routine yearly visit to the ICU (and all over the hospital), intubated her, gave her all kinds of medications, requested all modalities of imaging and labs tests, and attempted numerous invasive procedures, which the patient's family refused (on a sample case of course).

You need a process to follow to be successful on CCS and to avoid becoming lost and panicky:

1. **Read the history of the present illness (HPI).** Note the vital signs. Is the patient hemodynamically stable? If not, give emergent care such as CPR, intubation, and chest tubes. Always remember the ABCs (airways, breathing, circulation). In unstable patients, do *not* waste time with history and physical exam or diagnostic tests when immediate intervention is needed (i.e., intubation, IV access/fluids, chest tubes). These management scenarios are covered within *Strong Medicine*, especially in the Trauma section. You will be graded on the order in which you do things and not simply on whether you get them done. Intubating a corpse will score no points.

2. **Develop an initial differential diagnosis after you have read the presentation and vital signs.** You will be given quite a bit of information initially in the CCS scenarios. In my experience, these

were *classic* case presentations, and you should be able to rapidly form a differential diagnosis—if not nail the diagnosis—based on the initial information.

3. **Examine the patient.** The exam can be complete or focused. At any time, you can also retake the history, which is equivalent to asking the patient, "Now how are you doing?" Do a focused history and physical exam (H&P) in most cases. Some advocate a complete H&P for each patient, but the NBME/FSMB guidelines clearly state that CCS is "not designed to assess your ability to complete a history." I recommend a focused H&P based on your differential diagnosis. If the patient has come for a routine office visit, a complete exam may be warranted.

4. **Order tests.** Obtain laboratory tests, imaging studies, and other tests that most efficiently cover the differential diagnosis that you should have in your head. Cost is definitely an issue. If you are absolutely certain of the diagnosis, it is okay to take a highly efficient approach to managing the patient and not cover the entire differential. The NBME guidelines plainly state that neither approach will result in a lower score.

   a. Common CCS radiologic studies include chest x-ray (CXR), kidney-ureter-bladder study (KUB), ECG, echocardiogram (transthoracic [TTE] or transesophaeal [TEE]), CT, MRI, colonoscopy, barium swallow, bronchoscopy, VQ scan, arteriogram, Doppler ultrasound, and endoscopic retrograde cholangiopancreatography (ERCP).

   b. Common CCS lab tests include complete blood count (CBC), comprehensive metabolic profile (chem12), lipid profile, liver function tests, urinalysis/culture, cardiac markers/enzymes, urine sputum blood culture and sensitivity, creatinine phosphokinase (CPK), thyroid-stimulating hormone (TSH), free T_4, total T_3, drug levels, coagulation profile, D-dimer, stool guaiac, folate/vitamin B_{12} levels, peripheral smear, and iron, ferritin, and lipase, amylase levels.

5. **Treat the patient.** Manage the patient with the medications and other therapies that you deem necessary after getting the diagnosis. The case may end well before the allotted time if you know the diagnosis and manage the therapy very efficiently.

6. **Order consultations.** You can order consultations (e.g., ob/gyn or surgery), but these guys have a serious work aversion on Step 3. You do score points for ordering the consultation anyway. You have to type in the procedure that you want done (e.g., laparotomy). They may surprise you and step in if your patient goes down the tubes after you have placed a consultation.

7. **Move or discharge the patient.** Options include home, office, emergency department, ward, and intensive care unit (ICU). Generally, if the patient in your clinic becomes unstable, move the patient to the ED. If the patient is in the ED when you start treatment, you will admit the patient to the ward or ICU, depending on the severity of illness.

8. **Location, location, location.** The location in which you see the patient is generally a good indicator of the acuity of the situation: ED patients generally are admitted, and clinic patients generally go home.

9. **Move the clock.** Nothing will happen and your orders will not be carried out if you do not move the clock. Physical exam and procedures also advance the clock.

10. **Intervene.** If the patient becomes unstable at any time, intervene as stated above.

11. **Counsel the patient.** Be sure to counsel patients about safe sex and other important topics. These are easy points that you do not want to miss. You might recognize and treat the STD, but you still need to counsel the patient. Also be sure to order health maintenance tests as appropriate. These tests are covered in this text and include colonoscopies, mammograms, and lipid panels, among others.

SAMPLE CASE DEMONSTRATIONS

Here are possible inputs for the sample cases provided by the NBME/FSMB. Download these cases and follow along on your computer. http://www.usmle.org/CBT2004/menu.htm

Due to copyright regulations, I cannot print the text of the actual cases, but you can follow the order entry on your computer step-by-step.

CCS SAMPLE INPUT 2004 UNTIMED BLOCK 1:

65 yo male with pleuritic chest pain. The patient is tachycardic, hypotensive, and tachypneic. Differential diagnosis should include pneumothorax, cardiac disease.

1. Click Write Orders or Review Chart.
2. On Order Sheet, click Order button. We need some immediate orders.
3. Oxygen, inhalation, continuous.
4. IV access.
5. Cardiac monitor.
6. Blood pressure monitor.
7. Pulse oximetry.
8. Click on Interval Hx or PE button.
9. Check the Interval History, Gen appearance, Chest/lungs, Heart/cardiovascular boxes.
10. Click OK. A prompt will come up about advancing the clock. Click OK past this.
11. Note results of the focused exam, especially the tracheal deviation and lack of breath sounds on right. Click past this. We need to intervene right away. We will address immediate intervention throughout this text.
12. Click Write Orders or Review Chart.
13. On Order Sheet, click Order button.
14. Needle thoracostomy. Click OK. Note the whoosh.
15. Click Order button again.
16. Tube thoracostomy. Note CCS will allow you to skip the needle and directly insert a chest tube.
17. Click on Interval Hx or PE button.
18. Check the Interval History, Gen appearance, Chest/lungs, Heart/cardiovascular boxes. This will advance clock, and the chest tube will go in when you click OK.
19. Note the patient update that pops up and all of the interval information. Pat yourself on the back.
20. Click Write Orders or Review Chart.
21. On Order Sheet, click Order button.
22. CXR portable. Click OK. Defaults to STAT.
23. ECG 12-lead.
24. Click Obtain Results or See Patient Later. Click With Next Available Result. CXR results confirm your astute clinical intervention.
25. Click Change Location and select ICU. Review the Order will pop up. Click past.
26. The case will end in 5 minutes of "real time," which will pop up. We are all over this. Click OK. Let's gild the lily and add some orders to treat his asthma and address his lifestyle.
27. Albuterol inhalation, continuous.
28. Ipratropium bromide inhalation, continuous.
29. Counsel patient, asthma care.
30. Counsel patient, smoking cessation.
31. Enter your diagnosis: Tension Pneumothorax.

The ATLS guidelines say that you should insert the chest tube before the x-ray is done in patients with suspected pneumothorax, but you have multiple options for attacking this case. Depending on your training and background, you might be inclined to hold off the chest tube until the CXR is done and the patient will not die. Go ahead and try it. Emergency medicine and surgery physicians may be inclined to take the more aggressive approach that I have illustrated and that ATLS guidelines support. Also note that omitting the asthma treatments will not cause you to fail. You can exit the case, enter the diagnosis and move on with your life.

CCS SAMPLE INPUT 2004 UNTIMED BLOCK 2:

32 yo female with knee pain, fatigue. Note carefully that the history gives female with bilateral joint stiffness, worse in the morning. This is highly suggestive of rheumatoid arthritis (RA). The differential diagno-

sis should include RA immediately. Osteoarthritis (OA) is much less likely. Since loss of libido and fatigue can also be nonspecific symptoms of depression, screen for depression and go along with RA as well.

1. Click on Interval Hx or PE button.
2. Click Interval and Complete exam. Complete exam is generally a good idea on routine office scenarios.
3. Click Write Orders or Review Chart. Then Order Sheet. Then Order.
4. TSH, serum (hypothyroidism is very common and fatigue merits checking this possibility).
5. CBC, CMP (routine labs appropriate, especially with fatigue).
6. Rheumatoid factor (this will hopefully establish the diagnosis).
7. Lipid panel (for adults over 30 yo lipid screening is indicated health maintenance).
8. Depression screen (fatigue and loss of libido can be nonspecific for depression).
9. Pap smear (she is overdue if you look at history).
10. Enter all these labs and hit ENTER after each. Click through ROUTINE ONCE on all these selections.
11. Bextra or Celebrex or other NSAID of your choice. Click PO continuous.
12. Change location to Home. Schedule appointment in 2-3 weeks. Click OK. Lots of results will pop up now. Note the rheumatoid factor and patient update. Keep clicking through all the pop-ups.
13. The case will end in 5 minutes of "real time," which will pop up. You have nailed it! Click OK. Lets rack up some bonus points. Write new orders.
14. Counsel patient about breast self-examination.
15. Counsel patient about exercise program.
16. Order x-rays (for baseline measurement of disease progression and response to therapy).
17. Get erythrocyte sedimentation rate (ESR) and C-reactive protein (CRP) (may correlate with disease activity or signal presence of erosive disease).
18. American College of Rheumatology recommends starting disease-modifying antirheumatic drug (DMARD), such as methotrexate, early after diagnosis (to prevent progression of disease).
19. Exit the case.
20. Enter your diagnosis: RA.

CCS SAMPLE INPUT 2004 TIMED BLOCK 1:

5 yo boy with nosebleed and petechiae. Note that history includes preceding upper respiratory infection (URI). The differential should immediately include Henoch-Schönlein purpura, hemolytic uremic syndrome (HUS), idiopathic thrombocytopenic purpura (ITP), and thrombotic thrombocytopenic purpura (TTP). Vital signs appear stable.

1. Click on Interval Hx or PE button.
2. Check the Interval History, HEENT/Neck exam. He is still actively bleeding.
3. Click Write Orders or Review Chart.
4. On Order Sheet, click Order button. We need some immediate orders.
5. Pressure to nose. (Computer will automatically put phenylephrine on for you!)
6. Click on Interval Hx or PE button.
7. Check the Interval History, HEENT/Neck exam. You fixed him!
8. CBC, CMP, coagulation profile, urinalysis (UA), antiplatelet antibodies (these lab tests will give us a look at the patient's hemoglobin and kidney function).
9. If platelet count is low, get reticulocyte count.
10. While waiting on these labs, do a real exam. A complete exam will run the clock.
11. Click Interval and Complete exam. Complete exam is generally a good idea for routine office scenarios. Note the rectal exam for occult blood and petechiae on the skin.

continued

12. Click Obtain Results or See Patient Later. Click With Next Available Result. Look at all these lab tests! Note the platelet count and the blood in urine. Note that creatinine is normal. The mother is upset about the rash.
13. Move patient to ward. These are very low platelets, and the little guy needs some TLC. He may become hemodynamically unstable.
14. Continue to advance the clock. Note the antiplatelet antibody that finally pops up. Viola! ITP.
15. Counsel patient, avoid aspirin (affects platelets).
16. Order CBC every 24 hours. Keep advancing the clock, and note that platelets are improving. Otherwise we would have to consult surgery and remove the spleen.
17. The case will end in 5 minutes of "real time," which will pop up. Click OK.
18. Click on Interval Hx or PE button.
19. Enter your diagnosis: ITP

ITP resolves in 80% of patients without intervention, and if you type REASSURE PATIENT FAMILY, this case will end. The standard of care is to intervene if platelets are under 20,000 and the platelet count in this case is right at 20,000. You can also give platelet transfusions below this level.

CCS SAMPLE INPUT 2004 TIMED BLOCK 2:

25 yo male with diarrhea. Note stable vital signs and the key fact of a camping history.

1. Click on Interval Hx or PE button.
2. Check the Interval History, Complete exam. Note the hyperactive bowel sounds and lack of other symptoms.
3. Click Write Orders or Review Chart.
4. On Order Sheet, click Order button.
5. CBC, CMP, Giardia antigen stool.
6. Change location to Home.
7. Schedule appointment for 1 week. Lab results will start popping up, stating the diagnosis.
8. Metronizadole, continuous PO (after confirming Giardia on stool antigen test).
9. Loperamide PO.
10. Enter your diagnosis: *Giardia lamblia*

Note that you can order a stool O&P (ova and parasite) study, which will find *Giardia* in CCS.

CCS SAMPLE INPUT 2004 TIMED BLOCK 3:

65 yo woman with left-sided chest pain that radiates to the jaw and back. Note her blood pressure (BP) and tachycardia.

1. Click on Interval Hx or PE button.
2. Check the Interval History, Gen appearance, Chest/lungs, Heart/cardiovascular boxes.
3. Click Write Orders or Review Chart.
4. On Order Sheet, click Order button. We need some immediate orders. Remember MONA for possible ACS/MI.
5. Oxygen, inhalation, continuous.
6. Blood pressure monitor.
7. Cardiac monitor.
8. Pulse oximetry.
9. IV access.
10. Morphine IV, continuous.
11. Nitroglycerin IV, continuous (sublingual OK but she has HTN that NTG will help).
12. Aspirin therapy PO one time.
13. ECG, 12-lead STAT.
14. CXR, PA/Lateral STAT.
15. Cardiac isoenzymes.
16. Troponin I.
17. CBC, CMP, coagulation profile, lipid panel, TSH (all standard in possible MI).
18. Esmolol IV, continuous (any beta blocker works in this CCS Scenario. Esmolol is ultra-short-acting IV beta blocker than can be shut off quickly).
19. ECG results pop up. Kind of nonspecific . . . not really like an MI at all.
20. Advance the clock. CXR results pop up. Note the wide mediastinum. Oh yeah, the pain radiated to the back. Aren't you glad we did not start thrombolytics without the CXR? Just for fun and education, redo this case and give the TPA to get a feel for what happens when a case is badly mismanaged.
21. Order a CT of the chest,
22. Consult thoracic surgery (enter reason: aortic dissection). This guy won't help you, but enter this order anyway.
23. Move the clock forward.
24. Patient's BP has improved, which will pop up. (Good—medical management of HTN is continued up to emergent surgery.)
25. Move patient to the ICU (until we can get into OR. You could probably safely keep her in the ED until surgery).
26. Troponin I returns to within normal limits (WNL). We already suspected that it was not an MI, but it was smart to check this anyway.
27. Advance the clock some more. CT confirms that the aorta is dissecting.
28. Repair aortic aneurysm, thoracic STAT.
29. The case **will** end soon after this, no matter what you do.
30. Enter diagnosis: ascending aortic aneurysm.

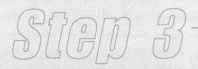

CHAPTER 1

Cardiovascular System

ARRHYTHIMIAS
Atrial fibrillation and flutter
First-degree heart block
Second-degree heart block/Mobitz I
(Wenckebach)
Third-degree heart block
Wolff-Parkinson-White syndrome
Ventricular tachycardia
Ventricular fibrillation
Asystole
Premature ventricular contractions
Tachycardia
Palpitations

HEART FAILURE
Cardiomyopathy
Congestive heart failure
Pericarditis

HYPERTENSION
Elevated blood pressure without
diagnosis of hypertension
Essential hypertension
Hypertensive heart disease
Hypertensive renal disease
Secondary hypertension

ISCHEMIA
Acute coronary syndrome/myocardial
infarction

VALVULAR DISEASE
Murmurs
Rheumatic heart disease
Aortic stenosis
Mitral regurgitation
Mitral stenosis
Aortic regurgitation
Endocarditis
Congenital anomalies of the heart
Patent ductus arteriosus
Ventricular septal defect
Atrial septal defect
Tetralogy of Fallot
Coarctation of the aorta

VASCULAR DISEASE
Aortic aneurysm
Arteriosclerotic disease/atherosclerosis
Arterial embolism/thrombosis
Peripheral vascular disease
Phlebitis/thrombophlebitis
Varicose veins
Venous embolism/thrombosis

ARRHYTHMIAS

Arrhythmias and conduction disorders. Expect a strip requiring recognition of the rhythm and then a next-step management question using the ACLS/PALS protocols.

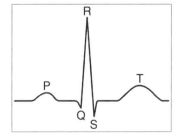

Figure 1. Normal ECG. (From Hampton JR: The ECG Made Easy, 6th ed., Edinburgh, Churchill Livingstone, 2003, p 4.)

Atrial Fibrillation and Flutter

Presentation: P waves absent, heart rate high (150–200 bpm); look for patient with history of lung disease or atrial enlargement, palpitations. Atrial flutter presents with a heart rate of about 150 and classic "sawtooth" pattern.

Management:

- Order the appropriate lab tests, including CBC, BMP, and TSH levels (thyroid disease can cause atrial fibrillation).
- You must rule out an ischemic event with cardiac panel, especially with first-time atrial fibrillation (a-fib). Prognosis is poor when a-fib is associated with myocardial infarction (MI). Ask about alcohol use to rule out "holiday heart."
- Get an ECG, of course.
- Chest x-ray is advised.
- Transesophageal echocardiogram is warranted to ascertain whether a thrombus may be floating around in the blood. If you decide to use cardioversion, this clot could float away and kill the patient.
- Rate control with IV diltiazem drip is standard, but use beta blockers if a-fib is related to thyroid storm or MI. Digoxin for heart failure.

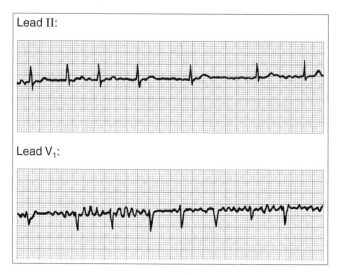

Figure 2. Atrial fibrillation. (From Hampton JR: The ECG Made Easy, 6th ed., Edinburgh, Churchill Livingstone, 2003, p 79.)

- If the patient is symptomatic and unstable, emergent synchronized cardioversion with 100 Joules is appropriate; increase energy if needed and repeat.
- Anticoagulate the patient if a-fib persists for longer than 48 hours with warfarin (INR of 2–3).
- Attempt to cardiovert patients with first-time a-fib that is either chemical or electrical. Amiodarone is not a bad choice for chemical conversion, but there is no consensus about the optimal choice.
- Patients with chronic a-fib should take warfarin as outpatients to prevent strokes. Aspirin can be used if warfarin is not tolerated.
- Heart rate is controlled with oral diltiazem in outpatients.
- Electrical ablative methods are available for treating a-fib but are rarely indicated.

First-degree Heart Block

Presentation: asymptomatic; see strip below.

Management:

- Do nothing unless it is associated with obvious pathology such as MI.
- Avoid beta blocker or calcium channel blocker.
- Follow-up ECGs to monitor progression.

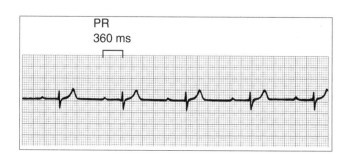

Figure 3. First-degree block. (From Hampton JR: The ECG Made Easy, 6th ed., Edinburgh, Churchill Livingstone, 2003, p 31.)

Second-degree Heart Block/Mobitz I (Wenckebach)

Presentation: presents with progressive PR interval increases; then QRS drops.

Management:

- Use atropine and transcutaneous pacing if the patient is symptomatic.
- Mobitz II (PPPQRS): associated with MI.
- Avoid AV blocking agents. This can easily progress to complete heart block.
- Transcutaneous pacing should be started. Atropine can be considered if the condition is not MI-related.
- Refer to cardiac care unit for placement of pacer.

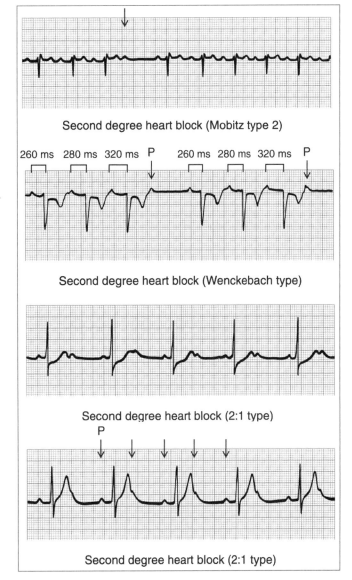

Second degree heart block (Mobitz type 2)

Second degree heart block (Wenckebach type)

Second degree heart block (2:1 type)

Second degree heart block (2:1 type)

Figure 4. Second-degree heart block. (From Hampton JR: The ECG Made Easy, 6th ed., Edinburgh, Churchill Livingstone, 2003, p 32-33.)

Third-degree Heart Block

Presentation: look for "escape" rhythm, 40-60 bpm, and complete AV dissociation.

Management:
- Patients are usually unstable on presentation.
- Pace them.
- Rule out MI and treat for MI if needed.
- A pacemaker is the definitive treatment.

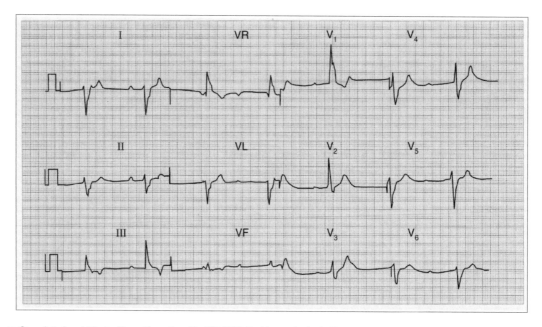

Figure 5. Complete heart block. (From Hampton JR: 150 ECG Problems, 2nd ed., Edinburgh, Churchill Livingstone, 2003, p 5.)

Wolff-Parkinson-White Syndrome

Presentation: delta waves with slurred upstroke QRS, short PR interval (0.12 sec), wide QRS (>0.12 sec).

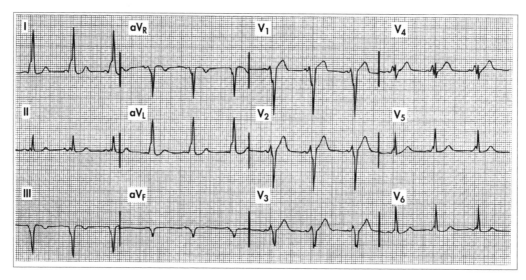

Figure 6. WPW. (From Goldberger AL: Clinical Electrocardiography, A Simplified Approach, 6th ed., St. Louis, Mosby, 1999, p 251.)

Management:

- Administer oxygen.
- Cardiovert if the patient is hemodynamically unstable.
- Treat a-fib first in WPW syndrome.
- Adenosine, 6 mg IV fast push; follow with 12-mg IV push.
- Procainamide is classic for slowing conduction through the accessory pathway.
- Ablation of the accessory pathway is the first-line option for recurrent or refractory tachyarrhythmia.
- Avoid digoxin because slowing AV transmission may increase the transmission through the WPW pathway.

Ventricular Tachycardia

Presentation: wide QRS, >150 bmp but less than 200, AV dissociation.

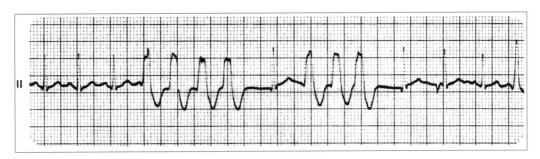

Figure 7. Ventricular tachycardia. (From Goldberger AL: Clinical Electrocardiography, A Simplified Approach, 6th ed., St. Louis, Mosby, 1999, p 167.)

Management:

- Unstable patient: immediate synchronized cardioversion followed by amiodarone.
- Stable patient: start lidocaine.
- Be aware that this can degenerate to v-fib quickly.
- Amiodarone can be given for refractory cases.

Ventricular Fibrillation

Presentation: pulseless, electrical chaos.

Management:

- Start CPR.
- Defibrillate with high energy: 200, 300 then 360 Joules.
- Check for pulse.
- Intubate.
- IV access.

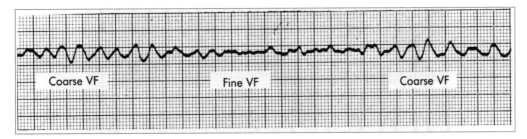

Figure 8. Ventricular fibrillation. (From Goldberger AL: Clinical Electrocardiography, A Simplified Approach, 6th ed., St. Louis, Mosby, 1999, p 172.)

- Resume CPR for 30 seconds.
- Give epinephrine every 3 minutes.
- Correct the 4Hs and 4Ts (from PALS): **h**ypoxia, **h**ypovolemia, **h**yperkalemia/**h**ypokalemia, **t**ension pneumothorax, **t**amponade, **t**oxic/therapeutic substances, **t**hromboembolic/mechanical obstruction
- Defibrillate at 360 J, give lidocaine, defibrillate, give lidocaine, defibrillate. . .
- Consider amiodarone at this point.
- This is the most common cause of sudden cardiac arrest along with ventricular tachycardia. In other words, if you see someone suddenly drop, it is most likely fatal arrhythmia—not asystole. Thus access to a defibrillator is most important.

Asystole

Presentation: flatline.

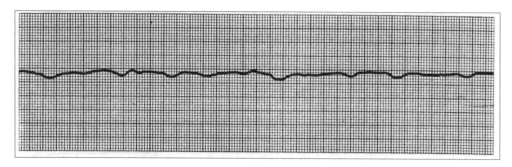

Figure 9. Asystole bordering on fine ventricular fibrillation. Asystole must be confirmed in at least two leads in order to exclude fine ventricular fibrillation. (From Seelig, CB: Simplified EKG Analysis, A Sequential Guide to Interpretation and Diagnosis, Philadelphia, Hanley & Belfus, 1992, p 76.)

Management:
- Check another lead on ECG to verify true asystole.
- Start CPR.
- Give epinephrine.
- Continue CPR.
- Give atropine (except in children).
- Do **not** shock patients in asystole despite what you see on television!

Premature Ventricular Contractions (PVCs)

Presentation: see strip below.

Management:
- PVCs are generally benign.
- Give lidocaine if the patient is unstable.

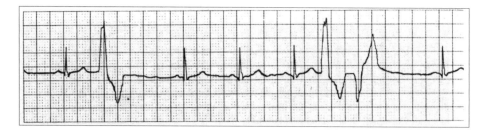

Figure 10. Multifocal PVCs with two occurring in a row (paired PVCs). (From Seelig, CB: Simplified EKG Analysis, A Sequential Guide to Interpretation and Diagnosis, Philadelphia, Hanley & Belfus, 1992, p 88.)

Tachycardia

Presentation: heart rate over 100 in teens/adults, greater than ~150 in children.

Management:

- Get lab tests, including BMP, especially for potassium and magnesium.
- Ask about fever, diarrhea, and vomiting preceding illness.
- Get ECG, of course.
- Differentiate sinus tachycardia from supraventricular tachycardia (SVT). Subtract age in years from 220 for maximal expected heart rate. If the heart rate exceeds this number, the patient does **not** have sinus tachycardia. Does the rate change with activity? If yes, the diagnosis is sinus tachycardia. SVT is fast and constant. Was the tachycardia sudden with no predisposing illness/dehydration? If yes, the diagnosis is SVT.
- SVT has no P waves on ECG. These ECGs can be hard to interpret in truth.

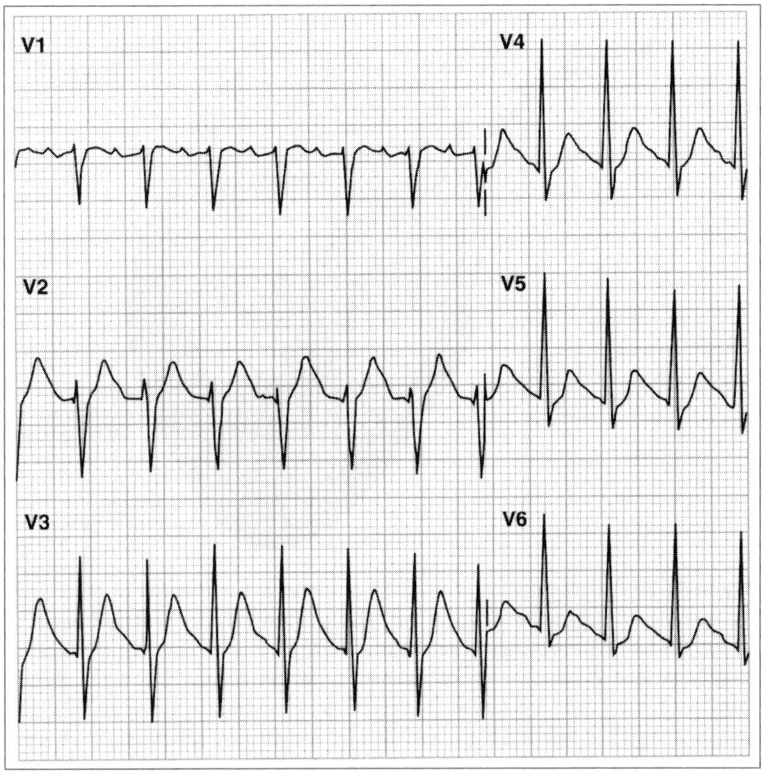

Figure 11. Sinus tachycardia; rate, 165 bpm. (From Khan, MG: Rapid ECG Interpretation, 2nd ed., Philadelphia, Saunders, 2003, p 287.)

- If the diagnosis is sinus tachycardia, give the patient a fluid bolus of isotonic fluid (lactate Ringer's or normal saline). The patient is likely to have a history of vomiting or diarrhea, and this is the first step in the protocol.

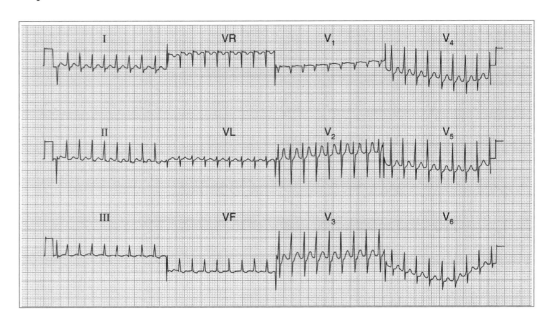

Figure 12. Supraventricular tachycardia. (From Hampton JR: The ECG Made Easy, 6th ed., Edinburgh, Churchill Livingstone, 2003, p 74.)

- If the patient is stable and has SVT, attempt vagal maneuvers with ice bag on face. Call for cardiologist. Do not rush to cardiovert or push adenosine right away. This is the sequence: vagal manuevers, adenosine, cardioversion.
- Proceed to load adenosine, 6 and 12 mg, for rapid IV infusion. (Since the patient will briefly flatline in asytole, **you** may need cardioversion! Then suddenly normal sinus rhythm is restored.)
- If the patient is unstable, cardiovert immediately. No one will fault you for cardioverting unstable patients, because this is protocol.
- If the diagnosis is ventricular tachycardia, cardiovert unstable patient or give lidocaine first to stable patient. See ventricular tachycardia (above) for more information.

Palpitations

Presentation: uncomfortable awareness of heartbeat.

Management:
- EKG.
- Ask about caffeine use as well as stimulants like ephedra and alcohol.
- Check TSH (the patient may be hyperthyroid).
- If palpitations are associated with chest pain, be sure that the problem is not an acute ischemic event such as MI.
- If the patient passes out or the event is prolonged, the problem may be a dangerous arrhythmia.

HEART FAILURE

Cardiomyopathy

Presentation: symptoms of congestive heart failure (CHF), as below.

Type	Presentation
Ischemic	After heart attack
Dilated	Affects men usually
Restrictive	Heart is stiff and cannot relax in diastole; may be caused by amyloid or sarcoid
Alcoholic	Direct toxic affect of alcohol on heart
Hypertrophic	Familial usually. Left ventricular hypertrophy is prominent. There is delayed ventricular relaxation in diastole.

Management:
- Treat as CHF, below.
- Consider dual chamber pacemaker in all cases.
- Cardiac transplant may be the only definitive cure.

Congestive Heart Failure (Failure of the Heart to Maintain Output)

Presentation: dyspnea on exertion, shortness of breath, lower extremity edema.

Management:
- In history ask how many pillows are used at night. Does the patient cough up frothy sputum?
- Look for jugular venous distention (JVD). Listen for S3 on cardiac exam. Listen for rales on pulmonary exam.
- 100% oxygen, NRM, elevate head of bed.
- Get routine lab tests such as BMP and TSH.

- Get BNP on admission.
- Cardiac markers are a wise choice.
- Get a chest x-ray, and look for cephalization, Kerley B lines.
- Admit the patient, possibly to ICU if the patient is hemodynamically unstable.
- Get an echocardiogram.
- Start diuretics (e.g., Lasix), and get the fluid off.
- Clear up pulmonary edema with initial use of nitrates (e.g., nitroglycerin drip).
- Consider morphine, which dilates the veins and reduces preload.
- Give inotropic agents such as dobutamine for patients with severe failure in the ICU.
- Nesiritide (Natrecor) is a new, expensive, effective therapy in CHF.
- Start an ACE inhibitor.
- Start digoxin, an inotropic agent, for a-fib or rapid ventricular rate, but be aware that it takes a long time to load and reach therapeutic levels.
- Beta blockers decrease mortality, but use with caution in acute failure and avoid calcium channel blockers.
- Ongoing care: sodium restriction is critical.

Pitfalls:
- Make sure that the patient did not have a heart attack recently; see the protocol for ischemic heart disease.

Pericarditis

Presentation: After a respiratory infection the patient presents with chest pain that may radiate to neck and is improved by leaning forward, JVD and Kussmaul respirations, which are JVD with inspiration. Pericardial friction rub is pathognomonic.

Management:
- Pericarditis is inflammation of the pericardium. It can be caused by a virus, especially adenovirus and coxsackie virus. Other possibilities include autoimmune disease, TB, and renal failure (hyperuremic).
- Get routine lab tests (CBC, basic metabolic panel [BMP]).
- Get ECG. It may show signs that mimic heart attack with ST elevation in many leads; get cardiac markers as well.
- Get blood culture and C-reactive protein (CRP) to rule out infectious cause.
- Get erythrocyte sedimentation rate (ESR), ANA, rheumatoid factor.
- Pericardiocentesis, using needle to withdraw fluid for analysis, may aid in diagnosis.
- Give NSAIDs to reduce the inflammation.
- In most patients, try corticosteroids if NSAIDs do not work.
- If no relief with above measures, pericardectomy (cutting pericardium) is the definitive cure but is associated with a 10% mortality rate.

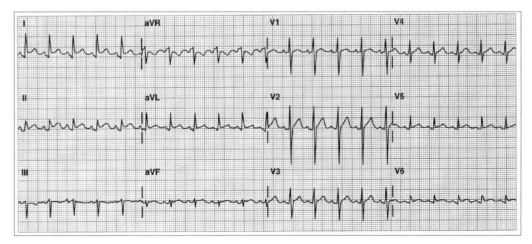

Figure 13. Acute perdicarditis. (From Khan, MG: Rapid ECG Interpretation, 2nd ed., Philadelphia, Saunders, 2003, p 241.)

HYPERTENSION

Elevated Blood Pressure Without Diagnosis of Hypertension

Presentation: patient shows up in clinic with less than ideal blood pressure for the first time.

Management:

- At least 2 separate readings over 2–3 months are needed to give the diagnosis of hypertension.
- Have patient return to your office at a later time and recheck blood pressure.
- You may then commence treatment for hypertension.

Essential Hypertension (No Cause Can be Found)

Presentation: systolic pressure over 140 mmHg or diastolic blood pressure over 90 mmHg (130/80 mmHg for diabetics or patients with renal disease, according to JNC 7). Usually **no** symptoms except perhaps headache. Accounts for over 90% of patients with hypertension.

Management:

- Measure BP at least 2 times on separate occasions. Be aware of "white coat" hypertension.
- CBC, BMP with electrolytes, creatinine, glucose, uric acid, and urinalysis.
- Order lipid profile; JNC also recommends EKG.
- Listen for S4 on cardiac exam.
- Lifestyle modifications at first: weight loss, exercise, sodium restriction, reducing alcohol consumption. DASH diet with lots of calcium and potassium from dairy, fruits, and vegetables.
- Thiazide diuretic or beta blocker is the initial therapy of choice.
- Calcium channel blockers, ACE inhibitors/ARBs are used stepwise. For pure systolic hypertension, calcium channel blocker is preferred.
- Tailor medication to other comorbidities. For example, if the patient has benign prostatic hypertrophy (BPH), consider terazosin to relax the prostate as well as lower blood pressure. If the patient is diabetic, certainly include ACE inhibitor for renal protection. Avoid diuretics in gout. Hydrochlorothiazide (HCTZ) is preferred for African Americans.

Pitfall:
- Excessive use of labs and tests (unless some primary cause is suspected).

Hypertensive Heart Disease

Presentation: Left ventricular hypertrophy (LVH) and enlargement of left atrium, AV arrhythmias, systolic/diastolic heart failure, ischemic heart disease, or MI.

Management:

- Prevent it: once LVH develops, risks of sudden death and arrhythmias increase dramatically.
- Order appropriate lab tests: CBC, BMP, TSH.
- Chest x-ray shows pulmonary cephalization, Kerley B Lines, and a big heart (cardiomegaly).
- Get an ECG. LVH manifests with multiple ECG criteria, but for the purposes of the Step 3 exam look for high voltage, especially in the precordial leads V4-V6. Look for tall R waves in V5 especially.
- Echocardiogram yields the most information. If Step 3 gives you a specific choice, select transthoracic echocardiography.
- Beta blockers and ACE inhibitors are the drugs of choice because of documented mortality benefits.
- Spironolactone and diuretics are added in heart failure.

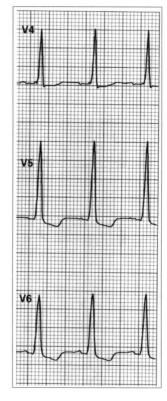

Figure 14. LVH on ECG. (From Khan, MG: Rapid ECG Interpretation, 2nd ed., Philadelphia, Saunders, 2003, p 181.)

Hypertensive Renal Disease

Presentation: hypertension is especially damaging to the kidneys in combination with diabetes, and the two tend to be found together. Blacks are more likely affected by hypertension-induced renal disease.

Management:

- Lab tests include BMP with electrolytes and creatinine.
- Look for microalbumin in urine.
- Give maximal dosage of ACE inhibitor.
- Avoid NSAIDs in renal disease.

Secondary Hypertension

Cause Diagnosis	Management	
Renal artery stenosis	Order ultrasound with Doppler of renal arteries Order renal angiography	Stenting renal arteries is definitive cure
Pheochromocytoma	Order metanephrine/catecholamine levels from urine and serum Order CT to visualize adrenals for tumor	Give prazosin and metyrosine and get to the OR to remove the tumor
Cushing syndrome	Look for other signs of Cushing syndrome on exam (obesity, hypertension, hirsutism) Check cortisol	Consult for adrenalectomy
Hyperaldosteronism	Elevated K+ on BMP is initial finding Get plasma aldosterone/plasma renin activity (PRA) ratio Can get captopril suppression test; in normal person aldosterone will drop Get CT with adrenal glands Adrenal venous sampling is gold standard	Adrenalectomy is definitive surgical procedure
Coarctation of aorta	Patient may report dizziness Check for high blood pressure upper body with low blood pressure lower body Chest x-ray may show notching of the ribs Order chest CT	Surgical repair is standard of care. Without surgical repair, patients usually die before middle-age.
Other causes	Hypo/hyperthyroidism Corticosteroids Estrogen Sympathomimetics like cocaine, MAO inhibitors Sleep apnea Immoderate alcohol use	

ISCHEMIA

Acute Coronary Syndrome/Myocardial Infarction

Presentation: retrosternal pain, diaphoresis, pain in arm/back/jaw, pain with exertion/exercise. Diabetics may present with abdominal pain rather than typical chest pain.

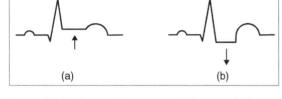

Figure 15. (a) Elevated ST segment. (b) Depressed ST segment. (From Hampton JR: The ECG Made Easy, 6th ed., Edinburgh, Churchill Livingstone, 2003, p 101.)

Management:

- Manage the risk factors to prevent it: dyslipidemia, diabetes, hypertension, obesity, smoking, hostile personality type.
- Get CBC, BMP, TSH, coagulation profile, and lipid panel on presentation in ED.
- Get chest x-ray.
- Get cardiac markers q 6h × 3. Troponin I is most sensitive and specific chemical cardiac marker of acute event.
- Get ECG. Look for Q waves, ST elevation/depression, or T-wave inversion. Depression in the ST segment is classic for ischemia. Elevation indicates infarction.
- Give oxygen.
- Give aspirin.
- Give morphine for pain.
- Nitroglycerin should be given sublingually or by drip unless BP <90 or HR <50.
- Start beta blocker therapy with low-dose metoprolol, 5 mg PO q 6 h.
- Start ACE inhibitor even if the patient is not hypertensive because of proven post-MI benefits.
- Start statin drug; even without knowing cholesterol, statins have proven post-MI mortality benefits.
- Heparin should be given by drip weight-based protocol with bolus and continuous infusion; or give enoxaparin (Lovenox), 1 mg/kg q 12 h.
- Admit to CCU.
- Rule out MI with cycled cardiac markers. Keep getting markers until peak is reached.
- Decision point is whether to start thrombolytic therapy (i.e., tissue plasminogen activator [tPA] or eptifibatide [Integrilin]). If cardiac enzymes rule in MI, start thrombolytics. Avoid thrombolytics without persistent ST changes or new-onset left bundle-branch block.
- Get cardiac catheterization as soon as possible. This information will lead to coronary artery bypass grafting (CABG) or percutaneous transluminal coronary angioplasty (PTCA.)
- CABG is open-heart surgery for treatment of coronary artery disease. PTCA and stenting are invasive treatments for coronary artery disease. Order if needed.
- If MI is ruled out, get stress test—either treadmill or chemical (if the patient cannot exercise). You may still wish to consider outpatient catheterization.

Pitfall:

- Missing MI/acute coronary syndrome is the most common cause of lawsuit for primary care physicians; do not attribute chest pain to reflux disease or some other cause without proper investigation.

CCS SAMPLE INPUT—Acute Myocardial Infarction

Oxygen, inhalation, continuous

Access, IV

Focused physical exam: HEENT/neck, chest/lungs, heart/vascular system, abdomen, extremities

ECG: STAT

continued

CCS SAMPLE INPUT—Acute Myocardial Infarction (*continued*)

Chest x-ray (posteroanterior and lateral): STAT

Cardiac isoenzymes, serum: STAT (note that troponin is not included in CCS panel) q 8 hr

Troponin I, serum: STAT q 8 hr

CBC, CMP, coagulation profile, lipid profile

Monitor cardiac function continuously

Sublingual nitroglycerin 1 time or IV nitroglycerin continuously

Aspirin, orally 1 time STAT

Morphine IV

Lisinopril, orally 1 time

Metoprolol, orally continuously

Atorvastatin (Lipitor), orally continuously

Consult cardiologist STAT → POPUP Enter: Patient with MI

Change location to ICU. When location changes, some orders will need reentry.

Place patient on NPO status.

If ruled in:

Alteplase

Echocardiography

Cardiac catherization, angiocardiography

Stent placement in coronary artery or CABG STAT

If ruled out:

Echocardiography

Stress test

Change location to home

Schedule appointment 1 week (button appears for change to home)

Aspirin, lisinopril, atorvastatin (Lipitor), metoprolol PO (as outpatient)

Counsel patient, including smoking cessation

Diet low in cholesterol and sodium

VALVULAR DISEASE

Murmurs

Presentation: turbulent flow of blood through the heart causes abnormal sound that may be due to valve stenosis, regurgitation, or innocent murmur. Murmur may be systolic, diastolic or continuous.

Management:

- An innocent murmur (especially in a child) may be asymptomatic but may get louder with physical activity or excitement.
- If accompanied with CHF or other symptoms such as chest pain, further work-up is needed.
- Get an ECG.
- Get an echocardiogram.

Rheumatic Heart Disease

Presentation: poststreptococcal throat infection.

Management:
- Rheumatic fever can lead to mitral stenosis.
- Prophylaxis is recommended for those at high risk of reinfection.

Aortic Stenosis

Presentation: angina, syncope, and heart failure

Management:
- Listen for harsh systolic ejection murmur.
- Tell patient: **no** exercise.
- Consider digoxin.
- Use caution with diuretics and **extra caution** with nitrates.
- Surgery is definitive treatment.

Mitral Regurgitation

Presentation: associated with rheumatic heart disease. Feel for enlarged maximal impulse, and listen for apical holosystolic murmur

Management:
- Give diuretics and nitrates for afterload reduction.
- Digoxin may be considered.
- Do not miss MI that causes mitral regurgitation secondary to papillary muscle dysfunction.
- Surgery is definitive treatment.

Mitral Stenosis

Presentation: during diastole listen for blowing murmur at apex.

Management:
- Generally no treatment is needed.
- Rate control is in order; use digoxin (if a-fib is present) or beta blocker.
- Anticoagulant should be used according to a-fib protocol if a-fib is present.
- Surgery is definitive option, but balloon angioplasty can open up the valve as well.

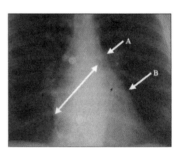

Figure 16. Mitral stenosis. (From Adelmann G, Ajani AE, Kleiber B: Valvular heart disease. In Weissman NJ, Adelmann GA (eds): Cardiac Imaging Secrets, Philadelphia, Hanley & Belfus, 2001, p 248.)

Aortic Regurgitation

Presentation: Listen for early diastolic decrescendo murmur

Management:
- Endocarditis prophylaxis is indicated for procedures.
- Vasodilators can be considered.
- Consider surgery.

Endocarditis

Presentation: patient may have artificial valve or be IV drug user.

Management:

- Look for/ask about fever, chills. Inquire about history of cardiovascular surgery, IV drug use.
- Listen for heart murmur, and look for petechiae.
- Get CBC, erythrocyte sedimentation rate (ESR).
- Get blood cultures; most common causative organisms are gram-positive cocci.
- Get echocardiogram (transthoracic for native valves, transesophageal for prosthetic valves). If Step 3 gives you one choice, pick this one.
- Start tailored antibiotic therapy as soon as possible.
  a. *Staphylococcus aureus* → oxacillin and gentamicin.
  b. Viridans streptococci → penicillin G.
  c. Enterococci → ampicillin and gentamicin.
  d. *Staphylococcus epidermidis* → vancomycin.
  e. **For empirical therapy,** give ampicillin + nafcillin + gentamicin.

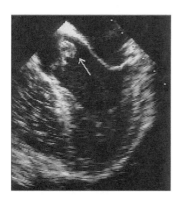

Figure 17. Endocarditis. (From Einhorn A, Adair OV, Voorhees DP: Endocarditis. In Adair OV (ed): Cardiology Secrets, 2nd ed., Philadelphia, Hanley & Belfus, 2001, p 132.)

Congenital Anomalies of the Heart

PATENT DUCTUS ARTERIOSUS (PDA): prenatal blood vessel that connects aorta with pulmonary arteries fails to close.

Presentation: Classic sign is machine murmur.

Management:
- Congenital rubella is frequent cause; prevent it with measles-mumps-rubella (MMR) vaccine.
- Can cause congestive heart failure.
- Close with indomethacin in premature babies (keep open with prostaglandin E1 if some other anomaly is present).
- Use surgery or catheterization to close in infants/adults.

VENTRICULAR SEPTAL DEFECT (VSD): hole in septum between ventricles that may lead to pulmonary hypertension, thrombus, right ventricular hypertrophy/dilation.

Presentation: Listen for holosystolic murmur.

Management:
- 50% close on their own by age 3; if not, treatment is needed.
- Surgery is definitive treatment.

ATRIAL SEPTAL DEFECT (ASD): hole in septum between atria that may lead to pulmonary hypertension, thrombus, right ventricular hypertrophy/dilation.

Presentation: Listen for split S2.

Management:
- Diuresis may be helpful.
- Surgical repair or catheterization is definitive treatment.

TETRALOGY OF FALLOT: VSD, right ventricular hypertrophy, pulmonary stenosis, and overriding aorta.

Presentation: Cyanosis is key sign, especially on exertion.

Management:
- Give oxygen, put in knee-chest position, and consider morphine.
- Beta blocker may prevent further tetany spells.
- Catheterization and early surgical repair are the standard of care.

COARCTATION OF THE AORTA

Presentation: frequent with Turner syndrome; look for varied blood pressure in upper extremity vs. lower extremity.

Management:

- Surgery is a must.
- Antibiotics should be used before procedures and after surgery.

VASCULAR DISEASE

Abdominal Aortic Aneurysm

Presentation: chest, belly or back pain, pulse in abdomen with abdominal aortic aneurysm (AAA).

Management:

- Control blood pressure, especially with beta blocker.
- Ultrasound is preferred screening tool.
- CT is tool of choice for suspected rupture or abnormal ultrasound.
- For aneurysm < 3.5 cm, monitor for 1 year with ultrasound or CT, consider beta blocker.
- For aneurysm of 3.5–5.0 cm, monitor for 6 months, consider beta blocker.
- For aneurysm > 5.0 cm, consider surgery.
- Prompt surgery is needed for ascending dissecting aneurysm.

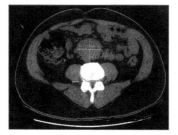

Figure 18. Abdominal aortic aneurysm. (From Baren JM, Alpern ER: Emergency Medicine Pearls, Philadelphia, Hanley & Belfus, 2004, p 97.)

Arteriosclerotic Disease/Atherosclerosis

Presentation: Stroke or MI may be the first presentation. Also causes peripheral vascular disease as well as AAA. Cholesterol and scar tissue build up inside the artery as plaque → plaque ruptures → thrombus forms → occludes vessel.

Management:

- Eliminate risk factors such as hypertension, hyperlipidemia, diabetes, smoking.
- Check lipid profile, and put the patient on a statin (lipid-lowering drug) or lifestyle modification, low cholesterol diet.
- A hot new risk factor is fibrinogen; check it out.
- Moderate alcohol is a **positive** risk factor.
- Physical activity is a **positive** risk factor.
- Vitamin E and other antioxidants may be helpful in preventing LDL from being oxidized.
- Consider aspirin daily as well to prevent the thrombus from forming in ruptured plaque.

Pitfall:

- Remember: if one artery is clogged, others are likely to be clogged also.

Arterial Embolism/Thrombosis

Presentation: blood clot or atherosclerotic plaque blocks artery, causing pain, loss of pulses, numbness in extremity; infarction or ischemia in organ (which may show loss of function).

Management:

- Prevent it. A-fib and valve problems are risk factors; make sure that the patient is anticoagulated if needed.
- Some lab tests may be helpful (e.g., D-dimer).
- Order Doppler ultrasound of extremity.

- Arteriography may be useful.
- Thrombolysis may be required.

Peripheral Vascular Disease

Presentation: most common in smokers, men over 50; symptoms include pulselessness, paralysis, paresthesia, pain, pallor.

Management:
- Prevent it with smoking cessation, cholesterol control.
- Get ankle-brachial index.
- Get Doppler ultrasound to ascertain flow.
- Arteriography is gold standard.
- Consider anticoagulation (aspirin).
- Angioplasty is a possibility.

Phlebitis/Thrombophlebitis

Presentation: erythema, tenderness, edema; clot may be palpable.

Management:
- Risk factors are pregnancy and estrogen use, surgery, immobilization.
- Superficial phlebitis in itself is not dangerous but should be a warning to investigate possible deep thrombosis, especially above greater saphenous vein above the knee.
- Get D-dimer level.
- Rule out factors that may predispose to clotting: factor V Leyden, protein C and protein S deficiency, antithrombin III deficiency, antiphospholipid antibodies, lupus anticoagulant.
- Get Doppler ultrasounds of extremity to rule out deep vein thrombosis (DVT).

Varicose Veins

Presentation: more common in women, especially in pregnancy as valves become incompetent under influence of progesterone and high-pressure flows into low-pressure system.

Management:
- Tell patient to raise legs and rest.
- Order duplex ultrasound.
- Make sure that no DVT is shunting into superficial circulation before commencing treatment, along with compression stockings.
- Sclerotherapy (injection with polidocanol or sodium tetradecyl sulfate) is the most popular treatment.
- Laser and radio ablation are other accepted treatments.

Venous Embolism/Thrombosis

Presentation: edema, leg pain/tenderness due to venous stasis, vessel wall injury, and hypercoagulable state cause clot/obstruction that may break loose. Risk factors include female sex, pregnancy, estrogen, surgery, smoking, and long trip on train, plane, automobile.

Management:
- Pulmonary embolism (PE) is caused by DVT.
- Prevent it with anticoagulation prophylaxis in hospital: heparin 5000 U SQ 2 times/day. Heparin is safe in pregnancy.
- Treat it with low-molecular-weight heparin (Lovenox), and start warfarin orally on the following day.
- Once the therapeutic international normalized ratio (INR) = 2.0 or greater, stop heparin.
- IVC filter for recurrent PE or if anticoagulants contraindicated.
- Get CT of chest to rule out PE, and keep the patient in the hospital if PE is suspected.

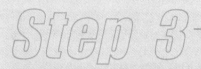
Dermatology

GENERAL ISSUES
    Contact dermatitis
    Decubitus ulcer
    Psoriasis
    Acne
    Folliculitis
    Urticaria
    Seborrhea
    Ingrowing nail
    Localized superficial swelling, mass, or lump
    Hyperhidrosis
    Keloid/hypertrophic scar

INFECTIOUS DISEASES
    Scabies
    Viral warts

MALIGNANCY/TUMORS
    Squamous cell carcinoma
    Basal cell carcinoma
    Malignant melanoma
    Keratoacanthoma
    Seborrheic keratoses
    Lipoma
    Keratoderma, acquired
    Sebaceous cyst
    Neurofibromatosis
    Manifestations of systemic disease

GENERAL ISSUES

Contact Dermatitis

Presentation: redness, itching, swelling.

Management:

- Contact dermatitis is usually type IV hypersensitivity.
- Ask about poison ivy exposure.
- Is the patient wearing jewelry that contains nickel?
- Tell patients that they must avoid allergen.
- Patch testing is gold standard for identification
- Steroids can be used for treatment.

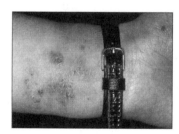

Figure 1. Allergic contact dermatitis to nickel in a watch strap buckle. (From Gawkrodger DJ: Dermatology, An Illustrated Colour Text, 3e. Philadelphia, Churchill Livingstone, 2003, p 31.)

Decubitus Ulcer

	Presentation	Management
STAGE I	Surface reddening of the skin	Air mattresses and frequent turning
STAGE II	Blister either broken or unbroken	Air mattresses and frequent turning, occlusive dressing
STAGE III	Through skin	Surgery, wound culture, and antibiotics
STAGE IV	Extends through the skin and involves underlying muscle, tendons and bone	Surgery, wound culture, and antibiotics

Management:

- Increase protein intake.
- Be alert to osteomyelitis.

Psoriasis

Presentation: skin lesions that are scaling and silvery (scalp, knees, elbows are most common sites).

Management:

- Ask about family history. A positive family history is common.
- Ultraviolet B light is used for severe, extensive psoriasis.
- Also use lubricants for mild psoriasis.
- Give topical steroids for short-term treatment of small areas.
- Prescribe keratolytics such as coal tar, salicylic acid for all types.

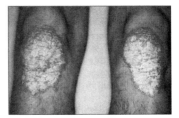

Figure 2. Psoriasis. (From Gawkrodger DJ: Dermatology, An Illustrated Colour Text, 3e. Philadelphia, Churchill Livingstone, 2003, p 27.)

Acne

Presentation: ranges from papules to nodular/cystic presentation that scars.

Management:

- Topical treatments are started first. Advise patient to wash with soap and water at least twice per day. Benzoyl peroxide is also commonly used.
- Then add systemic tetracycline or erythromycin (for pregnant women and children).
- Topical tretinoin (Retin-A) can be effective.
- Systemic isotretinoin (Accutane) is used for cystic acne, which is severely scarring.
- Consider low-dose birth control pill for girls with acne. Spironolactone also has anti-androgen properties and can be used instead.

Folliculitis

Presentation: red bumps around hair.

Management:

- Generally antibiotics are given first, and no other work-up is pursued initially. Cephalexin (Keflex) or dicloxacillin is an appropriate choice.
- If this approach fails, order culture and biopsy to rule out fungal infection or other bacterial causes.

Urticaria

Presentation: wheals; pruritic, erythmatous skin. Watch for progression to anaphylaxis with airway edema, hypotension, shock, plasma leakage into skin.

Management:

- If the patient is in anaphylaxis: intubate, give 100% oxygen, begin IV epinephrine, antihistamines, steroids, fluids, and vasopressors.
- Urticaria is triggered by extremes in temperature, exercise, food, stress, allergies to peanuts, shellfish, nuts, or aspirin.
- If anaphylaxis is not present, give diphenhydramine (cheaper) or fexofenadine (less sedating).

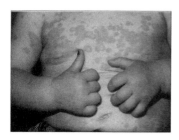

Figure 3. Urticaria in a child. (Courtesy of James E. Fitzpatrick, MD.) (From Nelson HS: Urticaria and angioedema. In Fitzpatrick JE, Aeling JL (eds): Dermatology Secrets in Color, 2e. Philadelphia, Hanley & Belfus, 2001, p 163.)

Seborrhea

Presentation: cradle cap in infants or scaling scalp, eyelids in adults.

Management:

- Shampoo for infants with cradle cap; weak corticosteroid cream/lotion may be added.
- For adults use dandruff/medicated shampoo. May also add topical corticosteroids. Shampoo may contain coal tar, zinc, sulfur or salicylic acid.

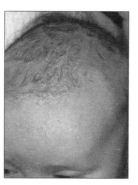

Figure 4. Seborrheic dermatitis. (From McGovern TW: Dermatits (eczema). In Fitzpatrick JE, Aeling JL (eds): Dermatology Secrets in Color, 2e. Philadelphia, Hanley & Belfus, 2001, p 55.)

Ingrowing Nail

Presentation: starts with redness, progresses first to purulence, then to granulation tissue. If left untreated, an ingrowing nail can form an abscess (paronychia).

Management:

- In first stage, warm water soaks may be effective.
- Resect the toenail if beyond this stage. Digital block to the toe is used to cut a wedge section out of toenail.
- Give cephalexin (Keflex) orally.
- If you neglect to treat, it can lead to osteomyelitis and systemic infection.

Localized Superficial Swelling, Mass, or Lump

Presentation: may be cancer, lipoma, abscess, cyst, infected hair follicle.

Management:

- Fine-needle biopsy is minimally invasive and quite sensitive.
- If cancer is found, CT scan is warranted to rule out deeper involvement.
- Excision can be pursued once the diagnosis is certain.

Hyperhidrosis

Presentation: excessive sweating, generally in the armpits, hands, soles of feet.

Management:

- Special topical antiperspirant aluminum chloride (Drysol) is applied at night.
- Surgical sympathectomy is last-resort treatment.

Keloid/Hypertrophic Scar

Presentation: Occur mainly on ear lobes, upper back, and chest (e.g., in African American woman after ear-piercing/surgery).

Management:

- Prevent keloids by meticulous surgical technique that follows lines of Langerhans.
- Steroids are injected into the area. Triamcinolone is the usual choice.
- Excisional surgery is frequently associated with recurrence.

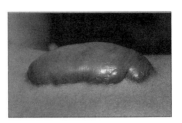

Figure 5. Keloid. (From Grammer-West NY: Special considerations in black skin. In Fitzpatrick JE, Aeling JL (eds): Dermatology Secrets in Color, 2e. Philadelphia, Hanley & Belfus, 2001, p 420.)

INFECTIOUS DISEASES

Scabies

Presentation: classic symptom is severe itching at night/bedtime.

Management:

- Ask the patient about itching, especially at night.
- Look for vesicles/papules along burrows.
- Scrape burrow track and look under microscope for mite, eggs, or feces.
- Prescribe permethrin, which should be applied from neck to feet. Leave on 12 hours and wash off.
- Gamma benzene hexachloride (lindane) can induce seizures and is not used much any more.
- Repeat in one week if no resolution.
- Advise patient to wash clothes and bedding in hot water and to dry on high cycle.
- Watch for secondary bacterial infection,
- Give hydroxine (Atarax) for itching. Diphenhydramine (Benadryl) also is effective.
- Systemic ivermectin can be given for immunosuppressed individuals.
- Use sulfur in petrolatum for pregnant women and children < 2 months old.

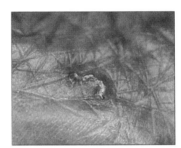

Figure 6. A scabetic burrow on the side of the finger in an elderly patient. (From Gawkrodger DJ: Dermatology, An Illustrated Colour Text, 3e. Philadelphia, Churchill Livingstone, 2003, p 59.)

Viral Warts

Presentation: growths that can be genital or nongenital.

Management:

- Salicylic acid is a common choice for treatment or observation.
- Burn it, freeze it.
- Podophyllum is a cytotoxic agent and must not be used in pregnancy or in women considering pregnancy.
- Imiquimod (Aldara) is the most popular treatment for genital warts.
- For genital warts, exclude other STDs.

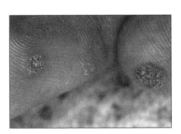

Figure 7. Common viral warts on the hand. (From Gawkrodger DJ: Dermatology, An Illustrated Colour Text, 3e. Philadelphia, Churchill Livingstone, 2003, p 48.)

MALIGNANCY/TUMORS

Squamous Cell Carcinoma

Presentation: white men, middle-aged to elderly; more common with immunosuppressive drugs, arsenic exposure, areas of sun exposure.

Management:
- Do skin biopsy.
- Consider cryosurgery if the lesion is well-circumscribed, or electro-desiccation and curettage.
- Excision.
- Radiation therapy.

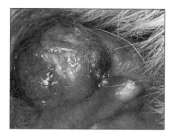

Figure 8. Squamous cell carcinoma. (From Gawkrodger DJ: Dermatology, An Illustrated Colour Text, 3e. Philadelphia, Churchill Livingstone, 2003, p 97.)

SAMPLE QUESTION:

A 65-year-old man comes to the office because of a lip lesion. He has had the lesion for a year. The patient is of Scottish heritage and has worked as a roofer. The most likely diagnosis is:

Basal cell carcinoma

Keratoacanthoma

Leukoplakia

Melanoma

Squamous cell carcinoma

The correct answer is found at the end of the chapter.

Basal Cell Carcinoma

Presentation: small round /oval area of skin thickening may be pearly looking

Management:
- Do skin biopsy.
- Consider cryosurgery if the lesion is well-circumscribed, or electro-desiccation and curettage.
- Excision.
- Radiation therapy is primary treatment.

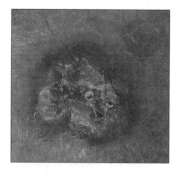

Figure 9. Basal cell carcinoma. (From Gawkrodger DJ: Dermatology, An Illustrated Colour Text, 3e. Philadelphia, Churchill Livingstone, 2003, p 96.)

Malignant Melanoma

Presentation: white adult presents with itchy mole that shows asymmetry, border irregularity, color change/variation, diameter larger than pencil eraser.

Management:
- Ask about changes in size or color. Change to white is an ominous sign.
- Biopsy must be done.
- Staging should be pursued.
- Surgery with wide excision is treatment of choice.
- Follow up with radiotherapy and chemotherapy.

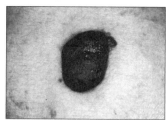

Figure 10. Malignant melanoma. (From Sahn EE: Dermatology Pearls, Philadelphia, Hanley & Belfus, 1999, p 128.)

Keratoacanthoma

Presentation: grows quickly for several weeks, then resolves in a few months. Round, red papules change to dome-shaped nodules, then form crater in center with a plug of keratin.

Management:

- Keratoacanthoma (KA) and squamous cell carcinoma (SCC) appear very similar.
- The risk factors for SCC and KA are the same.
- Surgical excision is almost always pursued.
- 5-Fluorouracil can also be effective if surgery is impossible.
- Examine patient carefully for other skin cancers.

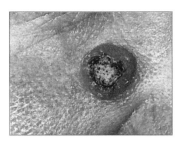

Figure 11. Keratoacanthoma. (From Gawkrodger DJ: Dermatology, An Illustrated Colour Text, 3e. Philadelphia, Churchill Livingstone, 2003, p 98.)

Seborrheic Keratoses

Presentation: classically described as "stuck-on" brown macules, most often found on the trunk.

Management:

- You can treat seborrheic keratoses (SKs) with cryotherapy.
- Surgical excision can also be performed; a shave biopsy is a clean removal technique.
- Ammonium lactate and trichloroacetic acid can be applied topically.
- No treatment is acceptable in absence of irritation, itching, and cosmetic concerns.
- SKs increase with age and are benign; they are generally not considered to have malignant potential. A sudden appearance has been associated with GI adenocarcinoma.
- You should send for biopsy because you do not want to mistake a malignancy for an SK.

Lipoma

Presentation: most likely a freely mobile mass that is subcutaneous; very common tumor that can be superficial or occur in almost any area of the body.

Management:
- Remove for cosmetic reasons or
- Send for biopsy to rule out liposarcoma if the lesion is very large or not freely mobile. Also order biopsy if the lesion is on the legs, which are the most common site of liposarcoma.
- Lipomas recur frequently.

Keratoderma, Acquired

Presentation: hyperkeratosis usually found on soles of feet or palms of hands. Associated with psoriasis, among other diseases; also common in postmenopausal women (climacteric).

Management:
- Topical keratolytic such as salicylic acid is used to soften skin.
- Etretinate is used to treat.

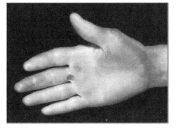

Figure 12. Keratoderma. (From Gawkrodger DJ: Dermatology, An Illustrated Colour Text, 3e. Philadelphia, Churchill Livingstone, 2003, p 86.)

Sebaceous Cyst

Presentation: firm, round, movable subcutaneous nodule; sometimes foul-smelling liquid is expressible when the nodule is squeezed.

Management:
- Inject triamcinolone into cyst.
- Incision and drainage are appropriate if the cyst appears infected. Follow up with PO antibiotics such as cephalexin (Keflex).

- These cysts have been associated with underlying malignancy; once excised, the cyst should be sent for biopsy

Neurofibromatosis (NF)

Presentation: presents generally in late adolescence.

NF1	Multiple neurofibromas, café-au-lait macules, Lisch nodules of the eye (hamartomas of iris), pheochromocytomas
NF2	Central neurofibromatosis, bilateral acoustic schwannomas

Management:

- Since NF is an autosomal dominant disease, genetic counseling is necessary.
- NF has variable expression in different families.
- MRI of brain, spinal cord is the most useful tool to evaluate for tumors.
- Neurosurgeon can excise tumors that are causing neurological problems.
- Watch for transformation in neurofibromas because they have malignant potential.
- Biopsy suspicious lesions.
- X-ray of skull and long bones to detect bony changes.

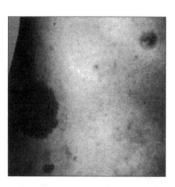

Figure 13. Cafe au lait spots. (From Sahn EE: Dermatology Pearls, Philadelphia, Hanley & Belfus, 1999, p 139.)

Manifestations of Systemic Disease

	Symptom	Cause
Acanthosis nigricans	Darkening of nape of neck, underarms	Hyperinsulinemia, malignancy
Amyloidosis	Easy bruising	Multiple myeloma
Cullen's sign	Purpuric discoloration of the umbilicus	Pancreatitis
Cutaneous lupus erythematosus	Malar butterfly rash across bridge of nose	Lupus
Dermatitis herpetiformis	Itchy vesicles on knees and elbows	Gluten sensitivity
Dermatomyositis	Muscle weakness and plaques. Look for rash around eyes.	Adenocarcinoma
Ehlers-Danlos syndrome	Hyperflexible skin	Collagen synthesis problems
Erythema chronicum migrans	Bull's-eye rash	Lyme disease

continued

Manifestations of Systemic Disease (continued)

	Symptom	Cause
Erythema multiforme/ Stevens-Johnson syndrome	Target lesions progress to desquamation of lips, vulva	Herpes or mycoplasma or drug reaction (usually to an antibiotic)
Erythema nodosum	Sores on shins	Sarcoid
Exfoliative dermatitis	Peeling and itching	Sézary cutaneous T-cell lymphoma
Leser-Trelat sign	Many pruritic seborrheic keratoses suddenly appear	Adenocarcinoma of GI system, lymphoma/leukemia
Necrolytic migratory erythema	Erythema, bullae	Glucagonoma
Osler-Weber-Rendu syndrome	Frequent nose bleeds. Telangiectases on the skin and oral mucosa	Autosomal dominant disorder
Paget's disease	Unilateral, eczemalike plaque of nipple	Intraductal carcinoma
Palpable purpura	Raised areas of hemorrhage normally on lower body	Henoch-Schönlein purpura, sepsis, infections
Pemphigus vulgaris	Mucosal blisters that erode and spread	Autoimmune with IgG deposition
Peutz-Jeghers syndrome	Freckles around lips/mouth	Hamartomatous polyps in small bowel
Porphyria cutanea tarda	Fragile skin that is photosensitive	Porphyria
Progressive systemic sclerosis	CREST syndrome with **c**alcinosis, **R**aynaud's phenomenon, **e**sophageal dysmotility, **s**clerosis/contractures of the digits, **t**elangiectasias	Autoimmune anticentromere
Pyoderma gangrenosum	Ulcer with blue border	Ulcerative colitis
Scleroderma	Erythematous patches change to hypopigmented plaques with purple borders. Step 3 classic is picture of hands with red, "tight"-looking skin.	Autoimmune antitopoisomerase
Sister Mary Joseph nodule	Umbilical metastases	Cancer in bowel/pelvis
Sweet's syndrome	Red plaques and papules	Leukemia/lymphoma
Grey-Turner's sign	Purpuric flank discoloration	Hemorrhagic pancreatitis (due to retroperitoneal bleed)
Vitiligo	Loss of skin color	Autoimmune disorder, hypothyroidism
Xanthomas	Skin tags	Hyperlipidemia

Answer to sample question:

E.

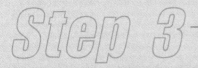

CHAPTER 3

Emergency Medicine and Trauma

BURNS/EXPOSURE
 Burns
 Frostbite
 Heat stroke

EARS, NOSE, AND THROAT EMERGENCIES
 Foreign body in ear
 Foreign body in nose
 Foreign body in trachea/aspiration
 Swallowed foreign body
 Epistaxis (nosebleed)

EYE EMERGENCIES
 Foreign body in eye
 Eye burn/flash burn
 Ocular injury

SURGICAL COMPLICATIONS
 Central nervous system complications
 Respiratory complications
 Gastrointestinal complications
 Hemorrhage complicating surgery
 Postoperative infections
 Other complications of devices/grafts

TOXICOLOGY
 Food poisoning
 Poisoning by drugs and medicinal
  substances
 Antidotes for medicinal substances
 Antidotes for nonmedicinal substances
 Adverse effects of drugs, medicinal and
  biological substances

TRAUMA
 General principles of management
 Primary survey: ABCDEs
 Secondary survey
 Rape/crisis adjustment
 Concussion, no loss or brief loss of
  consciousness
 Central nervous system trauma/cranial
  injuries
 Chest trauma
 Internal injuries: abdomen and pelvis
 Traumatic shock
 Wounds, including bites

BURNS/EXPOSURE

Burns

Presentation:

First-degree burn	Superficial: affects only epidermis. Looks like sunburn and is painful.
Second-degree	Partial-thickness: dermis is also involved. Look for blisters and extreme pain.
Third-degree	Full-thickness: look for charred eschar and painless area as nerves are burned away.

Management:

- Always mind the ABCs, especially with facial burns, and be alert for inhalation injury. Be prepared to give 100% oxygen.
- Management depends on extent of burns. Grading includes depth of burn and percentage of body surface area (BSA). One hand = 1% of body surface area.
- The first step is to cover the burn with sterile dressing and irrigate with cold saline.
- Then use topical antiseptic with iodine, and rinse it off.
- Do **not** pop blisters. Debride blisters if they are large.
- Update tetanus status.
- Apply topical antibiotics such as silver sulfadiazine only if the burn is minor and the patient is not being admitted to the hospital.
- Control pain aggressively. Morphine is a good choice.
- When the pain has subsided, gently cleanse the burn with povidone-iodine scrub, and rinse it off with normal saline.
- Admit to the hospital if the following criteria are met:
    - Third-degree burn over 5% BSA
    - Second-degree over 10% BSA
    - Either second- or third-degree burns of any BSA percentage involving the face, skin over joints, or genitals
    - Burns that are circumferential around chest (they may compromise breathing and may require escharotomy)
    - Coexisting problems such as inhalation injury or trauma
- Burn victims need aggressive fluid replacement. Follow urine output closely.
- Burn victims have increased protein needs as well. Supplement accordingly.
- Burn victims are at risk of hypothermia. Cover and keep warm.
- In burn units various techniques of skin grafting are performed.
- Never delay transfer of patient for definitive care.

Frostbite

Presentation:

Frostnip	Freezing of the epidermis only. Look for blanching and numbness. Becomes red and painful when rewarmed.
Mild frostbite	Involves freezing of dermis also. Appears white in appearance and feels like partially frozen bread dough. Also becomes red with more pain and edema when the patient is rewarmed. Blisters may form.
Severe frostbite	Different from mild frostbite and feels hard.

Management:

- Rewarm only if there is no possibility of refreezing. If you are in the ED and take a base station call, give this advice over the radio.
- Treat ABCs. Patients may have coincidental hypothermia and dehydration as well.
- Once the patient is in the ED a hot bath is an excellent choice.
- Start pain control. The injury is going to hurt once the patient is rewarmed.
- Update tetanus status.
- Antibiotics are not used routinely unless signs of infection are present.
- Many aspects of management are similar to those for treating burns. Cleanse and dress similarly.
- Sympathetic nerve drama may result in permanent cold sensitivity and abnormal fingernail growth.

- Advise the patient not to smoke and to avoid bars and other smoky areas to keep blood flow at maximum.
- Admit all cases of severe frostbite.

Heat Stroke

Presentation: an athlete who overdoes it in high temperatures, an elderly person who does not have air-conditioning. Fatigue, cramp, and weakness suddenly proceed to central nervous system dysfunction, including but not limited to seizures or coma. This progression differentiates heat stroke from milder heat injury. Patients may or may not be sweating.

Management:
- Mind the ABCs as always.
- Administer oxygen, ice packs, and fluids in the ED.
- Get lab tests including CMP, arterial blood gases, creatine phosphokinase (CPK). Look for liver function tests to be elevated in heat stroke.
- A CT of the head is warranted once the patient is stabilized.
- Spray water on the patient and turn on the fans—or consider an ice bath.
- Treat seizures with diazepam.
- Absence of sweating is a late and ominous sign.
- Admit for close monitoring.

EARS, NOSE, AND THROAT EMERGENCIES

Foreign Body in Ear

Presentation: child with a bug in the ear or something else that the child has stuffed there.

Management:
- Look in the ear.
- For a live insect, use mineral oil to drown the bug first; then proceed with definitive procedure.
- Techniques for removal:
  - Water irrigation or suction (for loose objects)
  - Alligator forceps (for soft objects)
  - Ear curette (for hard/round objects such as marbles, peas)
  - Cyanoacrylate glue on the end of Q-tip can be fixed to object, which is then pulled out.

Foreign Body in Nose

Presentation: pediatric patient or psychiatric patient with object stuffed in nose and possibly unilateral purulent nasal discharge.

Management:
- Look in the nose.
- Consider x-ray if you are not sure what is in the nose.
- Have patient try to blow nose.
- Restrain pediatric patients before attempting to mess with their nose.
- Apply topical anesthetic/vasoconstrictor such as phenylephrine and tetracaine/cocaine to inside of nose.
- Forceps, hooks, and clamps may be used in attempts to grasp the object. Do not push it in further.
- Positive pressure ventilation has also been used to blow out the object.
- You can also irrigate through the opposite nostril and wash out the object.

Foreign Body in Trachea/Aspiration

Presentation: preceded by eating peanuts/sunflower seeds. Patients usually present with coughing/choking, which can result in complete respiratory failure or almost no symptoms.

Management:

- Do a good history and physical exam, and figure out what was aspirated. Is it getting worse? Organic matter may swell over time. The object may be getting lodged deeper.
- Listen to breath sounds for wheezing and stridor.
- You may attempt to remove the object with forceps if you can directly visualize it and if it is high enough up.
- Get a chest x-ray with posteroanterior (PA) and lateral views.
- If you have to bet money on which side the object is in, it is probably the right mainstem bronchus.
- Extraction by bronchoscopy is the standard treatment. Steroids and antibiotics are given sometimes before the procedure to minimize infection and swelling/edema.
- If bronchoscopy fails after a second attempt, proceed to open thoracotomy.

Swallowed Foreign Body

Presentation: pediatric patient or drug "mule" (transporter).

Management:

- Make sure that the trachea is not also obstructed.
- Figure out where the object is with x-rays, including throat, chest, and abdomen .
- Consider barium swallow or metal detector if the object is radiopaque.
- Endoscopic removal is the standard of care.
- For blunt objects alternative techniques include:
  - Pushing the object into the stomach for elimination
  - Pushing a Foley catheter past the object, inflating it, and pulling the object out the mouth
- If the patient is a drug mule, consider Golytely to flush out the object. Such patients are at risk of poisoning if the condoms (or whatever they wrapped the drug in) bursts. Then you have a toxicology problem.

Epistaxis (Nosebleed)

Presentation: Frequently caused by nose picking; usually caused by trauma but also can reflect malignancy. In the ED worry only about management.

Management:

- Delay taking the history until bleeding is controlled. When you get the chance, ask about aspirin or wafarin use and find out whether the patient has had nosebleeds in the past.
- Make sure that the patient is hemodynamically stable and replace blood/fluids.
- Apply pressure to nostrils and ask the patient to sit up.
- Place anesthetic/vasoconstrictor solution into nasal cavity with cotton pledgets soaked with cocaine or epinephrine. Sometimes this approach is enough.
- Silver nitrate can be attempted to cauterize chemically.
- If these options fail, then pack the nose anteriorly.
- If you pack the nose, discharge the patient with an antibiotic to prevent sinus infection.
- CBC and coagulation profile if bleeding continues.
- The last-ditch option is inflatable posterior epistaxis balloons. You can even use a small female Foley catheter. If this strategy is needed, admit the patient and refer to an ENT specialist.

EYE EMERGENCIES

Foreign Body in Eye

Presentation: Construction worker struck by rust/particle while grinding/hammering metal.

Management:

- Apply anesthetic drops to eye.
- Check visual acuity.
- Examine anterior chamber with slit lamp.
- Perform funduscopy.
- Look for foreign body deep in the eye, especially if the object is a high-speed missile, which may barely ripple the surface of the eye. The worst mistake that you can make is to miss an intraocular foreign body. Consider CT of orbits to rule out foreign body.
- Scrape off foreign body.
- Residual rust rings must be scraped off with a burr.
- Fluorescein may be used to check for corneal defect.
- Flush the eye.
- Apply antibiotic and eye patch, and prescribe oral analgesics. This injury is going to hurt like the devil when the drops wear off.
- Schedule ophthalmologic follow-up in 24 hours.

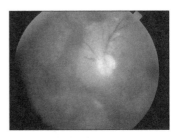

Figure 1. Foreign body in eye. (From Gault JA: Ophthalmology Pearls. Philadelphia, Hanley & Belfus, 2003, p 148.)

Eye Burn/Flash Burn

Presentation: The classic patient is a welder not wearing eye shields who gets splashed with chemicals or a skier who is exposed to bright sunlight and becomes snowblind after 8 hours.

Management of chemical burn:

- Water, water everywhere. Flush the chemical burn. This is the first-line treatment.
- Remove contact lenses if they are still in place.
- Alkali is more dangerous than acid.
- Consider calcium gluconate for acid burns, but do not be fooled: flushing is the mainstay of treatment. On Step 3, you should select that option above all others.
- Consider ascorbic acid drops for alkali burns, but do not be fooled: flushing is the mainstay of treatment. On Step 3, you should select that option above all others.
- Admit patients with serious penetration.

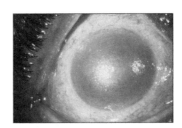

Figure 2. Chemical burn. (From Gault JA: Ophthalmology Pearls. Philadelphia, Hanley & Belfus, 2003, p 213.)

Management of flash burn:

- Do full exam, anterior and posterior, including fluorescein staining.
- Use systemic pain medicine—**not** topical.
- Give an antibiotic.
- Use a mydriatic agent to widen the pupils and decrease painful spasm.
- Apply patch to the eyes.
- Give tetanus booster.
- Advise patient to wear UV protective sunglasses/shield when exposed to the sun.

Ocular Injury

Presentation: blow to the eye from accident or sports (e.g., golf ball).

Management:
- Check visual acuity.
- Extraocular movement that is restricted vertically suggests orbital blow-out.
- Palpate the orbital rims for fracture.
- Check for papillary dysfunction, which may suggest optic nerve damage.
- Illuminate the anterior chamber to look for hyphema. A slit lamp is an awesome choice if you have that option.
- Do a fundoscopic exam, but if the patient has a head injury, do not dilate the eyes.
- Get a CT of the head.

SURGICAL COMPLICATIONS

- Retinal detachment or obital blowout requires an emergent ophthalmologic consult.

Central Nervous System Complications

Presentation: new onset of mental status changes may reflect hypoxia/hypercapnea, hypoglycemia, hypo/hypernatremia, hypercalcemia, uremia, pneumonia, sepsis, or simply reaction to general anesthesia.

Management:
- Give oxygen and get arterial blood gases/pulse oximetry.
- Get fingerstick, and give glucose if needed.
- Get lab tests to check electrolytes.
- Consider naloxone.
- Proceed with blood cultures, CT of head, and lumbar puncture as needed.

Respiratory Complications

Presentation: atelectasis, deep venous thrombosis (DVT)/pulmonary embolism, pneumonia.

Management:
- Give supplemental oxygen.
- Chest physiotherapy helps prevent respiratory complications.
- Postoperative DVT prophylaxis prevents clots in immobile patients, especially orthopedic patients.
- Incentive spirometer and deep breathing exercise are recommended postoperatively.

Gastrointestinal Complications

Presentation: swollen, distended abdomen. Paralytic ileus may occur after surgery; nausea and vomiting are also common.

Management:
- A nasogastric (NG) tube is passed into the stomach for suction to relieve distention until the bowel "wakes." Kidney, ureter, and bladder x-rays are used for follow-up.
- Nausea and vomiting are frequent reactions to anesthesia. This is why patients are kept on NPO status before surgery. Both should diminish on their own.

Hemorrhage Complicating Surgery

Presentation: decreasing hemoglobin, frank blood.

Management:
- Prevent hemorrhage: ask all preoperative patients about use of aspirin, ginkgo biloba.
- Get international normalized ratio (INR) before surgery; in general, do not operate if the INR is above 1.5. Give vitamin K to correct.
- Clopidogrel (Plavix) cannot be given prior to coronary artery bypass grafting, because tamponade can develop. Heparin generally is used and stopped on the day of the intervention in patients undergoing cardiothoracic surgery.
- Give packed red blood cells as needed.

Postoperative Infections

Presentation: timing of fever/other signs can indicate source of infection. Urinary tract infection (UTI) is usually first, followed by pneumonia, then wound infection.

Management:
- Suspect UTI if symptoms of infection appear very early after surgery. Culture and treat.
- Get chest x-ray to rule out pneumonia and atelectasis.
- Examine wound and consider culturing it.
- Get blood cultures to rule out sepsis.
- If you still have no answer, consider CT to look for deep abscesses, especially after abdominal surgery.

Other Complications of Devices and Grafts

Presentation: most common complications are infection of any indwelling device as well as clotting around stents or artificial valves.

Management:
- Know the guidelines for anticoagulation. For artificial heart valves, INR should be between 2.5 and 3.5.
- Consider antibiotics before dental/invasive procedures that can cause temporary bacteremia.

TOXICOLOGY

Food Poisoning

Presentation: patient with nausea, vomiting, cramps, and, diarrhea.

Management:
- Make absolutely sure that the problem is food poisoning; you need a solid history to support this diagnosis. Ask about other affected individuals. Make sure that the patient does not have obstruction, abdominal aortic aneurysm, mesenteric ischemia, myocardial infarction, pancreatitis.
- Check electrolytes if the problem has been present for some time.
- IV fluids (lactate Ringer's or normal saline) are appropriate.
- Antibiotics generally are not used, although there are some exceptions:
- For *Shigella* food poisoning, give trimethoprim-sulfamethoxazole (TMP-SMX).
- If typhoid fever is present (malaise, fever, abdominal pain, and bradycardia), treat *Salmonella* food poisoning with TMP-SMX. Do not treat otherwise because antibiotic prolongs carrier state.
- Initiate trial of oral fluids.
- Criteria for admission are hypotension and intolerance for oral intake.
- For outpatient care: oral rehydration therapy (ORT) is the standard, even if the patient is not yet dehydrated clinically. ORT is basically water, salt, sugar, fruit juice, and baking soda.
- You may give prochlorperazine suppository for continued nausea/vomiting or Imodium for diarrhea. However, do not give either right away as toxins are eliminated from the body.

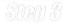

Poisoning by Drugs and Medicinal Substances

Many of these substances have been covered already.

Management:

- ABCs are always the priority. Follow the ACLS, ATLS, PALs protocols. You may badly want to give a particular antidote. But if the patient is in respiratory failure and needs to be intubated, you must intubate first. Otherwise the patient may not live long enough to get the antidote. Step 3 likes to test your clinical judgment in prioritizing care. Watch for **the next most appropriate step** on the exam.
- Supportive care is frequently all that can be offered. It includes intubation, fluids, pressors, seizure control, and/or pacemaker insertion, based on clinical need.
- Generally, charcoal is almost always safe to give in overdose patients, but too much can induce vomiting and cause aspiration. Sometimes multiple unknown substances have been ingested, and charcoal may be useful for some of them.
- Inducing vomiting/gastric decontamination is not advisable when aspiration risk is higher than the toxicity. If the patient is intubated and an NG tube is placed to suction, vomiting may be used for aromatics, hydrocarbons, heavy metals, and pesticides. In general, however, do not pick induction of vomiting.
- If a mother calls you, always err on the conservative side and tell her to go to the local ED. Expect a question like this. Do not offer reassurance.
- Call the local toxicology center for recommendations; the center is frequently located at the local children's hospital.
- Specific antidotes are listed below, but **do not forget to include supportive therapies**.

Antidotes for Medicinal Substances

TOXIN	ANTIDOTE
Acetaminophen	Acetylcysteine
Anticholinergic drug	Physostigmine
Antidepressant	Bicarbonate for TCAs
Antidysrhythmic drug	Hemodialysis, pacer, pressors
Antihistamine	Physostigmine, benzodiazepines, bicarbonate
Barbiturate	Bicarbonate
Benzodiazepine	Flumazenil
Beta blocker	Glucagon, then atropine, isoproterenol, or epinephrine
Calcium channel blocker	Calcium chloride, then glucagon
Carbamazepine (TCA)	Bicarbonate
Digoxin	Digibind; maintain optimal potassium level
Gamma-hydroxybutyrate (GHB), also known as date rape drug	Atropine in bradycardia Physostigmine in coma
Isoniazid	Pyridoxine (vitamin B6)
Lithium	Hemodialysis is definitive, but give GoLytely acutely
Narcotics	Naloxone

continued

Antidotes for Medicinal Substances (continued)

TOXIN	ANTIDOTE
Neuroleptic agents (neuroleptic malignant syndrome)	Dantrolene
Salicylate	Sodium bicarbonate
Sedative/hypnotics	Flumazenil
Thallium	Prussian blue
Theophylline	Hemoperfusion is definitive; give phenobarbital for seizures and increase excretion
Thyroid hormone	Beta blocker, propylthiouracil
Valproate	Hemodialysis
Warfarin	Vitamin K

Antidotes for Nonmedicinal Substances

TOXIN	ANTIDOTE
Methanol	Give ethanol or fomepizole
Arsenic	Dimercaprol
Carbon monoxide	Oxygen
Caustic ingestions	Methylprednisolone for lungs and ranitidine for gut
Chlorine gas	Bicarbonate and albuterol
Cyanide	Sodium nitrite
Ethylene glycol	Fomepizole or ethanol
Fluoride	Calcium carbonate
Heavy metals: lead, arsenic, and mercury	Dimercaprol
Hydrocarbon insecticides	Benzodiazepines and cholestyramine
Hydrogen sulfide	Sodium nitrite
Iron	Deferoxamine and GoLytely
Lead	Dimercaprol or EDTA
Mercury	Dimercaprol
Mushroom, Amatoxin	High-dose penicillin
Mushroom, Gyromitra	Methylene blue
Mushrooms	Pyridoxine and benzodiazepines for seizures
Nitrous dioxide	Prednisone and methylene blue
Organophosphates (insecticide)	Atropine and 2-PAM (pralidoxime)
Thallium	Prussian blue

Adverse Effects of Drugs and Medicinal and Biological Substances

DRUG	NOTE	SIDE EFFECT
Angiotensin-converting enzyme (ACE) inhibitors	Switch to angiotensin receptor blocker (ARB) for cough; check creatinine and stop if above 1.5	Cough, failure in renal artery stenosis, renal agenesis in first trimester
Acetaminophen (Tylenol)	Avoid alcohol with Tylenol	Liver damage, especially with alcohol
Acetazolamide (Diamox)	Can be used for altitude sickness	Metabolic acidosis
Alpha-1 blockers (terazosin)	Advise patient to take first dose lying in bed	Orthostatic hypotension
Aminoglycoside	Avoid loop diuretics	Ototoxicity and renal toxicity
Amiodarone	Get TSH, LFTs before commencing treatment	Pulmonary fibrosis, thyroid problems, corneal deposits
Aspirin	Never give with warfarin	GI bleed
Beta blockers	Avoid in asthma	Asthma exacerbation, AV block
Bleomycin		Pulmonary fibrosis
Bupropion		Seizures
Calcium channel blockers		Heart block
Chloramphenicol		Gray baby, aplastic anemia
Cisplatin		Liver damage
Clindamycin	Treat with metronidazole or vancomycin	Pseudomembranous colitis
Clozapine	Measure CBC regularly	Agranulocytosis
Dideoxyinosine (ddI)		Pancreatitis
Digoxin	Avoid in renal failure	GI upset, bradycardia
Diphenhydramine (Benadryl)	Used in elderly but should not be	Mental obstipation
Doxorubicin		Cardiomyopathy
Estrogen		DVTs, strokes, breast cancer
Ethambutol	Routine ophthalmologic exams	Optic nerve damage
Finasteride	Must avoid exposure in pregnant women	Genital malformation in male fetus
Fluoroquinolones		Cartilage damage in fetus
Halogen	Give dantrolene	Malignant hyperthermia
Heparin		Thrombocytopenia
HMG CoA reductase (Lipitor)	Measure CPK with pain, routine AST/LFTs	Liver damage, rhabdomyolysis, muscle aches
Isoniazid	Give with vitamin B6	Vitamin B6 deficiency
Isotretinoin (Accutane)	2 forms of birth control mandated	Teratogen

continued

Adverse Effects of Drugs and Medicinal and Biological Substances (continued)

DRUG	NOTE	SIDE EFFECT
Lithium		Hypothyroidism, diabetes insipidus
Loop diuretics		Hypokalemia, ototoxicity, hypocalcemia
Monoamine oxidase (MOA) inhibitors	Never give with SSRI	Tyramine crisis with aged cheese, sauerkraut, wine
Meperidine (Demerol)	Avoid prolonged use	Seizures and coma
Methyldopa		Depression, hemolytic anemia
Metronidazole	Avoid alcohol	Photosensitivity, disulfiram reaction with alcohol
Minoxidil		Excess body hair
Niacin	Give aspirin before niacin to reduce flush	"Flush" or itch
Oxytocin		Syndrome of inappropriate antidiuretic hormone
Penicillin		Allergic reaction
Phenytoin (Dilantin)	Do not stop in pregnancy if mother has serious seizure disorder	Possible birth defects
Procainamide		Lupus
Progesterone		Moodiness, weight gain, breast tenderness, bloating, depression
Pseudoephedrine/ephedra		Hypertension, dry mouth, urinary retention
Sildenafil (Viagra)	No nitrates	Blue vision, critical hypotension with nitrates
Selective serotonin reuptake inhibitors (SSRIs)		Gastrointestinal upset, delayed ejaculation
Sulfa-containing drugs		Allergies
Testosterone/anabolic steroids		Dyslipidemia, hirsutism, liver damage, testicular atrophy, clitoral enlargement
Tetracyclines		Tooth-staining in children, OCP failure, photosensitivity
Thiazide diuretics	Avoid in gout	Hypercalcemia, hyperglycemia, gout
Trazodone		Priapism
Vancomycin	Give antihistamine	Red man syndrome
Warfarin	Contraindicated in pregnancy	Birth defects

TRAUMA

Here is a quick overview of trauma/ATLS guidelines. This section may sound foreign to all but ED and surgery residents. There are certainly both MCQs as well as CCS scenarios in which these concepts come into play on Step 3.

General Principles of Management

- The ABCs **always** take precedence. Do not delay for any lab test or diagnostic study.
- Never delay transfer to a more appropriate trauma center for diagnostic tests such as CTs and x-rays. If you are in a small ED or someone carries a patient into your office after trauma, complete the primary survery and arrange immediate transfer.
- Doctor-to-doctor communication is required for transfers.

Primary Survey: ABCDEs

- **A**irway with cervical spine control:
  - Jaw thrust is best in case of presumed cervical injury.
  - Bag and tube the patient, do a cricothyroidotomy—whatever it takes get an airway because nothing else matters without it.
- **B**reathing
  - Every patient gets oxygen as soon as possible.
  - Bag or ventilate patient if needed. (Postive-pressure ventilation before needle decompression is a no-no in patients with a spontaneous pneumothorax because it can convert the problem to a tension pneumothorax.)
  - Do inspection, palpation, percussion, and auscultation of the thorax.
  - Look for distended neck veins, asymmetry in chest rise and fall, accessory muscle use, contusions, penetrating injuries, sucking wounds, dyspnea, tachypnea.
  - Feel for tenderness, crepitus, subcutaneous emphysema, tracheal deviation, or flail chest.
  - Listen for hyperresonance, dullness, asymmetry of breath sounds, or distant heart tones.
  - Proceed with needle thoracentesis and chest tube placement if you suspect hemo/pneumothorax. Both are quite common.
- **C**irculation/control of bleeding
  - Use direct pressure.
  - Give isotonic IV fluids, LR or NS (bolus 20 ml/kg in pediatric patients and 1–2 liters in adults)
  - Perform cardiopulmonary resuscitation (CPR).
- **D**isability/neurologic status
  - Look at the patient's pupils; they are the fastest neurologic sign.
  - Do not spend time on this step until the patient is resuscitated.
- **E**nvironment/exposure
  - Be aware of chemicals on the patient and protect yourself.
  - Undress the patient completely.
  - Roll the patient over to examine the back.
  - Prevent hypothermia.

Secondary Survey

- **AMPLE** history:
  - **A**llergies
  - **M**edications
  - **P**ast medical history

- □ Last meal: important information because trip to OR may be in patient's near future and aspiration is a risk after anesthesia
    - □ Environment /events related to patient's injury
- Musculoskeletal injuries require realignment and immobilization, which may require traction splint. Check for pulses. Order x-rays as needed later.
- The only x-rays generally done acutely after trauma are cervical, chest, and pelvic. Everything else can wait until transfer to the OR or SICU.
- Everybody gets a rectal exam for heme check.
- Do not insert a urinary catheter if blood is present at the urethral meatus or if the patient has a severely fractured pelvis or high-riding prostate on exam.
- Trauma is best managed in the OR, and the sooner you get the patient there, the better. Never delay for any test or study.

Rape/Crisis Adjustment

Presentation: female or male after sexual assault.

Management:
- Ask about the details of assault for law enforcement purposes.
- Maintain and collect evidence, including photographs, semen, hairs.
- Test and treat for STDs (gonorrhea and chlamydial culture, syphilis serology, HIV, hepatitis panel).
- Give female patients emergency contraception.
- Consider treatment for hepatitis B.
- Test for AIDS acutely and at 6 months.
- Get patient to counseling.
- Post-traumatic stress disorder is highly likely after this or any other traumatic event.
- Coping strategies after crisis include maintaining normal schedule, talking with friends and family, support groups.
- Emotional symptoms can persist for months or years.

Concussion, No Loss or Brief Loss of Consciousness

Presentation: patient comes to the ED with a bump on the head, perhaps while playing sports or after a motor vehicle accident.

Management:
- Know the mechanism of injury.
- On exam note any depression of skull.
- Do a neurologic examination.
- CT of the head is mandated with loss of consciousness, amnesia, CSF leak through nose/ear, bruising of the mastoid (Battle's sign), stupor/coma, or focal neurologic sign.
- Get skull films if the patient was hit with a hammer or a skull depression is noted.
- Observe patient for late signs of head injury including drowsiness, headache.
- Rules for return-to-play decisions in athletes after concussion are summarized below.

GRADE	SYMPTOMS	RETURN TO PLAY
Mild	No loss of consciousness Symptoms persist for under 15 minutes	May return to play after 15 minutes
Moderate	No loss of consciousness Symptoms persist for over 15 minutes	1 full week
Severe	Loss of consciousness	Withhold from play 1 month

Central Nervous System Trauma/Cranial Injuries

Presentation: frequently after a motor vehicle accident.

Management:

- Head trauma mandates CT of head. Slow bleeds may not be apparent for a day or so. Moderately hyperventilate the patient, treat shock with fluids **without** dextrose; in patients with elevated intra-cranial pressure, consider mannitol/Lasix after consulting with neurosurgeon.
- Spine trauma is best evaluated by neurologic exam.
- Do not clear collar until cervical x-ray shows all cervical vertebrae to T1.
- Document neurologic status so that change can be monitored.
- Steroids are given to prevent cord swelling and preserve function within 8 hours injury.
- Insert gastric and urinary catheters to prevent stomach/bladder distention if the patient is paralyzed.
- Scalp wounds bleed a great deal but are rarely life-threatening. Stapling is the most rapid way to close, but **never** close an area of depressed skull, which may hide something a neurosurgeon needs to see.

Chest Trauma

Presentation: unrestrained passenger strikes steering wheel in motor vehicle accident.

Management:

- In patients with thoracic trauma look for pneumo/hemothorax, pulmonary contusion, blunt cardiac injury, aortic disruption, diaphragmatic injury, mediastinal traversing wounds.
- Treatment often must be initiated before chest x-ray is done.
- A simple chest x-ray can show many of these injuries.
- Simple techniques such as intubation, ventilation, tube thoracostomy, and needle pericardiocentesis can be quite beneficial.
- Narrow pulse pressure, hypotension, increased JVP, and distant heart sounds may indicate tamponade; insert a needle and drain off the blood.
- Echocardiography is the gold standard, but tamponade is usually diagnosed on exam.

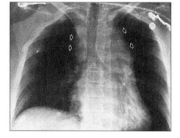

Figure 3. Traumatic aortic rupture. (From Groskin SA: Chest trauma. In Katz DS, Math KR, Groskin SA (eds): Radiology Secrets. Philadelphia, Hanley & Belfus, 1998, p 458.)

Internal Injuries, Abdomen and Pelvis

Presentation: seatbelt injury in motor vehicle accident, physical assault/battery.

Management:

- Abdominal trauma management is related to mechanism: penetrating vs. blunt injury.
- Celiotomy is mandated for penetrating injuries. Diagnostic peritoneal lavage is invasive but rapid and has a 98% sensitivity in finding bleeds in blunt injury. Serial exams or CT studies are slower alternatives in asymptomatic patients.
- Wrap a sheet around the patient's pelvis tightly to help control bleeding. A patient can hide a lot of blood in the pelvis.

Traumatic Shock

Presentation: frequently a motor vehicle accident, gunshot wound, or knife wound.

Management:

- One can hide many liters of blood in the abdomen, pelvis, and thighs.
- Initial fluid bolus: 20 ml/kg in pediatric patients and 1–2 liters in adult.

- Tachycardia is a late sign of hypovolemia, especially in young people and well-conditioned athletes.
- Be able to estimate blood loss and replace according to the 3:1 rule. If 1 liter is lost, give 3 liters of replacement.
- Type and cross–match as soon as possible, although crystalloid fluids are your first choice for resuscitation. It is safe to use type O negative blood if you do not have time to type and cross-match. Type O negative blood is especially advisable when you are presented with multiple trauma victims simultaneously because of the high risk that the wrong bag will be hung and lead to the nightmare of blood reactions in the middle of multiple traumas.
- Trauma in pregnant women is tricky because plasma volume increases and may mask signs of hypovolemia.

Blood Loss Adults	15%	15–30%	30–40%	>40%
Pulse	<100	>100	>120	>140
Urine output	>30	20–30	5–15	0
Systolic BP	>110	>100	<90	<90
Respirations	16	16–20	21–26	>26
Mental status	Anxious	Agitated	Confused	Lethargic
Capillary refill	<2 sec	>2 sec	>2 sec	>>2 sec
Replacement	Fluids	Fluids	Fluids + blood	Fluids + blood

Wounds, Including Bites

Presentation:

Presentation	
Cuts	Smooth
Lacerations	Jagged
Avulsions	Tissue is torn away

Management:
- Check the ABCs.
- Secure hemostasis. Direct pressure should be the first choice, not tourniquets.
- Ask how long ago the wound occurred and determine the mechanism of injury.
- It is essential to rule out tendon, nerve injury as well as retained foreign body. Consult an orthopedist for tendon or bone involvement.
- Consider x-rays to look for such problems as broken glass and/or bone involvement before sewing a wound closed.
- Anesthetize the patient, but do not use lidocaine with epinephrine in fingertips, nose, or penis. Consider digital block.
- Cleansing the wound is extremely important, but do not pour skin-cleansing solution directly into open wound.
- Do not close a wound if it is visibly infected; just dress it.
- Suture the patient, but staple scalp wounds.
- Consider cyanoacrylate for minor lacerations instead of sutures, especially in children.

- Apply antibiotic ointment and dressing.
- Give tetanus booster.
- Remove the sutures in:
    - 4 days (face)
    - 7 days (most places)
    - 9 days (back)
- Give antibiotic if the wound appears infected in few days or if it was a very dirty wound. Keflex is commonly used, but Augmentin is a better broad-spectrum antibiotic.
- Definitely give Augmentin for animal bites and consider rabies series. This problem is covered in the Neurology chapter.

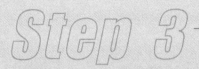
Endocrine and Related Issues

ENDOCRINE SYSTEM
  Malignant neoplasm of thyroid gland
  Hyperthyroidism
  Hypothyroidism
  Diabetes mellitus
  Gangrene, diabetes-related
  Hypoglycemia
  Hyperglycemia
  Hyperparathyroidism
  Endocrine discorders
  Disorders of adrenal gland

FLUIDS, ELECTROLYTES, ACID/BASE
  Disorders of mineral metabolism
  Electrolyte and fluid disorders
  Syndrome of inappropriate antidiuretic
    hormone

METABOLISM
  Phenylketonuria
  Disorders of lipid metabolism
  Gout
  Immunity deficiency

NUTRITION
  Malnutrition
  Vitamin and mineral deficiencies

ENDOCRINE SYSTEM

Malignant Neoplasm of Thyroid Gland

Type	Frequency	Presentation	Management
Papillary carcinoma	80%	Asymptomatic patient. Slow growing, usually present with cervical lymph node metastases	Excision, then radioiodine scanning and ablation
Follicular carcinoma	10%	Slow growing. Usually asymptomatic. Females age 50-60. Metastases via lymph and blood.	Excision, then radioiodine scanning and ablation
Medullary carcinoma	< 10%	Associated with MEN II. Elevated calcitonin levels. Rapid growth, invades locally, including recurrent laryngeal nerve, and leads to vocal cord paralysis. Very poor prognosis.	Excision, then radioiodine scanning and ablation

MEN = multiple endocrine neoplasia

Management:

- Feel for nodule on physical exam. Also palpate cervical lymph nodes.
- Initial screen is thyroid-stimulating hormone (TSH). Low TSH suggests hyperthyroidism, which is generally a good prognostic sign.
- Nuclear scan can find "cold" or "hot" nodules. Cold nodules with low uptake are bad.
- Ultrasound can locate nodules and assist in fine-needle aspiration (FNA) biopsy.
- Get FNA biopsy of any nodules. This key test cannot be skipped.
- Order CT of neck to detect metastases.
- Total surgical excision is the mainstay of treatment in all cases.
- Follow up with radioiodine scanning and ablation for residual disease and metastases.
- Start thyroid replacement.
- After ablation, follow up once or twice per year to look for increasing thyroglobulin level, which may indicate recurrence.

Hyperthyroidism

Type	Presentation
Graves' disease	Autoimmune disorder in which antibodies imitate TSH. By far the most common cause.
Subacute thyroiditis	Generally follows viral URI and resolves without problems
Struma ovarii	Pelvic mass (teratoma) with simultaneous hyperthyroidism caused by substances secreted by tumor

Presentation: Usually female with tremor/nervousness, tachycardia, palpitations, atrial fibrillation, goiter.

Management:

- Ask about diarrhea, weight loss with increased appetite.
- Look for exophthalmia on exam as well as lid lag, retraction.
- Check for brisk reflexes on exam; they are exaggerated in hyperthyroidism.
- Note blood pressure for high pulse pressure with high systolic relative to diastolic pressure.
- Make sure patient is not having a thyroid storm! Give propranolol to protect heart in this case. T_3 is elevated in this disorder.
- Initial labs to get are TSH, T_4, T_3, and T_3 resin uptake.
- TSH will be low, with all other elements elevated in Graves' disease.
- Start propylthiouracil (PTU) or methimazole. Both are definitely contraindicated in pregnancy, but PTU is used in breast-feeding mothers.
- Proceed to radioactive iodine ablation with I-131. This is also contraindicated in pregnancy.
- Thyroidectomy is rarely used but can be considered in pregnant woman. If Step 3 presents the case of a pregnant woman with severe hyperthyroidism, pick this answer.
- After destruction of thyroid, you need to commence thyroid replacement.

Hypothyroidism

Type	Presentation
Hashimoto's thyroiditis	Most common. Associated with microsomal antibodies against the thyroid gland itself
Iodine deficiency	Rare in U.S. due to supplementation, but consider in immigrants
Euthyroid syndrome	Chronic illness, malnutrition; look for normal TSH, low T_3, T_4.

Presentation: weight gain, cold intolerance, anemia, goiter.

Management:

- Ask about constipation, fatigue, menstrual disturbances.
- Ask about medication that affects thyroid: amiodarone, lithium are classic examples.
- Look for coarse hair and facial features on exam as well as hair loss, especially around the brow.
- Hypothyroidism is associated with carpal tunnel syndrome.
- Hypothyroidism can cause high cholesterol levels.
- Get a TSH first. Expect it to be elevated in hypothyroidism.
- Get a free T_4, total T_4, T_3, and expect levels to be low. They may be normal in early hypothyroidism with a high TSH level.
- Order autoantibodies: antimicrosomal and antithyroglobulin to ascertain the etiology.
- Prescribe levothyroxine with goal of getting TSH in normal range. This is synthetic T_4 that is converted to T_3 in the peripheral tissues of the body.
- Myxedema is the most severe manifestation. It is due to long-term, untreated hypothyroidism in patients affected by sickness, cold, or other stress. Look for all the other signs of hypothyroidism and a precipitating event. It can lead to coma.
- Mind the ABCs and be prepared to intubate the patient. Admit to ICU.
- Start stress dose steroids, liothyronine (T_3), and levothyroxine (T_4). If you suspect myxedema, start therapy before results of lab tests are reported.

Diabetes Mellitus

Presentation: classic is polydipsia, polyuria, weight loss.

Type	Presentation	Etiology
Type 1	Young, thin patient; ketoacidosis common, weak genetic component	Antibodies to beta cells of pancreas
Type 2	Patient over 30, obese; ketoacidosis is uncommon, but possible, strong genetic component. An American epidemic: one third of adults in U.S. are projected to have type 2 DM.	Insulin resistance

Management:

- Current criteria for diagnosis include either:
  a. Fasting blood sugar > 126 (on at least 2 occasions) or
  b. Random blood sugar > 200 with associated polyuria, polydipsia, and weight loss
     or
  c. 2-hour blood sugar > 200
- Adjust lifestyle factors. Weight loss is therapeutic in some obese type 2 diabetics.

	Mechanism	Side Effects
Sulfonylureas (glipizide, glyburide)	Stimulate beta-cell release of insulin	Can have hypoglycemia as side effect
Metformin	Blocks liver gluconeogenesis, increases glucose uptake muscle	Lactic acidosis Contraindicated in renal disease, CHF, liver disease. Stop before giving IV contrast!
Acarbose	Blocks carbohydrate digestion/absorption	Flatulence
Troglitazone	Increases glucose uptake in muscles	Hepatic damage

- Insulin therapy is mainstay of type 1 management.
- First-line option is to institute oral drug therapy for type 2.
- Insulin may eventually be required even in type 2 as the pancreas burns out.
- Insulin can always be safely used even if you must stop oral agents for use of contrast or acidosis.
- Diabetics require yearly foot exam as well as dilated exam by ophthalmologist. The leading cause of blindness in the U.S. is diabetes.
- Check urine microalbumin every year.
- Check lipid panel every year. Diabetes greatly accelerates arteriosclerosis. Diabetes is considered the CV equivalent of a prior heart attack. Put patients on statin if LDL ≥ 100.
- Check HgBA1c levels every year and keep under 7; a value of 6 ideal. A simple formula is 20 times the HA1c level = average blood glucose. HgbA1c reflects the blood glucose average of 3 months.
- Step 3 will expect you to tweak insulin regimens:
  - Generally a morning and evening dose of insulin are given, usually regular and NPH.
  - NPH has a peak effect over 12 hours after administration. If morning fasting blood sugar is high, increase evening NPH dose.
  - Regular insulin peaks 2 hours from administration.
  - Ask patients if they wake up in the middle of the night sweaty and tremulous; this is a sign that they are becoming hypoglycemic and need to reduce medications later in the day.
- Add ACE inhibitor to protect kidneys, regardless of the existence of hypertension. Patients should receive maximal dosage of ACE inhibitor if they have hypertension.
- Neuropathy is common in the feet and hands. Tricyclic antidepressants may help alleviate pain caused by such neuropathy.
- Neuropathy and vasculopathy in diabetes lead to impotence, gastroparesis, and silent myocardial infarctions.
- Diabetics are at risk for various infections, including rare fungal infections such as mucormycosis.
- When a patient is made NPO, give regular insulin dose.
- A patient with type I (rarely type II) may present in diabetic ketoacidosis (DKA); you should be prepared to manage this presentation on the CCS section of the exam:
  - Mind the ABCs as usual.
  - Draw arterial blood gases; expect metabolic acidosis.
  - Check for serum and urine ketones.
  - Get CMP; look for low serum bicarbonate and anion gap. Expect glucose to be high, but do not be surprised to find a patient in DKA with a fasting blood sugar in the 200-300 range.
  - Give IV fluids aggressively. Add bicarbonate if pH is less than 7.0.
  - Give bolus of normal saline or other isotonic fluid immediately.
  - Start IV insulin.
  - Get hourly fingersticks while the patient is on IV insulin.
  - Get frequent CMPs to check electrolytes, especially K+. Serum K+ will drop as it moves into the cells. Replace K+ as well as magnesium and phosphorus.
  - Get EKG.
  - Watch for the anion gap to close and ketones to disappear.
  - Panculture with urinalysis, blood cultures, chest x-ray to rule out infections, which often precipitate DKA.
- Similarly, a type 2 patient may present in nonketotic hyperosmolar hyperglycemic coma (NKHHC), which is quite similar to DKA but without the ketones and is managed similarly. NKHHC has a mortality rate of 50%.

Gangrene, Diabetes-related

Presentation: usually occurs after surgery in diabetic patient with crepitance, foul/sweet-smelling discharge, bullae, fever, tachycardia.

Management:

- ABCs as usual: give the patient fluids, oxygen, supportive care.
- If patient is septic and hypotensive, avoid pressors because the tissue is already underperfused. Increasing fluids would be a better option.
- Gangrene breaks down tissue and leads to hyperkalemia, myoglobinemia.
- Pencillin G and gentamicin should be given IV as soon as possible.
- CT may show tissue involvement or osteomyelitis, but do not delay antibiotic therapy to get a CT.
- Immediate surgical debridement/excision is the standard of care.

Hypoglycemia

Presentation: sweating, shakes, dizzy, fatigue, headache.

Management:

- Differential diagnosis is broad. Try to find clues in history and physical exam that point to cause: drugs, starvation, insulinoma, alcohol, hyperthyroidism, cortisol deficiency, glycogen storage diseases, disorders of metabolism.
- Determine whether the patient is stable. ABCs as usual.
- Give a patient who presents in coma D5 immediately, especially if the patient is a known diabetic and you do not know fasting blood sugar value.
- Glucagon is also beneficial to reverse hypoglycemia acutely. If this fails to increase fasting blood sugar, suspect a glycogen storage disease. Glycogen storage disease and other metabolic problems are likely to present in pediatric patients and are treated with special diets. Maple syrup urine disease is treated with restriction of amino acids such as leucine.
- Ask patients about dietary habits. Do they eat regularly? If they are diabetic, they should never skip meals and should eat frequent small meals.
- Ask about alcohol intake. This can cause hypoglycemia in diabetics on insulin.
- If patients are diabetic and on medications, carefully evaluate to make sure they are not overmedicated. Adjust medications as needed.
- To diagnose an insulinoma, measure insulin, C-peptide and get a 72-hour fast to induce hypoglycemia. This is the gold standard for diagnosing insulinoma. Diazoxide is the initial treatment of insulinoma; it blocks insulin release from the pancreas.
- Get TSH level to rule out hyperthyroidism.
- If the patient has cortisol deficiency due to primary or secondary adrenal insufficiency (Addison's disease or chronic users), give glucocorticoids.

Hyperglycemia

Presentation: high glucose on fasting blood sugar test or metabolic panel.

Management:

- See diabetes mellitus section above.
- Stress, infection, cortisol, and growth hormone increase glucose in the blood.
- Check for overnutrition in patients on TPN or with D5 in their IV fluids.

Hyperparathyroidism

Presentation: fractures/osteopenia, kidney stones, abdominal pain/constipation/pancreatitis, depression/mental status changes.

Type	Etiology
Primary	Adenoma of parathyroids
Secondary	Renal failure as PTH increases with rising phosphorus

Management:

- Get serum Ca2+ and expect it to be elevated
- Get PTH levels and expect elevation.
- Expect phosphorus to be normal or low in primary hyperparathyroidism and high in secondary hyperparathyroidism due to failure of renal excretion.
- Be alert to calcification/obstruction of kidneys and get imaging if suspected.
- IV fluids combined with furosemide can help excrete more calcium through the kidneys acutely.
- Calcitriol is used for secondary hyperparathyroidism.
- Add a bisphosphonate to protect bone from further destruction.
- Surgical removal of parathyroid is treatment of choice for primary hyperparathyroidism.
- Watch for calcium to plummet after removal of parathyroid because the bones absorb much needed calcium that has been unavailable in the hyperparathyroidism state. Give calcium supplement.

Endocrine Disorders (diabetes and thyroid covered above; adrenals covered below)

Name	Presentation	Diagnosis	Management
MEN I	Hyperparathyroidism, VIPomas, gastrinomas/Zollinger-Ellison syndrome, prolactinomas. It may include all or some of the above.	Order lab tests for each affected system, including MRI of head, CT of pancreas	1. Proton pump inhibitor for gastrinoma 2. Octreotide for VIPoma, but surgical removal is definitive treatment 3. Bromocriptine for prolactinoma 4. Surgery for hyperparathyroidism
MEN II	Medullary thyroid cancer (MTC), pheochromocytoma, and hyperparathyroidism	Order lab tests for each affected system, including calcitonin, 24-hour urine for vanillylmandelic acid (VMA) and metanephrine	1. Surgery to remove thyroid for MTC 2. Parathyroidectomy for hyperparathyroidism 3. Possible unilateral or total adrenalectomy
Diabetes insipidus, central	Many liters of dilute urine, thirst. Head injury. Compulsive water drinking can mimic signs of DI. Low urine osmolarity with high serum osmolarity.	Water deprivation test under supervision where patient is dehydrated and given vasopressin, which causes big increase in urine osmolarity in DI patients. (Normal not much change.)	Desmopressin or vasopressin
Diabetes Insipidus, renal	Many liters of dilute urine, thirst. Medications like lithium. Also X-linked disorder of males. Low urine osmolarity with high serum osmolarity.	Water deprivation test under supervision in which patient is dehydrated and given vasopressin, which causes big increase in urine osmolarity in DI. (Normal patients: not much change.)	Free water orally and hydrochlorothiazide
SIADH	Hyponatremia with normal potassium and bicarbonate. High urine osmolarity with low serum osmolarity. Frequently psychiatric medications are culprits. Also seen in head trauma and as a paraneoplastic syndrome.	After getting lab tests, order chest x-ray and head CT to locate primary causes.	Water restriction mainstay of therapy; if it fails, then use demeclocycline If the patient is severely symptomatic, then slowly correct with isotonic NS but not too fast to avoid the dreaded central pontine myelinolysis

Disorders of Adrenal Gland

Name	Presentation	Diagnosis	Management
Addison	Hyperpigmentation, syncope, dizziness, hypotension, nausea/vomiting, hyperkalemia, hyponatremia, mild nongap metabolic acidosis. Can lead to death under stressful conditions.	Adrenocorticotropic hormone (ACTH) stimulation test with cosyntropin. Expect cortisol to rapidly elevate in normal individual, remain flat in Addison disease.	Steroids with fluids
Secondary adrenal insufficiency	Long-term steroid user under stress (surgery/ICU) who develops hypotension, hyperkalemia, hyponatremia	Cortisol low and ACTH high	Steroids—never delay giving steroids to obtain lab tests
Cushing's syndrome	Central/truncal obesity, buffalo hump, striae, osteoporosis, diabetes	Expect ACTH and cortisol to be high but get dexamethasone suppression test, which should give low cortisol the next day in normal patient but remain elevated if Cushing's syndrome is present. Can measure 24-hour urine cortisol alternatively.	MRI of the pituitary and CT of the adrenals to find source; then surgery followed by replacement steroids
Conn syndrome	Hypernatremia, hypokalemia, metabolic alkalosis leading to fatigue/weakness, cramps, headache, palpitations	Check renin levels; expect them to be low and aldosterone to be high. CT of abdomen, adrenal venous sampling	Spironolactone can be used to correct hypokalemia initially, but surgery is standard of care
Pheochromocytoma	Fluctuant hypertension, tachycardia	Metanephrines and VMA in 24-hour urine test. CT of abdomen	Phenoxybenzamine, propranolol, and metyrosine; then surgery after catecholamines have cooled off. Acute crisis usually treated with phentolamine or nitroprusside
Androgen-secreting tumors, congenital adrenal hyperplasia	Virilization in girls, precocious puberty in boys	Expect decreased serum aldosterone and cortisol with increased 17-ketosteroids in urine	Corticosteroids

FLUIDS, ELECTROLYTES, ACID/BASE

Disorders of Mineral Metabolism

Disorder	Presentation	Cause	Management
Hypocalcemia	Tetany/cramps, QT prolongation, convulsions, psychosis	Parathyroid removal most common cause. Others: pancreatitis/short bowel, poor vitamin D intake, renal failure, diuretics, low magnesium	Make sure calcium corrected for albumin is normal or measure ionized calcium; then give IV calcium gluconate acutely, followed by oral calcium with vitamin D
Hypercalcemia	Old med school mnemonic: bones, stones, groans, psychiatric overtones, i.e.: fractures/osteopenia, kidney stones, abdominal pain/constipation/pancreatitis, depression/mental status changes. Also short QT with long PR.	C = Calcium IV (excess) H = Hyperparathyroidism/ hyperthyroidism I = Thiazide M = metastases/milk alkali P = Paget's disease A = Addison's disease N = Neoplasm Z = Zollinger-Ellison syndrome E = Excess of vitamin D E = Excess of vitamin A S = Sarcoid	PTH is the most important initial test. Give IV normal saline (NS) to dilute, Lasix, prednisone/steroids, calcitonin/phosphate; dialysis acutely, then restrict calcium and give steroids and phosphate chronically. If not severe, the drug of choice is pamidronate
Hypomagnesemia	Tetany, increased deep tendon reflexes, arrhythmias/ tachycardia, constipation; potassium will likely be awry also	After prolonged diarrhea/ vomiting, hyperaldosteronism, celiac disease, renal failure	IV magnesium sulfate, followed by oral magnesium oxide
Hypermagnesemia	Patient likely presents as OB/GYN case. Respiratory failure, CNS depression, deep tendon reflexes depressed	Renal failure, too much IV magnesium	Calcium IV, insulin + glucose, furosemide, dialysis if severe
Hypophosphatemia	Muscle weakness (including diaphragm)	Diabetic ketoacidosis	IV phosphorus if severe, but try to use oral form
Hyperphosphatemia	Metastatic calcification, hypocalcemia	Renal failure, too much IV phosphours	Calcium carbonate will bind phosphorus

Electrolyte and Fluid Disorders

Disorder	Presentation	Cause	Management
Hyponatremia	Mental status changes, seizures	Dehydration, diuretics SIADH, polydipsia CHF, renal failure	If glucose is high, sodium will be falsely elevated Hypovolemic: give normal saline Euvolemic: water restriction Hypervolemic: water restriction and diuretics, hydrochloro-thiazide (HCTZ)
Hypernatremia	Mental status changes, pulmonary edema	Urine sodium gives a lot of information Diabetes insipidus Excess sodium Diarrhea/dehydration	Dehydration: give NS until volume rehydrated Diabetes insipidus central: Vasopressin (DDAVP) Diabetes insipidus renal: HCTZ and free water Almost never will you pick free water. NS is almost always a better choice, given over 2-3 days. Too fast a rate of delivery causes cerebral edema.
Hypokalemia	Weakness/tetany, flat T waves, atrial fibrillation/PVCs	Lasix/diuretics, alkalosis, insulin (while treating DKA), GI fistulas/diarrhea	Give potassium chloride (KCl) IV, then orally (be careful with IV KCl)
Hyperkalemia	Peaked T waves with wide QRS, ventricular fibrillation	Renal failure, rhabdo-myolysis, blood transfusion, hemolysis	IV calcium gluconate to protect the heart Move K+ into cells (fast) · Bicarbonate · Insulin + glucose · Albuterol breathing treatment Repeat blood metabolic panel (BMP) if lab confirms hyper-kalemia Remove K+ (takes time) · Kayexalate · Lasix · Dialysis (do not forget this option)
Hypovolemia	Dry mucous membranes, skin turgor decreased, tachycardia, increased diastolic relative to systolic pressure	Dehydration, underhydration especially in burn/trauma patients	Isotonic fluids such as normal saline (NS) or lactate Ringer's solution (LR) are initial choice because they can be safely bolused.
Hypervolemia	Weight gain, rales/crackles, jugular vein distention, hypertension	Overhydration, renal failure	Diuresis Dialysis if severe
Metabolic acidosis	pH low, bicarbonate low, CO_2 normal	Diarrhea, renal tubular acidosis/acute renal failure, diabetic ketoacidosis	Correct underlying causes IV fluids with bicarbonate if pH under 7.1 Dialysis if critical

continued

Electrolyte and Fluid Disorders (continued)

Disorder	Presentation	Cause	Management
Metabolic alkalosis	pH high, bicarbonate high, CO_2 normal	NG suction or vomiting, diuretics; classic example is patient who swallows too much bicarbonate in the form of antacids	Correct underlying causes
Respiratory acidosis	pH low, bicarbonate normal, CO_2 high	Hypoventilation, classic example is heroin addict who is barely breathing	Prepare to intubate If on ventilation, increase ventilation after you make sure tube has not moved and get chest x-ray to rule out sudden pneumothorax
Respiratory alkalosis	pH high, CO_2 low	Hyperventilation	Turn down the ventilator Calm the patient with some sedatives
Hypochloremic alkalosis	pH high, chloride low	NG suction or vomiting	IV normal saline

Syndrome of Inappropriate Antidiuretic Hormone (SIADH)

Presentation: hyponatremia with normal potassium and bicarbonate on CMP.

Management:

- When you check the urine, expect high urine osmolarity with low serum osmolarity.
- Frequently psychiatric medications are culprits.
- Also seen in head trauma and as a paraneoplastic syndrome. After getting lab tests, order chest x-ray and head CT to locate primary causes.
- Water restriction is mainstay of therapy; if it fails, give demeclocycline.
- If the patient is severely symptomatic, slowly correct with isotonic normal saline, but not too fast to avoid the dreaded complication of central pontine myelinolysis.

METABOLISM

Phenylketonuria (PKU)

Presentation: infant with mousy smelling urine/skin, pale skin.

Management:

- PKU is an inherited error of metabolism caused by deficiency in the enzyme phenylalanine hydroxylase, which normally converts phenylalanine to tyrosine. Phenylalanine can build up to toxic levels.
- All babies should be tested at birth. Testing is done with heel stick.
- PKU is autosomal recessive and can lead to mental retardation. You can run tests in parents to see if they are carriers; both have to be carriers for children to be affected.
- Chorionic villus sample can rule out PKU in womb.
- Key to management is dietary restriction of certain proteins; this means no aspartame/Nutrasweet, milk, dairy products.
- Adult women with PKU should adhere to the diet if they are planning to become or already are pregnant.
- Lofenalac is given to PKU infants.
- Prognosis is good if diet is adhered to as child.

Disorders of Lipid Metabolism

	Presentation	Management
Pure hypercholesterolemia	High LDL, high total cholesterol	HMG-CoA reductase inhibitors with or without bile acid sequestrants (such as cholestyramine) with or without niacin
Pure hypertriglyceridemia	High triglycerides (TGs)	Gemfibrozil. Avoid bile acid binders because they increase TGs.
Mixed hyperlipidemia	High TGs, high LDL	Niacin lowers TG, increases HDLs, and normalizes LDLs
Low HDL	Metabolic syndrome, male sex	Exercise, 1-2 glasses red wine per day, and estrogen

Management:

- Diet and exercise are first-line changes unless cholesterol profile is extremely high (LDL > 190 with 0–1 risk factors, >130 with 2 or more risk factors, or >100 with CAD or diabetes and total cholesterol over 240); then intervention is merited right away. LDL should be <160 in all cases, but goal drops to <100 in patients with 2 or more risk factors. This guideline continues to be revised downward in the literature.
- Other medical conditions/causes affect lipids, especially diabetes, hypothyroidism, nephrotic syndrome, and steroids (both anabolic and corticosteroids). Treat underlying cause.
- More and more evidence suggests that diabetics should take a statin if LDL > 100. Diabetes is considered by some cardiologists to be the equivalent of a prior MI.
- HMG CoA-reductase inhibitors generally should not be combined with clofibrates to avoid rhabdomyolysis. If proximal muscle pain/weakness develops, then check creatinine phosphokinase (CPK) to rule out this complication.
- Niacin causes severe flushing, and some patients cannot tolerate it, even though it is the nearly perfect lipid drug. Give aspirin beforehand to reduce flushing.
- Bile acid sequestrants raise triglycerides and interfere with absorbing other medications in the gut.
- Monitor liver function test yearly in patients taking any lipid medication.

Gout

Presentation: joint pain classically in the big toe (podagra) or other monoarticular joint pain, tophi in ear helix or Achilles tendon. Usually has sudden onset in obese male with purine-rich diet.

Management:
- Take history and ask if problem has ever occurred before.
- Take joint fluid sample and send for analysis. Gout is a crystal-induced arthritis diagnosed by the finding of needle-sharp crystals with negative birefringence. Pseudogout is positive birefringence with rhomboid shaped crystals.
- Joint sample is important to rule out other cause of joint pain (i.e., infection).
- Treat with NSAIDs such as indomethacin or colchicines acutely. Avoid aspirin.
- Also increase fluids to get rid of uric acid.
- Allopurinol is used to ward off attacks later once patient is asymptomatic, but generally not started after only one incident. Measure the uric acid excreted in urine to decide whether to start allopurinol.
- Colchicine can be used for prophylaxis as well as acute treatment.
- Get the patient to quit drinking and make lifestyle changes to avoid future attacks.

SAMPLE CCS INPUT: Acute Gout Attack

Focused exam of extremities/spine

Elevate foot of bed

CBC, CMP, uric acid

X-ray of foot/toes

Aspirate joint fluid

Joint fluid crystals, culture, Gram stain, glucose, cell count

Low protein diet (low purine not in CCS orders) or, if patient is overweight, weight loss diet

Indomethacin PO

Probenecid PO

Allopurinol PO (continuous after attack)

Counsel patient to limit alcohol intake

Immunity Deficiency

Type	Presentation
DiGeorge syndrome	Hypocalcemia/tetany, lack of thymus is responsible for immunodeficiency
Humoral immunodeficiencies	
X-linked agammaglobulinemia (Bruton's disease)	Boys with few B cells and frequent upper respiratory infections (URIs)
IgG subclass deficiencies	Low subclass of IgM, IgG, IgA
Hyper-IgM syndrome, autosomal or X-linked	High IgM, no IgA or IgG
Selective IgA deficiency	IgA levels low, frequent URIs
Aberrant lymphocyte activation	
Wiskott-Aldrich syndrome	Boys with low platelets, frequent URIs
Hyper-IgE syndrome	High IgE, frequent staphylococcal infections
Idiopathic disseminated mycobacterial infections	Frequent mycobacterial infections
Defects in lymphocyte development	
Severe combined immunodeficiencies	Missing T or B cells
Other	
Complement deficiency	Low C5-C9. Frequent *Neisseria* infections.
Chronic granulomatous disease	Boys with nitroblue tetrazolium test show poor activation. Frequent and severe bacterial and fungal infections.

Management:

- Get serum protein electrophoresis (SPEP) for breakdown of IgA, IgG, IgM, IgE. This test covers many of the above disorders.
- Intravenous immunoglobulin should be given for a specific deficiency.
- Granulocyte colony-stimulating factor can sometimes be used for neutropenia.
- Antibiotics are frequently given to treat infections or for prophylaxis.
- Review the HIV section regarding opportunistic infections and management.

NUTRITION

Malnutrition

	Presentation	What to Check/Management
Undernutrition	Patient post-surgery, alcoholic	Body mass index (BMI), midarm muscle area, cholesterol, albumin, prealbumin, and transferrin
Overnutrition	Patient on TPN, IV fluids with dextrose, sedentary patients	BMI, serum glucose, midarm muscle area, cholesterol, albumin, prealbumin, and transferrin
Marasmus	Low carbohydrates and low protein. Very thin with poor growth.	Electrolytes. Correct with whole milk-based formula with added oil for calories.
Kwashiorkor	Carbohydrates without protein. Edema (low albumin) with poor growth.	Electrolytes. Correct with whole milk-based formula with added oil for calories.

Vitamin and Mineral Deficiencies

Deficiency	Source	Presentation
Thiamine (vitamin B_1)	Numerous	Alcoholics, peritoneal dialysis Paresthesias/neuropathy, cardiac failure Wernicke/Korsakoff syndrome
Riboflavin (vitamin B_2)	Meat and dairy	Vegetarians, malabsorption Aphthous ulcers, corners of mouth bleed, dermatitis
Niacin (vitamin B_3)	Cereals, nuts, fish/meat	Pellagra = dementia, dermatitis, diarrhea Weight loss, fatigue
Pyridoxine (vitamin B_6)	Meat, vegetables, whole grains	Alcoholics, pregnant women, isoniazid users Seborrheic dermatitis, chapped lips, stomatitis: burning sensation of tongue, neuropathy
Cobalamin (vitamin B_{12})	Kidney, eggs, and milk	Neurologic symptoms and macrocytic anemia Impaired gastric absorption (e.g., celiac sprue)
Vitamin C	Vegetables and fruits	Scurvy, bleeding gums, poor wound healing, skin hemorrhages
Folic acid	Leafy green vegetables	Pregnancy, megaloblastic anemia; similar to B12 deficiency except no neurologic symptoms, which is why you replace both.
Vitamin A	Organ meats, yellow vegetables	Night blindness, corneal ulcers, dry eyes
Vitamin D	Dairy products, sunlight	Rickets, osteomalacia, muscle weakness/cramps due to hypocalcemia
Vitamin K	Leafy green vegetables	Elevated prothrombin time, excessive bleeding
Chromium		Poor glucose tolerance, peripheral neuropathy
Copper		Rare; mental retardation and kinky hair
Iodine		Goiter and hypothyroidism, myxedema, cretinism in infants
Iron		Microcytic anemia; patient with GI bleed or menstruating women
Manganese		Dermatitis, hypocholesterolemia
Selenium		Very rare; cardiomyopathy
Zinc		Poor wound healing, delayed sexual maturation

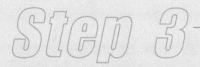
Gastrointestinal System

GENERAL ISSUES
Dyspepsia/indigestion
Constipation
Diarrhea
Hemorrhage of rectum and anus
Gastrointestinal hemorrhage
Nausea and vomiting
Abdominal pain
Abnormal stool contents
Heartburn/gastroesophageal reflux disease
Ascites
Hepatomegaly
Splenomegaly
Dysphagia
Esophageal varices
Achalasia/esophagitis
Gastric ulcer/peptic ulcer/gastritis
Duodenal ulcer/duodenitis
Hemorrhoids
Anal fissure
Anal abscess
Rectal prolapse
Appendicitis
Other noninfectious gastroenteritis
Intestinal obstruction
Diverticula of colon/small intestine

Irritable colon/irritable bowel syndrome
Peritonitis
Intestinal abscess
Inguinal hernia
Other hernias with obstruction
Ventral hernia
Diaphragmatic hernia
Calculus of gallbladder
Cholecystitis
Cirrhosis of liver
Stricture of the common bile duct
Pancreatitis

ONCOLOGY
Benign neoplasm of pancreas
Malignant neoplasm of pancreas
Malignant neoplasm of liver
Malignant neoplasm of colon/recto-
   sigmoid junction/rectum
Benign neoplasm of duodenum/
   jejunum/ileum
Benign neoplasm of rectum
Malignant neoplasm of stomach
Benign neoplasm of stomach
Malignant neoplasm of esophagus

GENERAL ISSUES

Dyspepsia/Indigestion

Presentation: pain/discomfort in upper part of the belly, "chronic indigestion," belching, heartburn.

Management:

- Lifestyle changes: smoking cessation, weight loss, avoidance of nicotine, caffeine, alcohol.
- Stepwise approach:
  - Antacids
  - H2 blocker (e.g., ranitidine)
  - Proton pump inhibitor (e.g., omeprazole)

- If dyspepsis/indigestion is associated with unintentional weight loss, patients with dysphagia must undergo endoscopy.
- Order endoscopy if symptoms persist.
- *Helicobacter pylori* infection may be seen as ulcers on upper GI endoscopy. If so, begin triple therapy: metronidazole + amoxicillin + omeprazole **or** clarithromycin + amoxicillin + omeprazole.

Constipation

Presentation: age over 65, women, children; defined as less than 3 bowel movements per week.

Management:
- In history and physical exam make sure that the patient really fits the definition of constipation.
- Ask about/increase water and fluid intake.
- Ask about/increase fiber in diet.
- Ask children if they ignore the urge to go to the bathroom and then become constipated. This behavior is very common.
- Ask about/limit chronic laxative use.
- Review medications, especially opioids, antacids, calcium channel blockers (especially verapamil).
- In physical exam, check rectal tone and look for masses. Checking for blood in stool is appropriate.
- Be aware of any neurologic problem (e.g., diabetic neuropathy/gastropathy).
- Get lab tests and make sure that potassium and magnesium are not too low and that calcium is not too high. Also check TSH because hypothyroidism can cause constipation.
- Get x-ray of abdomen and look for fecal impaction/bowel obstruction as well as stool in colon.
- Report of cramp-like pain in lower abdomen or back should make obstruction a particular concern. Obstruction becomes a surgical case. Do not forget hernias; look for obturator hernia, especially in elderly.
- Barium enema followed by x-ray may give good information.
- Consider colonoscopy to rule out masses and similar problems.
- Disimpact rectum manually if needed.
- Stepwise approach for acute relief:
  □ Bisacodyl, magnesium citrate.
  □ Fleet enemas (make sure to bring doughnuts to your nursing staff to maintain your popularity).
  □ GoLytely is a strong medicine. Before using it, make certain that no obstruction is present.
- Stepwise approach for maintenance:
  □ Increase fiber and water in diet.
  □ Bowel retraining (sit on toilet right after meal when gastrocolic reflex is peaking).
- Approach to narcotic bowel (add each one at a time):
  □ Docusate
  □ Senna
  □ Lactulose or sorbitol
  □ Bisacodyl

Pitfall:
- Do not miss sigmoid volvulus—a serious complication of constipation. Beware of cecal volvulus and intussusception.

Diarrhea

Presentation: loose, watery, soft stools, > 200 g total stool weight/daily. Vast differential diagnosis, but basically categorized as osmotic, secretory, malabsorptive, exudative, or infectious. Acute diarrhea is usually of infectious origin.

Presentation	Etiology
Nonenteric/systemic causes of diarrhea	Include hyperthyroidism, otitis, urinary tract infection, appendicitis, lower lobe pneumonia, and irritable bowel syndrome.
Children	Commonly rotavirus or *Campylobacter* sp. with fever, nausea/vomiting, pain.
Salmonella infection	Presents with watery diarrhea.
Shigella infection	Presents with watery diarrhea and tenesmus.
Escherichia coli infection	Accounts for most case of traveler's diarrhea.
Giardiasis	Campers

Management:

- Check electrolytes if diarrhea has been present for a significant time.
- Oral rehydration therapy is the standard of care, even if the patient is not yet dehydrated clinically.
- Admit dehydrated patients and treat with IV fluids.
- Get stool culture and culture for ova and parasites if you suspect bacterial/parasitic infection.
- Do not forget *Clostridium difficile* infection, especially in hospitalized patients receiving antibiotics. Get cultures and prepare to start metronidazole. For resistant strains use vancomycin.
- Antibiotics are generally not used with some exceptions:
  - *Shigella* infection: give trimethoprim-sulfamethoxazole (TMP-SMX).
  - Giardiasis: give metronidazole.
  - If typhoid fever is present (malaise, fever, abdominal pain, and bradycardia), treat *Salmonella* infection with TMP-SMX. Do not treat otherwise because antibiotics prolong carrier state.
- Begin normal diet as soon as possible.
- Go after other causes with colonoscopy, and consider food allergy or lactose intolerance if the problem continues or is frequent.

Hemorrhage of Rectum and Anus

Presentation: hematochezia or melena (black tarry stools).

Etiology	Presentation
Hemorrhoids	Constipation and pregnancy are common risk factors. Give stool-bulking agents.
Fistulas	History of Crohn's disease should tip you off. Surgery may be needed. Openings visualized in perineum.
Fissures	Hard stool passage is risk factor. Prescribe stool softeners, bowel retraining.
Diverticulosis	Diverticula can pouch outward and bleed all at once. Surgery may be needed.
Colon cancer	Must rule out colon cancer with bleeding from the rectum, especially in males over 50.
Prolapsed rectum	Rectum bulges outward through anus and bleeds. Surgical case.

Gastrointestinal Hemorrhage

Presentation: see table below.

Type	Source	Presentation
Upper	Esophagus, stomach, or duodenum Upper part of the small intestine	Look for black tarry stool, but extreme upper GI bleed can have bright red appearance because it moves through GI tract so fast.
Lower	Angiodysplasia, colon cancer, diverticulosis	Look for frank blood in stool.

Management:

- **Always** make sure that the patient is stable. Resuscitate if needed; remember the ABCs.
- Active and symptomatic GI bleed merits admission to MICU.
- Insert 2 large-bore IV lines—you need access right away.
- Give fluids and/or packed red blood cells as needed.
- Check hemoglobin. It is not a bad idea to check prothrombin time (PT), partial thromboplastin time (PTT), and international normalized ratio (INR) at this time.
- Type and cross-match blood just in case.
- Notify surgery if you have a bleeder; an urgent trip to the OR may be required
- Gastric lavage through nasogastric tube can help find upper GI bleed.
- Call GI to visualize upper and lower GI tract: esophagogastroduodenoscopy (EGD) and colonoscopy.
- Tagged red blood cell scan can be helpful if endoscopy yields nothing; sometimes bleeding is intermittent.
- If brisk bleeding is present, mesenteric angiography may be able to localize the source as well.

Nausea and Vomiting

Presentation: see table below.

Presentation	Etiology
Minor	Food poisoning/gastroenteritis, hangover, pregnancy, medications
Serious	Obstruction, pancreatitis, cholecystitis, appendicitis, diabetic ketoacidosis, atypical myocardial infarction

Management:

- Main priority is to separate serious from minor causes.
- Put the patient on NPO status.
- Treat dehydration and get electrolyte panel.
- Get kidney-ureter-bladder (KUB) and abdominal films.
- The Step 3 exam does test therapeutics. Below are some common choices for this problem:
  - Give promethazine as initial choice in nausea and vomiting. It is a general antiemetic, but watch for dystonic reactions along with sedation because it works synergistically with opioids.
  - Give metoclopramide, which is especially good for diabetic gastroparesis, but be aware of extrapyramidial reactions.

□ Ondansetron is the classic choice for chemotherapy-induced emesis, but watch for constipation.

□ Insert nasogastric tube to suction for obstruction or ileus.

■ Treat the cause.

Abdominal Pain

Presentation: see table below.

Presentation	Etiology
Right upper quadrant (RUQ)	Cholecystitis, pancreatitis. Cholecystitis radiates to right shoulder and presents with postprandial pain that waxes and wanes and positive Murphy's sign. Also, right lower lobe pneumonia is often seen on Step 3.
Right lower quadrant (RLQ)	Appendicitis (classic presentation moves from umbilicus to RLQ), pelvic inflammatory disease, ectopic pregnancy, ovarian torsion, ruptured cyst, endometritis.
Left upper quadrant (LUQ)	Spleen rupture with Kerr's sign; pain radiates to left shoulder.
Left lower quadrant (LLQ)	Diverticulitis, pelvic inflammatory disease, ectopic pregnancy, ovarian torsion, ruptured cyst, endometritis.
Epigastric	Abdominal aortic aneurysm (AAA), pancreatitis, atypical myocardial infarction in women or diabetics, peptic ulcer disease, Zollinger-Ellison syndrome, gastroesophageal reflux disease
General/diffuse	Gastroenteritis, diabetic ketoacidosis

Management:

■ Sort quickly into medical or surgical causes. You must rule out acute abdomen. Assess for peritoneal signs.

■ Testicular/ovarian torsion, ectopic pregnancy, obstruction, appendicitis, peritonitis, perforated ulcer, perforated diverticulitis, AAA, and mesenteric ischemia require rapid clinical intervention.

■ Surgery must be performed as soon as possible for appendicitis, bowel infarct, AAA, spleen rupture, ectopic pregnancy, and testicular/ovarian torsion and after 2 days of antibiotics for acute cholecystitis.

■ Determine time of onset and severity of pain, trend toward increasing or decreasing pain, past occurrences, factors that alleviate pain. Ask about associated symptoms such as nausea/vomiting, diarrhea, and burning with urination.

■ Do rectal and pelvic and abdominal exams.

■ Abdominal exams should be repeated multiple times. Rebound tenderness may indicate peritoneal inflammation and requires surgery. RLQ tenderness implicates the appendix, RUQ tenderness the gallbladder. LUQ pain with no trauma implicates the spleen.

■ Get CBC. A high white cell count may be a sign of inflammation (e.g., appendicitis).

■ A high lactate level may indicate mesenteric ischemia (e.g., dead bowel).

■ A low bicarbonate level on BMP may indicate diabetic ketoacidosis; get serum ketones and glucose levels as well.

■ Liver function tests may be elevated in hepatitis, gallstone pancreatitis, central bile duct stones, or similar problems.

■ Get urinalysis.

■ Amylase and lipase levels can help rule out pancreatitis.

■ All women are pregnant until proved otherwise. Get a pregnancy test in the ED: urine (quicker) or serum beta human chorionic gonadotropin (b-HCG).

- First get abdominal x-rays to look for free peritoneal air under the diaphragm or obstruction. If present, emergent surgery is needed. You may also see renal stones.
- Next get ultrasonography to rule out AAA, pyloric stenosis, intussusception, appendicitis, and gallbladder problems. Ultrasound is usually a good choice on Step 3 for initial evaluation of abdominal pain.
- Get CT for better look at pancreas, spleen.

Pitfall:

- Abdomens can degenerate in a hurry. Observe the patient for several hours to make sure that he or she is truly stable before discharge.

Abnormal Stool Contents

Presentation: see table below.

Presentation	Etiology
Fat in stool	Cystic fibrosis, malabsorption, maldigestion from pancreatic/bile duct obstruction, and post-surgical resection; also do not forget the new fat-blocking drugs for weight loss.
Mucus/pus in stool	Ulcerative colitis, Crohn's, infectious colitis or diverticulitis. WBCs suggest invasive bacteria.
Occult blood	Melena or black stool suggests that the bleeding is proximal to the cecum; look for upper GI bleeds such as peptic ulcer disease. Maroon blood suggests that the bleeding is in the distal small bowel. Bright red blood per rectum suggests that the bleeding is anorectal/colonic. You need to rule out colon cancer (colonoscopy).

Heartburn/Gastroesophageal Reflux Disease (GERD)

Presentation: burning sensation in the throat from stomach acid refluxing into esophagus. GERD and heartburn can also be caused by esophageal spasm, lower esophageal sphincter (LES) relaxation, and/or hiatal hernia.

Management:

- Focus on history; ask if symptoms occur after meals, especially when lying down.
- Get EGD with biopsy for H. pylori.
- 24-hr pH is the gold standard for diagnosis and highly sensitive and specific for GERD.
- Stepwise approach:
  - Lifestyle changes: smoking cessation, weight loss, avoidance of nicotine, caffeine, alcohol
  - Antacids
  - H2 blockers
  - Proton pump inhibitor (PPI)
- Laparoscopic Nissen fundoplication may be needed to create solid LES function.
- Complications of GERD include strictures or Barrett's esophagus (precancerous). Note that simply controlling acid reflux will not prevent Barrett's esophagus because **bile reflux** is also part of the disease process. Fundoplication is the only way to prevent reflux of acid and bile.
- EGDs should be ordered in patients who present with GERD for first time if it has been present for years to rule out metaplastic changes.

Ascites

Presentation: fluid accumulation within abdominal cavity. Look for alcoholic man complaining that trousers no longer fit around the waist.

Management:

- Anything that lowers albumin and increases portal vein pressure/peritoneal fluid production can cause ascites. Common causes: portal hypertension, cirrhosis, hepatitis, liver disease in general, and cancer.
- Check metabolic panel, liver panel, and albumin levels.
- Get chest x-ray and KUB study. Make sure that the patient really has ascites and that fluid is visible.
- Ultrasound is a better choice; choose it if given the option.
- Do diagnostic paracentesis.
- Send fluid to lab for cell count, albumin, culture and sensitivity, total protein, Gram stain, and acid-fast test.
- Get cytology to find malignant cause, especially for first-time case.
- Do therapeutic paracentesis if needed (e.g., if the patient cannot breathe).
- You can give albumin if levels are extremely low, especially after tapping off much fluid.
- Certainly put patient on sodium restriction and fluid restriction, if needed.
- You can add spironolactone for medical therapy. Watch for hyperkalemia.
- Give furosemide (Lasix) and later add metolazone if Lasix is not enough. You must follow creatinine levels because you can squeeze the kidneys fairly hard.
- If medical therapy fails, a transjugular intrahepatic portacaval shunt (TIPS) procedure can reduce portal pressure. Consult interventional radiology. TIPS is contraindicated in patients with hepatic encephalopathy.
- Watch for spontaneous bacterial peritonitis (SBP) in patients with ascites because the fluid becomes infected and the patient becomes septic. Sudden fever is a tip-off. Get cultures of fluid and start antibiotics.
- If SBP is present, start ceftriaxone (Rocephin) as soon as possible; it is the initial drug of choice.
- Control portal hypertension with propranolol.

Hepatomegaly

Presentation: enlargement of the liver.

Presentation	Etiology
Metabolic	Fatty liver can occur after alcoholic binges, Wilson disease, amyloid/sarcoid, hemochromatosis
Malignant	Metastases or primary tumor
Nonmalignant	Adenoma, focal nodular hyperplasia
Infectious	Mononucleosis, hepatitis
Other	Biliary obstruction

Management:

- View an enlarged liver in the context of patient history: jaundice, travel history, alcohol ingestion, fever.
- Get basic lab tests, including liver function tests: aspartate aminotransferase (AST), alanine amino-transferase (ALT), alkaline phosphatase, gamma-glutamyl transpeptase (GGTP), total and direct bilirubin.
- Get INR, albumin, and cholesterol level, which are also markers of liver function.
- Consider ammonia level if the patient has signs of encephalopathy, which is treated with lactulose, neomycin, and protein restriction.

- Order an ultrasound of the liver.
- CT of liver is likely to be the highest-yield imaging study.
- If the AST:ALT ratio is > 2, alcohol is the likely cause.
- Consider hepatitis panel.
- High level of direct bilirubin points to obstruction in the biliary system.

Splenomegaly

Presentation: enlarged spleen, usually palpated on physical exam. Kerr's sign is referred left shoulder pain.

Management:

- Causes are numerous, but the most common are viral infection (cytomegalovirus [CMV], Epstein-Barr virus [EBV]), sickle cell disease, portal hypertension, and end-stage liver disease secondary to hepatitis C.
- Check CBC, get a manual smear, and check platelet count.
- Get antibody titers for EBV, CMV, toxoplasmosis, HIV.
- Splenic sequestration crisis in a child with sickle cell disease requires fluids and packed red blood cells as soon as possible.
- Ultrasound is not a bad initial choice, but CT gives the most information.
- Consider removal of the spleen in sickle cell disease.
- Immunize against encapsulated organisms before spleen is removed: pneumococcal, meningococcal, and HIB vaccines.
- Be aware that after mononucleosis infection rupture of spleen is possible. Patients should avoid contact sports while the spleen is still enlarged.

Dysphagia

Presentation: disruption in swallowing process due to impaired function of the tongue, palate, pharynx, and/or esophagus.

Management:

- Ask about weight loss. Is it harder to swallow food or liquids? This is a very important question. Liquids point to a neurologic cause and solids to an obstructive cause. Neurologic causes include stroke, diabetic gastroparesis, Parkinson's disease.
- If the dysphagia is progressive, order an upper GI endoscopy. Progressive dysphagia points to a tumor. The classic patient is a middle-aged man with long-standing GERD who presents with difficulty in swallowing meat that first occurred occasionally and now is worse.
- Barium swallow can be a good approach if you anticipate finding a stricture or pouch.
- Get a swallow study from speech therapy.
- Treat associated dehydration.
- Get a chest x-ray to rule out aspiration.

Esophageal Varices

Presentation: caused by portal vein hypertension or superior vena cava (SVC) obstruction

Management:

- In the presence of massive hemorrhage, start fluids and blood (treat as any GI bleed).
- Note general signs of liver disease on exam.
- Get lab tests, including hemoglobin, INR, liver function tests. Blood urea nitrogen (BUN) may be high if the patient is digesting blood.
- Put on gloves, insert a finger in the anus, and do a heme check. Look for melena.
- Order endoscopy.

- If the patient has no bleeding but varices are found, start beta blockers to prevent bleeding. Propranolol is the first choice.
- If the patient is bleeding acutely, give octreotide before endoscopy.
- The next step is banding or sclerotherapy. If given both choices, choose sclerotherapy.
- Proceed to TIPS if above approach fails.

Achalasia/Esophagitis

Presentation: combination of loss of peristalsis in the esophagus and constriction of the LES.

Management:
- Barium swallow: look for classic "bird's beak" sign.
- Perform manometry of LES.
- Give nifedipine sublingually to relax LES.
- Order balloon dilation of the LES.
- Surgical myotomy with partial fundoplication is needed if above approach fails.

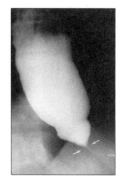

Figure 1. Bird beak achalasia. (From Zeligman BE: Radiography and radiographic fluoroscopic contrast studies. In McNally PR (ed): GI/Liver Secrets, 2e. Philadelphia, Hanley & Belfus, 2001, p 525.)

Gastric Ulcer/Peptic Ulcer/Gastritis

Presentation: a patient reports pain **after** meals with little relief from antacids, or a patient with chronic arthritis presents with anemia.

Management:
- Ulcer disease is usually caused by NSAIDs or H. pylori.
- Patients must undergo endoscopy so that biopsy can be done. Peptic ulcer disease (PUD) is a risk factor for cancer.
- Breath testing for urease produced by H. pylori can be helpful.
- Decrease acid if the cause is not H. pylori:
  - □ H2 blocker (e.g., ranitidine)
  - □ Proton pump inhibitor (e.g., omeprazole)
  - □ Sucralfate to protect lining
- For H. pylori infection, begin triple therapy: metronidazole + amoxicillin + omeprazole or clarithromycin + amoxicillin + omeprazole.
- Perforation requires surgery.

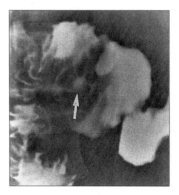

Figure 2. Duodenal ulcer. (From DeCorato DR, Raia CL: Peptic ulcer disease. In Katz DS, Math KR, Groskin SA (eds): Radiology Secrets. Philadelphia, Hanley & Belfus, 1998, p 108.)

Duodenal Ulcer/Duodenitis

Presentation: pain **decreases** with meals; very similar to gastric ulcer in that NSAIDs and H. pylori are the usual suspects.

Management:
- Be aware that duodenal ulcers can erode into pancreas.
- Treat as above for gastric ulcer.

Hemorrhoids

Presentation: straining on the toilet, pregnancy, or pulmonary venous hypertension (PVH) with liver disease. External hemorrhoids are painful; internal hemorrhoids have no innervation and may only bleed.

Management:
- Examine area around the anus.
- Use anoscopy to view internal hemorrhoids. Look for skin tags and thrombosis.

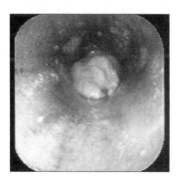

Figure 3. Internal hemorrhoid seen on slotted anoscopy. (From Gralnek IM,, Jensen DM: Lower gastrointestinal tract bleeding. In McNally PR (ed): GI/Liver Secrets, 2e. Philadelphia, Hanley & Belfus, 2001, p 380.)

- Prevent with high-fiber diet.
- Stool softeners, ice, and sitz baths may relieve symptoms.
- For internal hemorrhoids, rubber band ligation is effective.
- Surgical resection is needed if above approach fails.

Anal Fissure

Presentation: history of hard stools with extreme pain on defecation.

Management:
- Do anoscopy in clinic.
- Give stool softeners and analgesics.
- Recommend sitz baths.

Anal Abscess

Presentation: dull "pain in the butt," irritable bowel syndrome, diabetes.

Management:
- The gland becomes obstructed.
- Start bowel flora antibiotics.
- The standard of care is incision and drainage as soon as possible.

Rectal Prolapse

Presentation: in adults, the female-to-male ratio is 6:1, but in children it is 1:1; associated with cystic fibrosis.

Management:
- Reduce with finger.
- Incarceration requires emergency surgery.

Appendicitis

Presentation: classically pain is felt initially in the umbilical area, then migrates to the RLQ with fever, nausea/vomiting, and anorexia.

Management:
- Put the patient on NPO status; you do not want the appendix to perforate.
- Get IV access and start fluids.
- Get CBC; look for elevated white blood cell count.
- Abdominal CT with contrast is the best diagnostic choice if Step 3 forces you to pick a test.
- You can get an ultrasound, but even if it is negative, you still need to get CT.
- White blood cell scanning may be useful if you cannot see the problem on CT, but if your clinical suspicion is this high, you need to get to the OR.
- Start antibiotics: metronidazole and a cephalosporin.
- Laparoscopic appendectomy is the next step.
- Remember that the appendix changes location in pregnancy.
- A good surgeon will remove some healthy appendices. This means that they are not missing any cases of appendicitis. Err on the side of overly aggressive removal.

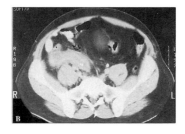

Figure 4. Acute appendicitis. (From Fox MG, et al: Nonivasive GI imaging: ultrasound, computed tomography, magnetic resonance scanning. In McNally PR (ed): GI/Liver Secrets, 2e. Philadelphia, Hanley & Belfus, 2001, p 568.)

Other Noninfectious Gastroenteritis

Presentation: mercury, lead, antibiotics, caffeine, NSAIDs, laxatives, lactose intolerance, or food allergy.

Management:
- Check electrolytes.
- Treat dehydration.
- Take detailed history, including exposure at work, food intake, coffee usage.

Intestinal Obstruction

Presentation: distended, painful abdomen with partial or complete blockage of bowel and no passing of flatus. Cause may be mechanical or ileus. Patient may have undergone recent surgery or be taking narcotics.

Management:
- KUB is quick initial choice for imaging study; look for air/fluid levels.
- Upper GI and small bowel series are next choices.
- Insert nasogastric tube to decompress bowel.
- If no resolution, head to the OR.

Diverticula of Colon/Small Intestine

Presentation: fever, elevated white cell count, LLQ pain. Outpouchings of bowel usually occur at mesenteric border at site of vascular inflow.

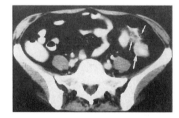

Management:
- Prevent diverticula with high fiber diet.
- CT of abdomen and pelvis is the diagnostic tool of choice.
- Ultrasound should be picked only if CT is not available.
- Diverticulitis is inflammation; perforation is a complication.
- Avoid irritant foods in simple diverticulosis.
- Surgery may be required in diverticulitis.

Figure 5. Diverticulitis on CT. (From Fox MG, et al: Nonivasive GI imaging: ultrasound, computed tomography, magnetic resonance scanning. In McNally PR (ed): GI/Liver Secrets, 2e. Philadelphia, Hanley & Belfus, 2001, p 568.)

Irritable Colon/Irritable Bowel Syndrome

Presentation: cramping, bloating, gas, diarrhea alternating with constipation. Much more common in women (like most autoimmune disorders). Symptoms must be present for at least 12 weeks during a 12-month period, or the patient must have two-thirds of the symptoms listed.

Management:
- Ask if pain is relieved with defecation. Does stool consistency change with pain? These are considered key questions to suggest the diagnosis.
- Studies have found that the colon is more sensitive/reactive to stress than normally, but stress is not the cause. The cause is unknown.
- Get CBC, sedimentation rate, TSH.
- Do stool heme check and stool ova and parasite culture.
- This is a diagnosis of exclusion after ruling out food allergy/lactose intolerance, Crohn's disease, and ulcerative colitis.
- Colonoscopy is mandatory.
- Consider barium swallow or imaging of the gallbladder if you suspect other etiology.
- Increase fiber and eliminate caffeine from the diet for relief of diarrhea.

Peritonitis

Presentation: fever, sepsis, abdominal pain, abdominal wall rigidity. Caused by perforation, ruptured appendix, pelvic inflammatory disease. Forceful vomiting with full belly can cause esophageal rupture (Boerhaave's syndrome) and Mallory-Weiss tear. Also spontaneous bacterial peritonitis (SBP) in patient with ascites.

Management:

- Get x-ray and look for free air below diaphragm.
- CT is the gold standard in peritonitis.
- **A silent abdomen demands a laparotomy**.
- Peritonitis can lead to multisystem failure and has a poor prognosis.
- Get CBC, urine and blood cultures.
- Send peritoneal fluid to lab for studies.
- Start antibiotics:
- Ceftriaxone (Rocephin) or levofloxacin (Levaquin) + metronidazole are good initial choices for community-acquired disease.
- Piperacillin/tazobactam + metronidazole are used for hospital-acquired disease.
- Get the patient to the OR, especially if there is an abscess that needs to be drained.

Intestinal Abscess

Presentation: *Entamoeba histolytica* is as frequent culprit, but bacterial abscesses are common as well.

Management:

- Give oral metronidazole.

Inguinal Hernia

Presentation: more common in men than women; may be direct or indirect.

Management:

- Rule out strangulated intestine as soon as possible.
- Is the hernia reducible manually? Be careful to avoid en masse reduction, which is reduction of a strangulated hernia within its sac without relief of strangulation.
- Reduce the hernia; prepare for emergent surgery if you cannot reduce.
- Surgical repair is standard of care in all cases.
- Trusses, belts, and other such options are **not** the standard of care.

Other Hernias with Obstruction

Presentation: bowel can develop gangrene in less than 6 hours if it is strangulated. Femoral hernias are especially common in women (most common type of hernia in women) and can easily become incarcerated.

Management:

- These hernias require emergent surgery.

Ventral Hernia

Presentation: patient complains of "bulge" in the abdominal wall with incisional hernias after a surgical procedure. Very obese persons can have ventral hernias as well.

Management:

- Treatment depends on severity, but surgery is probably needed to place mesh to hold everything in place.

Diaphragmatic Hernia

Presentation: mother may have signs of polyhydramnios (excessive amniotic fluid). Look for respiratory distress at birth.

Management:
- Get fetal ultrasound and look for abdominal contents in chest cavity.
- 90% are found on the **left** side of the chest.
- Surgery is required.

Calculus of Gallbladder

Presentation: distended gallbladder with positive Murphy's sign (tender RUQ); may lead to obstruction of cystic duct by stones.

Management:
- Insert nasogastric tube.
- Put patient on NPO status.
- Get basic lab tests (CBC, CMP); look for left shift on CBC.
- Ultrasound has the highest sensitivity and specificity for diagnosing gallstones. Get hepato-iminodi-acetic acid (HIDA) scan for acute pain. Ejection fraction (EF) < 48% is considered positive.
- Use IV antibiotics (ampicillin and gentamicin).
- Use IV pain medication (meperidine, morphine).
- Remove gallbladder within several days.

Cholecystitis

Presentation: remember the 4 Fs: female, fat, fertile, and forty. The classic symptom is pain after fatty meals.

Management:
- Look for Murphy's sign (RUQ tenderness).
- Get CBC, including white blood cell count, and liver function tests, including AST, ALT, bilirubin, alkaline phosphatase. Levels may be elevated.
- Also get amylase and lipase levels; look for gallstone pancreatitis.
- Blood cultures are advised as well as a urinalysis, especially if the patient is febrile.
- Put patient on NPO status and start IV fluids.
- Start pain control. Meperidine (Demerol) IM used to be considered a good choice because sphincter of Oddi constriction was thought to be exacerbated by morphine. However, it turned out to be just the opposite: use morphine.
- Ultrasound is the best initial test of choice; HIDA is second-line choice.
- Endoscopic retrograde cholangiopancreatography (ERCP) can be used to remove stones as well as provide good endoscopic visualization.
- Order ERCP if no stones are visualized but the duct is dilated and LFTs remain elevated.
- Pancreatitis is frequent complication of ERCP; be alert to it.
- Because the bladder needs to come out, surgery should be scheduled at a later time after the patient is stabilized.

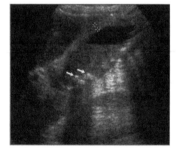

Figure 6. Acute cholecystitis on ultrasound. (From Harrow AR: The gallbladder and biliary tree. In Dogra V, Rubens DJ (eds): Ultrasound Secrets, Philadelphia, Hanley & Belfus, 2004, p 121.)

Cirrhosis of Liver

Presentation: portal vein hypertension, hepatic encephalopathy, ascites, esophageal varices, hepatorenal syndrome, bleeding.

Management:

- Causes include alcohol, viral infection (especially hepatitis C), hemochromatosis, alpha-1 antitrypsin deficiency, Wilson's disease.
- Get liver function tests, check coagulation profile.
- Order CT of the abdomen.
- Liver biopsy is the definitive diagnostic tool and yields the most information.
- Advise against use of acetaminophen (Tylenol).
- Suggest that the patient stop drinking alcohol.
- Treat portal hypertension with beta blocker.
- Treat hepatic encephalopathy with lactulose and low protein diet.
- Give antihistamine for itching due to bile salt build-up.
- Give vitamin K for coagulopathy as well as fresh frozen plasma.
- Liver transplant is the only cure.
- Be on the look-out for cancer to develop in cirrhosis.

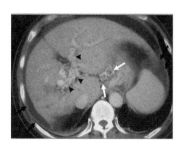

Figure 7. CT of cirrhosis of liver with ascites (arrows). (From Katz DS: Liver disease. In Katz DS, Math KR, Groskin SA (eds): Radiology Secrets. Philadelphia, Hanley & Belfus, 1998, p 131.)

Stricture of the Common Bile Duct

Presentation: most common after laparoscopic cholecystectomy procedure.

Management:

- Get serum chemistry panel.
- Compatible with obstructive jaundice: alkaline phosphatase (AP) and gamma-glutamyl transferase (GGT) levels typically rise.
- Order ERCP.
- Watch for postprocedure pancreatitis.

Pancreatitis

Presentation: 9 out of 10 cases are alcoholic pancreatitis. Other causes include biliary colic, certain drugs, sarcoidosis, hypercalcemia, hyperlipidemia, idiopathic disease, trauma, scorpion bites.

Management:

- Initiate bowel rest (i.e., place patient on NPO status).
- Start IV fluids and check electrolytes.
- Check amylase and lipase, which may be low in burned-out chronic pancreatitis.
- Evaluate Ranson criteria for increased mortality:
  - Age > 55 yr
  - White blood cell count >16,000
  - Glucose level ≥ 200
  - Lactate dehydrogenase (LDH) > 350
  - Asparate aminotransferase (AST) > 250.
  - Other: calcium < 8.
- Watch for frequent pulmonary complications, renal failure, infection, pseudocyst, necrotizing pancreatitis.
- In patients with chronic pancreatitis measure exocrine function with Chymex test. Ascertain endocrine function by looking for diabetes.
- May require pancreatic supplements to offset malabsorption caused by loss of exocrine function.
- May require insulin for lost endocrine function.

ONCOLOGY

Benign Neoplasm of Pancreas

Presentation: found in older/middle-aged women mostly commonly. Microcystic adenomas are cysts filled with glycogen with stellate calcifications seen on CT. These are exocrine tumors.

Management:

- Follow-up serial CTs are used for monitoring.

Malignant Neoplasm of Pancreas

Presentation: middle-aged person with pain and/or jaundice, depression. Painless jaundice is classic. Risk factors include smoking.

Management:

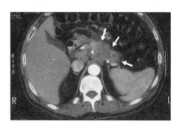

Figure 8. Unresectable pancreatic cancer. A mass (arrows) envelops the celiac artery and its branches. (From Katz DS: Imaging of pancreatic disease. In Katz DS, Math KR, Groskin SA (eds): Radiology Secrets. Philadelphia, Hanley & Belfus, 1998, p 129.)

- Check routine lab values, including liver function tests and bilirubin levels.
- CA19-9 may be elevated.
- The prognosis is dismal. Once big enough to see, the tumor is usually inoperable; < 20% are resectable. Adenocarcinoma is the most common and the most deadly.
- Get CT first.
- ERCP is the next step.
- Biopsy is needed for definitive diagnosis. Fine-needle aspiration may be done using ultrasound or CT.

Malignant Neoplasm of Liver

Presentation: risk factors include cirrhosis, hemochromatosis, aflatoxins, schistosomiasis, and glycogen storage disease.

Management:

- AFP is used to monitor.
- Surgery is needed.
- Chemotherapy: doxorubicin (Adriamycin), VP-16, cisplatinum, mitomycin, 5-FU, and leucovorin.
- CT is used for staging.
- Malignancy spreads to lungs and lymph nodes classically.

Malignant Neoplasm of Colon/Rectosigmoid Junction/Rectum

Presentation: heme-positive stool or obstruction, abdominal pain. Risk factors: family history, ulcerative colitis, advanced age, polyps. Most tumors are adenocarcinomas.

Management:

- Colorectal cancer is number-one most deadly cancer in nonsmokers.
- Routine colonoscopy is best method to find it early.
- Monitor levels of carcinoembryonic antigen (CEA) pre- and postoperatively.
- Get CT of chest as well as abdomen/pelvis to stage disease.
- Surgery options: right or left hemicolectomy, depending on site of cancer, or total colectomy in patients with familial polyposis.
- 5-FU and leucovorin are classic chemotherapy choices.
- Radiation requires an oncology consult.

Benign Neoplasm of Duodenum/Jejunum/Ileum

Presentation: usually asymptomatic; some patients report bleeding, constipation. Benign neoplasms include polyps, benign adenomas, lipomas, hemangiomas.

Management:
- Initial study: barium swallow.
- Do upper endoscopy.
- Consider arteriography if tumor appears to be bleeding.
- Laparotomy with excision is the standard of care.

Benign Neoplasm of Rectum

Presentation: soft tissue polyps vs. the harder carcinoma on exam; entirely limited to mucosa.

Management:
- Benign villous (remember villous = villainous) adenoma has great metastatic potential.
- Remove by local submucosal resection.
- Endoscopic microsurgery is an alternative.

Malignant Neoplasm of Stomach

Presentation: classic patient is an elderly Japanese person who smokes and eats smoked fish. Other risk factors include atrophic gastritis.

Management:
- Look for Virchow nodes (left supraclavicular).
- Order barium swallow.
- Order gastrointestinal endoscopy.
- Follow up with CT for staging.
- Consider bone scan.
- Remove the stomach surgically.
- Classic example is Krukenberg tumor (stomach-to-ovary metastases).

Benign Neoplasm of Stomach

Presentation: this diagnosis is histologically determined. An example is leiomyoma, which is differentiated from leiomyosarcoma.

Management:
- Benign neoplasm does not undergo metastasis and can be removed by surgical excision.

Malignant Neoplasm of Esophagus

Presentation: classic patient is a middle-aged man with long-standing GERD who presents with difficulty in swallowing meat that first occurred occasionally and then became worse.

Management:
- Order endoscopy with biopsy. Look for adenocarcinoma secondary to Barrett's esophagus or a squamous cell carcinoma.
- Surgery is the main treatment.
- Radiation is palliative.

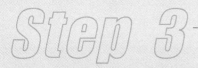
Gynecology

GENERAL ISSUES
   Endometrial hyperplasia
   Endometriosis of uterus
   Uterine prolapse
   Abnormal uterine bleeding/irregular
      menstrual cycle
   Abnormal Pap smear
   Prolapse of vaginal walls
   Imperforate hymen
   Dyspareunia
   Ovarian cyst
   Other ovarian failure
   Noninflammatory disorders of ovary/
      fallopian tube/broad ligament
   Dysmenorrhea
   Premenstrual tension
   Amenorrhea
   Excess menstruation
   Menopausal symptoms

Signs and symptoms in breast
Female infertility
Cervicitis/endocervicitis
Vaginitis/vulvovaginitis
Acute parametritis/pelvic cellulitis/pelvic
   inflammatory disease

ONCOLOGY
   Malignant neoplasm of uterus
   Leiomyoma of uterus
   Malignant neoplasm of cervix
   Malignant neoplasm of vagina
   Malignant neoplasm of vulva
   Malignant neoplasm of ovary
   Benign neoplasm of ovary
   Malignant neoplasm of breast
   Benign neoplasm of breast
   Fibrocystic breasts

GENERAL ISSUES

Endometrial Hyperplasia

Presentation: obese, diabetic women with abnormal vaginal bleeding.

Management:

- Late menopause is a risk factor.
- Unopposed estrogen without progesterone increases the risk.
- Order ultrasound to check for enlarged endometrial stripe (correlated with age).
- Obtain an endometrial biopsy.
- If the biopsy shows simple hyperplasia:
  □ If the woman is young/premenopausal or desires further children, give cyclic progestin to reverse hyperplasia, and repeat biopsy in 3 months.
  □ If the woman is postmenopausal or does not want any more children, the treatment is total hysterectomy.
  □ If the woman is anovulatory and insulin-resistant with polycystic ovarian syndrome (PCOS), regulate with metformin and birth control pills.

Endometriosis of Uterus

Presentation: tissue that normally lines the uterus (endometrium) grows in other areas of the body. If it penetrates the tough covering of the ovary, it causes an ovarian blood cyst (endometrioma).

Management:

- Laparoscopy/laparotomy is necessary for definitive diagnosis.
- Pseudopregnancy can be induced using oral contraceptives containing estrogen and progesterone.
- Pseudomenopause (a state resembling menopause) was developed as a means of treatment because of the observation that endometriosis regresses after menopause.
- Danazol, a weak androgenic (male characteristic) hormonal drug, may be used to reduce natural levels of estrogen and to decrease progesterone to low levels.
- Managing infertility
  - □ In patients under the age of 35 years, surgery may be undertaken to correct fallopian tubes, followed by induction of ovulation.
  - □ In vitro fertilization is the treatment of choice, especially in women over 35 years of age.

Uterine Prolapse

Presentation: uterus slides into the vagina; occurs typically in women who have given birth to many children vaginally.

Management:

- Ask the patient about pain with intercourse, backache, pain in the upright position.
- Perform a pelvic exam. In severe cases the uterus may actually protrude out of the vagina. Look for associated cystocele, rectocele, enterocele.
- Uterine prolapse is associated with low estrogen states and weak pelvic muscles.
- Consider estrogen replacement (intravaginal or oral).
- Kegel exercises should be prescribed as well as strengthening of muscles with weighted vaginal cones.
- Vaginal pessaries can be inserted into the vagina to hold organs in correct anatomic position.
- Surgery is definitive cure. Options include hysterectomy in women who no longer can or desire to bear children or colporrhaphy, particularly in patients with cystocele/rectocele.

Abnormal Uterine Bleeding/Irregular Menstrual Cycle

	Presentation
Regular cycle	Cycle of 21–35 days with regular frequency and flow less than 80 ml and duration of 2–7 days
Oligomenorrhea	Cycle length over 35 days
Polymenorrhea	Cycle length over 21 days
Amenorrhea	Absence of menses for 5 months or 3 cycles
Menorrhagia	Regular cycles with excessive flow/duration
Metrorrhagia	Irregular cycles
Menometrorrhagia	Irregular cycles and excessive flow/duration

Management:

- Obtain a pregnancy test, regardless of age. All women are pregnant until proved otherwise.
- Mind the ABCs. Get CBC to check hemoglobin levels.
- Admit to hospital for transfusion and IV fluids if needed.
- Consider heme work-up (PT/PTT, platelet count) to rule out some type of coagulopathy.

- Perform a bimanual pelvic exam to feel for masses/irregularly shaped uterus, which may indicate leiomyoma.
- Endometrial biopsy is done to rule out malignancy.
  - Not appropriate in very young (teenaged) women because their cycles are frequently irregular.
  - Biopsy must be done in women who are over 35, obese, diabetic, or postmenopausal.
- If patient has irregular cycles, do a progesterone trial: give progesterone for 10 days, and watch for bleeding to stop by day 2 of trial (and to remain stopped for the entire trial). Bleeding should restart once progestin withdrawn.
- If the above criteria are met, bleeding is anovulatory.
  - Consider checking TSH because hypothyroidism can cause metrorrhagia or menorrhagia.
  - Consider checking prolactin level to rule out prolactinoma.
- If the above criteria are not met, bleeding is ovulatory.
  - Get hysteroscopy to rule out lesions in the endometrium.
  - Biopsy the endometrium.
- If the above approach yields no definitive diagnosis, you can call it dysfunctional uterine bleeding (DUB), which is a diagnosis of exclusion. Administer NSAIDs, birth control pills, and progesterone to regulate cycles.
  - In acute DUB, give high doses of estrogen (3 times/day $\times$ 7 days) to stop the bleeding.
  - In chronic DUB, give birth control pills in usual daily dose.
  - In patients with chronic DUB who are trying to become pregnant, give clomiphene.

Abnormal Pap Smear

Presentation	Management
Normal	Repeat every year, or, if no risk factors after 3 normal Pap smears, repeat every 3 years
Atypical squamous cells of undetermined significance	Repeat Pap smear in 4–6 months or go directly to colonoscopy if patient is HPV-positive
Inflammation without atypia	Treat inflammation; repeat PAP smear in 1 year
Inflammation with atypia	Treat inflammation; repeat Pap smear in 1 month
Atypical glandular cells of uncertain significance	Colposcopy with biopsy or repeat Pap smear in 3 months
Low-grade squamous intraepithelial lesions (CIN II-III)	Immediate colposcopy with biopsy or repeat Pap smear every 4–6 months
High-grade squamous intraepithelial lesions	Colposcopy and direct biopsy except in adolescents and pregnant women. If the entire lesion and transformation zone are visualized, either excisional or ablative therapy is indicated.
If the entire lesion or the transformational zone cannot be seen	Cone biopsy
Squamous cell cancer	Colposcopy and direct biopsy. If the entire lesion and transformational zone are visualized, either excisional or ablative therapy is indicated.

Prolapse of Vaginal Walls

	Prolapse Location	Presentation
Cystocele	Anterior vaginal wall	Bladder is involved. Look for urinary incontinence.
Enterocele	Upper posterior vaginal wall	Small bowel is involved. May not have symptoms.
Rectocele	Lower posterior vaginal wall	Rectum is involved. Patient may insert finger in vagina when defecating.

Management:

- Ask about child-bearing history.
- Ask about pressure when standing up that is relieved by lying down.
- Do a pelvic exam.
- Vaginal wall prolapse is associated with low estrogen states and weak pelvic muscles.
- Consider estrogen replacement (intravaginal or oral).
- Kegel exercises should be prescribed as well as strengthening of muscles with weighted vaginal cones.
- Vaginal pessaries can be inserted into the vagina to hold organs in correct anatomic position.
- Surgery is definitive cure. Options include hysterectomy in women who no longer can or desire to bear children or colporrhaphy, particularly in patients with cystocele/rectocele.

Imperforate Hymen

Presentation: young woman in puberty who presents with abdominal pain.

Management:

- Hymen opening in virgins should be 1 mm per year of age; if it does not open at all, obstructed blood will be trapped inside during menses.
- Do a pelvic exam. You may note the hymen bulging from internal pressure.
- Hymenotomy should be performed.
- Progressive dilators can also be attempted as an alternative to surgery if the hymen is not completely imperforate.

Dyspareunia

Presentation: pain with intercourse.

Management:

- Ask the patient if pain occurs when the penis is first inserted or with deep penetration.
- If pain is superficial, vaginismus is likely psychological due to lack of desire or fear. Psychosexual counseling may be recommended.
- Pain with deep penetration probably indicates pelvic inflammatory disease, endometriosis, cervicitis, infection, or atrophic vaginitis.
- Vulvodynia is treated with amitriptyline through its effect on the pudendal nerve.

Ovarian Cyst

Etiology	Presentation	Management
Functional ovarian cysts	Usually unilateral	Most disappear within 30–60 days
Polycystic ovarian syndrome (PCOS)	Bilateral with hirsutism, infertility. Many cysts on ultrasound. Insulin resistance	Oral contraceptives, spironolactone, flutamide, and clomiphene citrate Metformin for insulin resistance

continued

Ovarian Cyst (*continued*)

Etiology	Presentation	Management
Endometriomas (chocolate cyst)	Unilateral. Can be quite large.	Ovary is the most common site of endometriosis; treat underlying condition

Management:
- Get a pregnancy test (always mandated).
- Get an ultrasound of the pelvis.
- Observation is usual course of action.
- If the cyst does not resolve, consider:
  - Laparoscopy for benign tumor
  - Laparotomy for malignant tumor

Other Ovarian Failure

Presentation	Cause
Premature - Amenorrhea - Hypoestrogenism - Elevated FSH - Under 40 years of age	Smoking cigarettes Trisomy X Autoimmune disorder Addison's disease Thyroiditis Diabetes
Induced	Radiotherapy Chemotherapy Surgically induced—i.e., total abdominal hysterectomy and bilateral salpingo-oophorectomy (TAH-BSO)

Management:
- Check level of follicle-stimulating hormone (FSH); expect it to be elevated in premature menopause.
- Estrogen supplementation is frequently given.

Noninflammatory Disorders of Ovary/Fallopian Tube/Broad Ligament

Cause	Presentation
Ovarian/tube torsion	Sudden pain in lower abdomen and mass. This is surgical emergency.
Broad ligament laceration syndrome	Pain, menstrual disturbances, pain with sex, backache. Cervix becomes hypermobile after damage to ligament from surgery, delivery, or induced abortion.

Dysmenorrhea

Presentation: pain/cramping with menses.

Management:

- Ask about associated nausea, vomiting, headache.
- Do a pelvic exam. Expect normal exam in primary dysmenorrhea. Be on the lookout for possible endometriosis, mass, cervical stenosis in secondary dysmenorrhea.
- Get ultrasound for patients with abnormal pelvic exam.
- Treat primary dysmenorrhea with NSAIDs (COX-2 preferred), birth control pills, and indomethacin to inhibit prostaglandins.
- Treat underlying cause in secondary dysmenorrhea.

Premenstrual Tension

Presentation: headache, bloating/weight gain, breast tenderness, back/abdominal pain, irritability/aggression, depression/anxiety/mood swings, and fatigue.

Management:

- Ask about symptoms and their timing in regard to menstrual cycle. Have the patient keep a diary of symptoms and their timing in cycle.
- A more severe manifestation is premenstrual dysphoric disorder with pronounced mood swings, anxiety/tension.
- Selective serotonin reuptake inhibitors (SSRIs), especially fluoxetine (Prozac, Sarafem), can improve symptoms, particularly in premenstrual dysphoric disorder.
- Exercise and limitation of caffeine, sugar, salt are helpful in relieving symptoms and should be tried first.
- Bromocriptine can help with breast tenderness.
- Spironolactone can be used for bloating.
- Birth control pills can regulate ovulation.
- In severe cases danazol (androgenic hormone) may be used.

Amenorrhea

Etiology	Presentation	Common Causes
Primary	No menses by age 16	Turner syndrome Androgen insensitivity Imperforate hymen
Secondary	Menses cease in women 20-40 years after regular established cycle	Pregnancy! PCOS Athletes undergoing severe training with low body fat Anorexia Hypothyroidism

Management:

- Do pelvic exam.
- Pregnancy test first.
- Progesterone challenge should result in bleeding.
- If it induces bleeding, conclude that estrogen is normal and check levels of luteinizing hormone (LH):

□ High = PCOS

□ Normal = prolactinoma, exercise/anorexia

- If the progesterone challenge does *not* induce bleeding, conclude that estrogen is inadequate and check follicle-stimulating hormone (FSH):

  □ High = premature ovarian failure (i.e., menopause). Rule out autoimmune disorder, Addison's disease, thyroiditis, diabetes as causes.

  □ Normal/low = order MRI or CT of brain to rule out hypothalamic tumor.

Excess Menstruation

Presentation: very heavy periods.

Management:

- Ascertain the quantity. One pad can hold about 5 ml of blood. Ask how many pads are used.
- Pregnancy test: Is this an abortion?
- Consider bleeding work-up (factor VIII, von Willebrand factor) in young women to rule out von Willebrand's disease.
- Ask about use of aspirin, anticoagulants
- Most cases are anovulatory in older women.
- See *Abnormal Uterine Bleeding* for more management details.

Menopausal Symptoms

Presentation: mean age is 51 years; symptoms include hot flashes, depression, mood swings, irritability, decreased vaginal lubrication, atrophy of vaginal epithelium. Preceded by perimenopause (3-5 years) with shorter and possibly irregular cycles.

Management:

- Women can become pregnant in perimenopause. Birth control is still needed.
- Risk of osteoporosis increases greatly. Do DEXA scan. Increase intake of calcium and vitamin D, and add weight-bearing exercise. Bisphosphonates also may be added.
- Cardiovascular risk after menopause is equivalent to that of a man. Check lipids and treat.
- Recommend lubricants for sexual comfort. Local estrogen may be required to treat atrophic vaginitis.
- Hormone replacement therapy (HRT) is quite controversial at this time due to the 1998 Heart and Estrogen/Progestin Replacement (HERS) Study, which was stopped short because of increases in mortality from HRT.
- Weigh the risks vs. current symptoms in deciding about HRT. Is the family history positive for breast cancer or endometrial cancer? Is the patient a smoker? Has she ever had deep venous thombosis? If answer is no to these questions, the woman may be candidate for HRT, at least for a short period, if quality of life has severely deteriorated. Progestin may be considered only in some cases. Estrogen is not given alone unless the patient has had a hysterectomy.

Signs and Symptoms in Breast

	Presentation	Management
Mastitis	Painful mass while breast-feeding, redness, fever	Continue breast-feeding. It is therapeutic. Moist heat Amoxicillin
Abscess	Swelling, redness, pus from nipple, fever	Moist heat Amoxicillin Drainage
Fat necrosis	Trauma to the breast	Breast exam, mammogram, fine-needle aspiration cytology

Female Infertility

	Cause
Anovulation	Polycystic ovarian syndrome (PCOS) Prolactinoma Hypothalamic-pituitary dysfunction Hypothyroidism
Fallopian tube disease	Pelvic inflammatory disease (PID) Endometriosis
Uterine factors	History of D&C Fibroids Endometriosis
Cervical factors	Cervicitis Cone biopsy/conization

Presentation: Inability to conceive within 12 months of unprotected sex.

Management:

- In 60% of cases female factors contribute to infertility but may only be partially responsible. The male should be tested at the same time with a semen sample.
- A woman's ability to become pregnant drops rapidly as she ages, especially after 30. One of the first tests to order is follicle-stimulating hormone (FSH) on the third day of her cycle. If the value exceeds 12, the ovaries are going to reach failure soon.
- The first step is to check for ovulation:
  - Are the patient's cycles regular and predictable? Keep a diary.
  - Have the patient record temperature. Her temperature should be elevated during midcycle.
  - Rule out prolactinoma, hypothyroidism: Check prolactin level, TSH.
  - Rule out PCOS: Check testosterone, LH/FSH. Testosterone levels may be elevated, and LH:FSH ratio exceeds 3 in PCOS.
  - Clomiphene can induce ovulation if you determine that the patient is anovulatory.
  - If clomiphene fails, the next step is human menopausal gonadotropin combined with midcycle human chorionic gonadotropin.
- The second step is to identify possible fallopian tube disease.
  - Ask the patient if she has had PID or ectopic pregnancy in the past. Both can scar the fallopian tubes.
  - Hysterosalpingogram can establish tubular patency.
  - Proceed to laparoscopy if this test shows a problem. Laparoscopy can help find adhesions/disease that can be surgically corrected.
- In vitro fertilization can be used if tubal disease cannot be repaired, if endometriosis is the problem, or if no obvious reason can be found.

Cervicitis/Endocervicitis

Presentation: discharge from vagina, symptoms of urinary tract infection (UTI), bleeding after sex.

Management:

- Take sexual history, and ask about Pap smear history/abnormal results in past.
- Causative agents include *Chlamydia* sp., *Neisseria gonorrhoeae*, *Trichomonas* sp., herpes simplex virus (HSV), or human papillomavirus.

- Other causes include trauma or cancer.
- Look carefully on external exam for blisters, warts.
- On pelvic exam look for red, swollen, friable cervix and note any purulent discharge.
- On bimanual exam note tenderness when you move the cervix.
- Do a Pap smear if not done recently.
- Culture for gonorrhea/chlamydial infection.
- Collect any discharge and look at it under microscope. Do the whiff test with KOH.
- Treatment agents:
  - Ceftriaxone IM or azithromycin PO for gonorrhea
  - Doxycycline for chlamydial infection (always give doxycycline when treating gonorrhea; chlamydial coinfection is found in 50% of gonorrhea infections).
  - Give metronidazole for trichomonal infection.
  - Give acyclovir for HSV.
  - Give imiquimod for genital warts.
  - Amino acid cervical cream is used for chronic cervicitis.
- Consider testing for other STDs, especially syphilis, that can affect the cervix.
- Counsel about sexual practices (do not forget this step on the CCS section of Step 3 exam).

Vaginitis/Vulvovaginitis

Presentation: discharge, burning, and itching,

Management:

- *Candida* sp. is a frequent culprit, especially in diabetics or after course of antibiotics, but remember that "not everything that itches is yeast."
- Bacterial vaginosis (BV) and trichomonal infection can also present with discharge.
- You should consider sexual abuse in children and should also look for foreign objects.
- Do KOH and wet-mount. Vaginal pH < 4.5 = normal or yeast; pH > 4.5 = BV.
- Treat candidal infection with oral fluconazoles or topical antifungals.
- Treat BV with metronidazole or clindamycin in patient only (not her partner).
- Treat trichomonal infection with metronidazole in both patient and partner.

SAMPLE CCS INPUT—Trichomonas vaginitis

Focused PE: abdomen, genitalia
Gonorrhea/chlamydial culture, urinalysis, syphilis serology
Wet mount, vaginal secretions
KOH preparation, vaginal secretions
PH, vaginal secretions
Metronidazole, oral
Treat sexual partner
Counsel about safe sex techniques
Change location to home
Counsel patient to avoid alcohol (disulfiram-like reaction with metronidazole)

Acute Parametritis/Pelvic Cellulitis/Pelvic Inflammatory Disease

Presentation: sexually active young woman with lower abdominal pain.

Management:

- Take a sexual history and be sure to ask about pain with intercourse. Also ask about any vaginal discharge. Has she had any fever, chills, or nausea/vomiting?

- Observe the patient: is she walking bent over, holding her abdomen and shuffling her feet? This finding is strongly suspicious for pelvic inflammatory disease (PID).
- Pelvic and abdominal exams are mandatory. Expect adnexal tenderness as well as cervical motion tenderness (known as the "chandelier sign" because the patient jumps off the exam table to the roof due to pain). Expect lower abdominal tenderness.
- If infection has ascended to liver capsule, the patient may have right upper quadrant tenderness (known as Fitz-Hugh–Curtis syndrome).
- Get a pregnancy test as soon as possible. It is so easy to miss an ectopic pregnancy.
- Get a urinalysis to rule out urinary tract infection.
- Get CBC; with PID expect the WBC count to be elevated over 10,000.
- Get erythrocyte sedimentation rate and C-reactive protein level; expect both to be elevated.
- Obtain cultures for gonorrhea and chlamydial infection, but do not wait for results to commence treatment.
- Consider STD work-up for syphilis and HIV.
- Consider ultrasound to rule out ovarian cyst/torsion or diverticular disease.
- Consider CT to rule out appendicitis.
- Do not wait for results of tests to start empirical treatment!
- Treat suspected cases while awaiting diagnostic confirmation.
- Admit the patient if she has high fever, uses an intrauterine device (IUD), is an adolescent or primigravida or appears unstable/septic. Treat with IV antibiotics:
  □ Cefoxitin IV plus doxycycline IV *or*
  □ Clindamycin IV plus gentamicin IV
- Normally treat on an outpatient basis:
  □ Mild: ceftriaxone IM plus doxycycline PO
  □ Severe: ceftriaxone IM plus doxycycline PO plus metronidazole
- PID increases risk for infertility and ectopic pregnancy; tell the patient so.
- Treat the partner.
- Counsel about safe sex.

ONCOLOGY

Malignant Neoplasm of Uterus

Presentation: postmenopausal woman with abnormal vaginal bleeding. Endometrial cancer is the most malignant neoplasm.

Management:
- Late menopause is a risk factor.
- Unopposed estrogen without progesterone increases the risk.
- Fractional D&C and hysteroscopy are needed for diagnosis.
- Staging is surgical. Uterine cancer spreads to lymphatics as well as surrounding tissues in pelvis and abdomen.
- Total abdominal hysterectomy and bilateral salpingo-oophorectomy (TAH-BSO) are used in all cases. Remove the uterus and ovaries.
- Radiation and chemotherapy are added for invasion/metastases.

Leiomyoma of Uterus

Presentation: often black women in their 50s who have children. This is the most common uterine tumor.

Management:

- Leiomyomas are usually asymptomatic but can cause abnormal bleeding, loss of fetus in second trimester.
- Do a bimanual pelvic exam, and expect to find large, firm, asymmetrical uterus.
- Leiomyomas are classified by location within the uterus.
- Get hysterosalpingogram to diagnose submucosal myomas.
- Get ultrasound to diagnose intramural or submucosal myomas.
- You can attempt to resect individual lesions after giving GnRH agonists to shrink them, but hysterectomy is definitive cure.

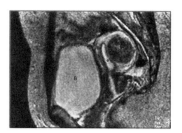

Figure 2. Leiomyoma of uterus. (From Poster RB: Uterine and cervical imaging. In Katz DS, Math KR, Groskin SA (eds): Radiology Secrets. Philadelphia, Hanley & Belfus, 1998, p 252.)

Malignant Neoplasm of Cervix

Presentation: vaginal bleeding, especially postcoital or on routine Pap smear.

Management:

- Smoking, human papillomavirus, and sex early in life with multiple partners are risk factors.
- Get Pap smear.
- If cervical cancer is suspected, go to colposcopy with biopsy; you need cervical biopsy to diagnose.
- Once you get the diagnosis, proceed as follows:
    - Cryotherapy or loop electrosurgical excision procedure (LEEP) for highly localized disease.
    - Cone biopsy for women who are not yet done with child-bearing if the disease is confined to the cervix.
    - Otherwise the treatment is hysterectomy.

Malignant Neoplasm of Vagina

Presentation: painless vaginal bleeding.

Management:

- Malignant neoplasm of the vagina is very rare, and unfortunately the diagnosis is often delayed.
- Most vaginal cancers are metastases, frequently from the cervix or vulva. You should determine the source.
- Diethylstilbestrol (DES) usage presents with clear cell carcinoma in female offspring. Such girls should be screened very early in adolescence.
- Examine the vagina and take punch biopsies of lesions. Lesions are usually ulcers but may be a mass also.
- Generally treated with surgical excision, including hysterectomy, vaginectomy, and lymph node dissection.
- Radiotherapy can also be used in some cases.

Malignant Neoplasm of Vulva

Presentation: woman in her 60s with itching.

Management:

- Human papillomavirus and obesity are considered risk factors.
- Squamous cell cancer is the most common tumor.
- Take a punch biopsy of any lesions. This is absolutely essential.

Malignant Neoplasm of Vulva (*continued*)

Presentation	Management
Squamous hyperplasia	Fluorinated steroid cream
Lichen sclerosis	Testosterone cream
Moderate dysplasia	Surgical excision, local
Carcinoma in situ	Skinning vulvectomy
Invasive squamous cell carcinoma	Radical vulvectomy and lymph node dissection

Malignant Neoplasm of Ovary

Presentation: usually no symptoms, although advanced disease can present with mass. Krukenberg tumor may be found when stomach/colon cancer metastasizes to the ovaries.

Management:
- Ask about family history/BRCA 1 gene, infertility, nulliparity. All are risk factors.
- You can help prevent it by having children or taking birth control pills, both of which reduce the number of ovulations.
- Check CA125, CEA to find epithelial tumors, which are by far the most common.
- Check alpha fetoprotein (AFP), beta human chorionic gonadotropin, lactate dehydrogenase to find germ cell tumors.
- Check estrogen and testosterone levels to find gonadal stromal tumors.
- Histology is needed for definitive diagnosis.
- Surgical removal is mainstay of treatment with adjunctive radiation therapy.

Benign Neoplasm of Ovary

	Presentation
Serous cystadenoma	Can grow very large
Mucinous cystadenoma	Can rupture and cause pseudomyxoma peritonei
Benign cystic teratomas (germ cell)	Usual patient age: 20–30 yrs. Consist of teeth, hair, and bone.

Management:
- In women under 40 the tumor is most likely benign; in women over 40 it is rarely benign.
- Get a pregnancy test. This is always mandated.
- Order an ultrasound.
- Do laparoscopy.
- Surgical resection is the treatment.

Malignant Neoplasm of Breast

Presentation: patient may have no symptoms. Be highly concerned in women over age 35 with new breast mass, nipple changes, or new calcifications on mammogram.

Management:
- Yearly breast exams are recommended; teach patient self-exams.
- Order baseline mammogram at age 35–40, then get mammogram every year after 40.

- Biopsy any suspicious mass.
- Treatment options vary with disease from lumpectomy to radical mastectomy and generally a lymph node dissection under the armpit.
- Commence radiation and chemotherapy, including hormonal therapies for estrogen and/or progesterone receptor-positive varieties.

Benign Neoplasm of Breast

Presentation: rubbery mass that grows with high estrogen states such as use of birth control pills or pregnancy; usually fibroadenoma.

Management:

- Observation is preferred approach in young women under 35 without family history of breast cancer.
- Ultrasound is preferred diagnostic method in young patients. Mammogram is not used because breast tissue is so dense.
- In older women get a mammogram.
- If any doubts remain, order biopsy, especially with rapid change in size.

Fibrocystic Breasts

Presentation: most common cause of breast lumps in women aged 30–50 years. Common symptom is bilateral breast tenderness that fluctuates with menstrual cycle.

Management:
- Recommend monthly self-breast exams after age 20.
- Breast exam should also be done by health care professional.
- Do mammogram at 35–40 years of age.
- Biopsy should be ordered if you are at all suspicious.
- Tell patients to avoid caffeine.
- Bromocriptine or danazol can be given for severe pain. Watch for side effects such as weight gain, amenorrhea, masculinizaton, infertility, nausea.
- Surgical removal of lumps is the last resort.

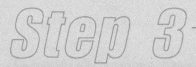
Health Maintenance

GENERAL ISSUES
   Community-related prevention
   Routine child/infant health check
   Other counseling
   Follow-up exams
   General medical exam
   Laboratory exam
   Child behavioral/developmental disorders
   Counseling for contraception
   Sterilization
   Surveillance of prescribed contraception
   Contraceptive management
   Genetic counseling
   Antenatal screening
   Gynecologic examination
   Routine cervical Pap smear
   Postpartum follow-up
   Breast cancer screening
   Dietary surveillance
   Cardiovascular risk screening

   Exercise
   Influenza vaccination
   DTP and polio vaccinations
   Other vaccinations
   Desensitization to allergens
   Prophylactic chemotherapy
   Skin sensitization tests

SUBSTANCE ABUSE
   Alcohol abuse
   Tobacco use disorder
   Hallucinogen abuse
   Sedative, hypnotic, or anxiolytic abuse
   Withdrawal
   Opioid abuse/overdose
   Opioid withdrawal
   Cocaine abuse
   Amphetamine abuse
   Antidepressant-type abuse
   Mixed, nonspecified drug abuse

GENERAL

Community-related Prevention

Management: Prevent, detect, and treat:
- Drug/alcohol use
- Abuse
- Helmet/seatbelt use
- Abstinence/sex education
- Safe storage of firearms
- Violence/suicide prevention
- Tobacco use

Routine Child/Infant Health Check

Management:
- Do complete physical exam.
- Update immunizations.
- Test for anemia and lead at 1 year.
- Check height, weight, and development.
- Nutrition check (ask about eating habits).
- Screen vision, dental status, and hearing.
- Ask about behavior and psychological development, including potty training, walking, talking.
- Babies basically need to be checked every 1–2 months during first year.
- Toddlers should be checked every 3–4 months.
- After age 2 annual check-up is appropriate, including teens.

Other Counseling

Management: Ask about:
- Marriage and family concerns
- Elder care
- Parenting
- Advance directives

Follow-up Examinations

Management:
- Generally after outpatient surgical procedures the standard follow-up is the next day, 1 month, then 1 year.
- For medical problems, it is a judgment call. Tailor follow-up to severity of patient's condition. If you start the patient on a new medication, consider 3-6 month follow-up to monitor progress. If everything checks out, 12-month schedule may be adequate.

General Medical Examination

Management: In the United States, certain format/components of the history and physical exam should be reflected in the physician's notes. This list may appear elementary to some readers:
- Record chief complaint.
- Elicit history of present illness.
- Include past medical and surgical history.
- Document allergies.
- Ask about medications, including over-the-counter drugs and herbals.
- Elicit family and social history.
- Conduct review of systems.
- Assess vital signs, including temperature, pulse, blood pressure, respirations.
- Assess general appearance.
- Address specific organs/systems: skin, head, eyes, ears, nose, throat, neck, chest, breasts, heart, vascular system, abdomen, rectum, genitalia, musculoskeletal system, neurologic status.
- Record assessment and plan for management.

Laboratory Examination

Management:
- Hemoglobin/CBC once before 2 years of age, then again between 10 and 18 years of age.
- Urinalysis at 5 years, then once between 11 and 18 years.
- Pap and pelvic exams in women at age 21 or at first sexual activity, then annually.

- Lead screening from birth to 18 years. Evaluate first with questions, then get lab test if the patient is at risk
- Tuberculosis test from birth to 18 years. Evaluate first with questions, then get lab test if the patient is at risk.
- Cholesterol and lipid profile every 3 years from 18–39 years of age, every 2 years from 40–49 years, and annually from 50–64 years. This is the only exam mandated in all adults.
- Colonscopy every 10 years after 50 years of age.
- PSA/prostate screening every 2 years from 40–49 years of age, then annually from 50-64 years.
- Obviously if the patient has other medical conditions, other lab tests will be mandated; for example, a hemoglobin A1C in diabetics at least yearly as well as metabolic panel to monitor renal function/creatinine and urine microalbumin. Other lab tests, including liver function tests and CBC, may be needed, especially if patient is on certain drugs. If the patient is hypothyroid, you should get a TSH level.
- Many physicians order too many unneeded and expensive lab tests. Step 3 will penalize for this practice.

Child Behavioral/Developmental Disorders

Presentation: includes autism, retardation, mental/emotional problems, delinquency, substance abuse, coping difficulties, developmental concerns, poor grades.

Management:
- Rule out medical/physical contribution to problem.
- Refer to child psychiatric services.

Counseling for Contraception

Management:
- Take complete sexual history.
- Do complete history and physical exam and make sure blood pressure is not elevated before giving oral contraceptive pills (OCPs). Also rule out pregnancy, history of thromboembolic disease, stroke, history of breast cancer, liver dysfunction.
- Pap smear and cervical screening are mandatory, certainly within 3 months of starting OCPs.
- Recommend nonbarrier methods only to married/monogamous women.
- Consider implants for women who may be noncompliant in taking OCPs.
- If the woman is over 35 and a smoker, OCPs are contraindicated because of risk of deep venous thrombosism (DVT).
- Know the findings of the latest Women's Health Initiative study when counseling patients about the benefits and risks of hormone replacement therapy:
    - 41% increase in strokes
    - 29% increase in heart attacks
    - 100% increase DVTs/blood clots
    - 22% increase in total cardiovascular disease
    - 26% increase in breast cancer
    - 37% reduction in cases of colorectal cancer
    - 33% reduction in hip fracture rates
    - 24% reduction in total fractures
    - 0% difference in total mortality

Sterilization

Management:
- Rarely done in anyone under 30 because so many change their minds later.
- Options include tubal ligation or vasectomy or hysterectomy.
- Counsel patients that sterilization techniques are considered permanent and not easily reversed.

Surveillance of Prescribed Contraception

Management:
- Frequent follow-ups maximize compliance.
- Quarterly visits recommended in adolescents to discuss utilization, compliance, and complications.

Contraceptive Management

Management: Know common side effects of OCPs:
- Nausea: take pill at bedtime or with meal or take low-estrogen OCP.
- Fluid retention, migraines, moodiness: consider change to low-estrogen OCP.
- Weight gain: change to low-estrogen OCP with low androgenic activity.
- Hypertension: switch to progestin-only pill.
- Depression: decrease progestin dose.
- Decreased libido: increase androgenic activity.
- Dry eyes: switch to progestin.

Genetic Counseling

Management:
- Create a family history/pedigree of medical problems.
- Look for genetic conditions in family.
- Explain these conditions, especially if heredity is involved.
- Refer to genetic counselor.
- Lay out the options to the family with risks/benefits.

Antenatal Screening

Management: Purpose is to determine early in pregnancy whether the unborn child possibly has a major disorder:
- Amniocentesis and chorionic villus sampling are mainstays of antenatal screening.
- Down's syndrome and cystic fibrosis are the most commonly screened disorders, along with various neural tube defects.
- Provide information to help couple in decision making.
- Do not push the couple into this testing, and do not pressure them to have an abortion.

Gynecologic Examination

Management: Similar to general medical exam but includes some new elements:
- Sensitivity to patient's embarrassment: have a chaperone for this sensitive exam.
- Take a menstrual history.
- Past medical history should include obstetric, gynecologic, contraceptive, and sexual issues.
- Take care while performing the abdominal exam
- Pelvic exam should include the vulva, vagina, cervix, uterus, adnexa, and rectal-vaginal area. Obtain appropriate cultures and screening for Pap smears.

Routine Cervical Pap Smear

Management:
- Start screening within 3 years of onset of sexual activity or at age 21, then every 3 years thereafter.
- Stop after 65 years of age if all exams have been negative in the recent past.

Postpartum Follow-up

Management:

- 2 and 6 weeks are typical follow-up intervals.
- Counsel all mothers about care of baby and breastfeeding, hygiene/healing, nutrition.
- Look for signs of infection, especially after C-section.
- Common problems include bladder incontinence/urinary tract infections, hemorrhoids, and constipation. These problems should be addressed.
- Depression and exacerbation of mental illness are very common in this period. Be alert.
- Sex may be resumed after 6 weeks if the patient is comfortable.
- Contraception should be discussed.
- Domestic abuse is quite high after childbirth; be alert to this possibility.

Breast Cancer Screening

Management:

- All women should be taught breast self-exam.
- A breast exam should be part of yearly gynecologic exam.
- Women over age 40 should have yearly mammogram.
- Begin at earlier age if the patient is at high risk, and consider genetic testing.

Dietary Surveillance

Management:

- Minimize saturated fats and simple carbohydrates and excessive calorie intake in general.
- Prenatal vitamins with folate are recommended for women of child-bearing age.
- Lots of fruits and vegetables are recommended for everyone.
- Encourage milk/calcium intake, especially among young women.

Cardiovascular Risk Screening

Management:

- Check lipids in all adults.
- For patients aged 40 to 64 years, get a baseline ECG.
- After age 65 get ECG annually.
- Consider stress test if angina is reported.
- Consider catheterization if stress test is not reassuring.

Exercise

Management:

- Guideline: at least 3 times per week of cardiovacular exercise for 30 minutes.
- Weight-training is becoming more appreciated by the medical community. Recommend 3 times per week with day off between sessions. Weight-bearing exercise can stave off lean body mass loss and osteoporosis.
- Emphasize swimming for arthritic patients who cannot endure joint stress.
- Walking is generally a safe recommendation.

Influenza Vaccination

Management:

- Not routine in children unless they are immunocompromised.
- Immunocompromised adults and those around them, including health care workers, should have the vaccine every year.

DTP and Polio Vaccinations

Management:

- Diphtheria, tetanus, and pertussis at 2, 4, 6, 12 months, then at about 5 years and 11 years of age. Tetanus booster alone should be given every 10 years no matter the age.
- Oral polio vaccine at 2, 4, 6 months, then at about 5 years of age.

Other Vaccinations

Management:

- HIB (Influenza B) at 2,4 months, then 12–15 months of age.
- Measles, mumps, rubella (MMR) at 12–15 months, then age 4–6 years.
- Hepatitis B at 2,4, 6–18 months.
- Chickenpox (varicella) at 12–18 months; consider second dose in adolescence if the patient is not immunized by titer.
- Pneumococcus at 2, 4, 6, 12–15 months, and about 5 years of age.

Desensitization to Allergens

Management:

- Give gradually increasing doses (shots) of the allergens, which reduce the strength of the IgE and its effect on the mast cells. This protocol induces tolerance.

Prophylactic Chemotherapy

Management:

- One example is malaria prevention in travelers to endemic areas.

Skin Sensitization Tests

Management:

- Use to identify specific substance causing allergy symptoms or to screen for TB.
- Usually done on back with various allergens injected into the skin with controls. These sites rise like mosquito bites for positive reactions. Be sure to hold antihistamines before the test and be alert to anaphylaxis reactions. Useful especially in hay fever, asthma, suspected penicillin allergy, or bee sting allergy.
- Mantoux intradermal tuberculin skin test is used to identify those exposed to TB. Reaction is read 48 hours after injection. The site will be raised in exposed individuals unless they are anergic, immuno-compromised.

SUBSTANCE ABUSE

Alcohol Abuse

Management:

- Problem drinkers may have legal problems, engage in drinking and driving or binge drinking.
- Do the CAGE survey to evaluate patients: Have you felt that you should **c**ut down on your drinking? **A**ngry when confronted? Feel **g**uilty? Need **e**yeopener?
- Other questions that may be helpful: Do you drive when drinking? Do you have blackouts after drinking? Have you missed work or lost a job because of drinking? Is your tolerance going up—are you drinking more than before to become intoxicated?
- Recommend that women have no more than one drink per day and men no more than two per day.

- An initial trial of moderation is not out of the question in problem drinkers. If this approach fails, then lifelong abstinence may be required.
- Proceed to recommend alcohol treatment programs with detoxification.
- Follow with support group such as Alcoholics Anonymous.

Tobacco Use Disorder

Management:

- Tobacco causes heart disease, cancer, emphysema, birth defects, vascular disease, asthma in children.
- Smoking causes more preventable death in the U.S. than anything else.
- Three minutes of physician intervention can increase by 50% the chances of quitting.
- Ask about tobacco use, including chewing tobacco.
- Advise to quit. Counsel patient about the risks of smoking, including to unborn children, others in the household.
- Assess willingness to make attempt to quit.
- Assist in quit attempt. The antidepressant Zyban (Wellbutrin) combined with nicotine patches is fairly effective at helping cessation.
- Follow up.

Hallucinogen Abuse

Presentation: extremely dilated pupils, warm skin, perspiration, distorted senses of sight/hearing/touch, distorted time perception, mood/behavior changes, flashbacks. PCP adds an extra dose of violence and paranoia.

Management:

- Common hallucinogens include mescaline/peyote, psilocybin mushrooms, LSD, MDMA/ecstasy, STP, PCP.
- Talk to family and friends if possible, because it may not be obvious what is going on. Drug screens are limited in value and cannot detect LSD but order a drug screen anyway. Here are some notable characteristics that may assist in the diagnosis:

	Presentation
LSD	Really big pupils, 12-hour trips, flashbacks (in people who have dosed > 10 times), small pieces of paper on tongue.
Ecstasy	Hottest new rave drug: hypertension, bruxism (grind teeth) are common. The patient may wear pacifier around neck for bruxism. Look out for rhabdomyolysis, pills.
PCP	Violence, vertical/horizontal/rotary nystagmus. The patient feels no pain (PCP used to be used as an anesthetic curiously). Cigarettes dipped in PCP liquid are smoked commonly.
Peyote/mushrooms	Native Americans: GI pain is quite common, along with respiratory depression.

- Make sure that another treatable condition is not the cause for the presentation. Get lab tests, arterial blood gases, CT of head, lumbar puncture, as judgment dictates.
- From a management perspective, talking the patient down is the first step.
- Put patients in a dark, quiet room and do not bother them excessively.
- Benzodiazepines are generally safe to give with all the hallucinogens.
- Physical restraints may be used if needed.
- Observe and discharge after intoxication wears off unless the patient is unstable or has other associated symptoms. Definitely consult psychiatrist if psychotic symptoms do not wear off with the intoxication.

- Generally the psychiatry resident on-call has to come to the ED to see the patient.
- Watch for hyperthermia, hypertension, seizures, or cardiac arrhythmias, especially with ecstasy. Admit patients with arrhythmias to MICU.

Sedative, Hypnotic, or Anxiolytic Abuse

Presentation: Overdose leads to sedation, respiratory depression.

Management:
- Flumazenil is the antidote.
- Toxicology screen should look for other substances; get other lab tests to rule out other physiologic contribution.
- Consider CT of head to rule out other organic causes.
- Get routine lab tests.
- Consider IV fluids for possible rhabdomyolysis.
- Admit and observe.

Withdrawal

Presentation: sweating, tachycardia, tremors, nausea/vomiting, hallucinations, agitation, seizures.

Management:
- Manage the airway,
- Initiate benzodiazepine taper.
- Order gastric lavage.
- Admit and observe.

Opioid Abuse/Overdose

Presentation: pinpoint pupils, constipation, respiratory depression, euphoria/drowsiness.

Management:
- Manage the airway.
- Give fluids.
- Get an ECG.
- Naloxone is the antidote.
- Be alert to comorbidities associated with needles (HIV, endocarditis) and talc (pulmonary fibrosis).

Opioid Withdrawal

Presentation: symptoms are opposite of overdose: diarrhea, rhinorrhea, nausea/vomiting/cramping, emesis, hunger for the drug. Generally the patient looks poorly.

Management:
- Methadone is used for withdrawal.
- Clonidine can reduce autonomic symptoms in withdrawal.
- Naltrexone in combination with clonidine can drastically shorten withdrawal.
- Provide psychotherapy and ongoing assistance.

Cocaine Abuse

Presentation: big pupils, headache, anorexia, euphoria, agitation/paranoia, tachycardia, hypertension, sweating, tremors, confusion, seizures, stroke, cardiac arrhythmias, hyperthermia.

Management:

- Urine drug screen, TSH, creatinine kinase (CK), cardiac markers.
- Treat symptoms acutely; they may lead to hypertension, seizures, myocardial infarction.
- CT scan of brain for patients with focal neurological deficits.
- ECG for patients with chest pain.

Pitfalls:

- Do not miss cocaine-induced rhabdomyolysis with elevated CK and consequent renal failure.
- Be careful not to misdiagnose thyroid storm.
- Do not give neuroleptics in agitated long-term cocaine users. They can lead to malignant hyperthermia.
- Do not give beta blockers (including labetalol) for cocaine-induced hypertension. Unopposed alpha-adrenergic activity will predominate and worsen hypertension.

Sample question:

His family brings a 19-year-old man to the ED because he says that the police and drug dealers are following him and are going to kill him. Vitals signs: temperature, 38°C; pulse, 112 bpm; blood pressure, 180/100 mmHg. His pupils are dilated. He has needle-tracks on his forearms. He most likely ingested which substance?

A. Alcohol
B. Heroin
C. Cocaine
D. Diazepam
E. Ecstasy

The correct answer is at the end of the chapter.

Amphetamine Abuse

Presentation: Patients generally present similarly to those on cocaine with added psychosis. Signs of use include weight loss, hypertension, big pupils, hypervigilance. Ecstasy (MDMA) is a mixed hallucinogen/amphetamine derivative; crystal meth is the other popular "speed."

Management:

- See *Hallucinogens* for ecstasy information.
- Give IV fluids.
- Give benzodiazepines for agitation.
- Give haloperidol (Haldol) for psychotic reactions.
- Ammonium chloride hastens urinary excretion.
- Get toxicology screen to look for other drugs.
- Get an ECG.
- As always, check for some other metabolic/organic cause of this presentation.
- You can use beta blockers for hypertension with amphetamines, but be sure cocaine is not the culprit!
- Order gastric lavage.
- Give supportive outpatient therapy.

Antidepressant Type Abuse

Presentation: suicide attempt in depressed patient. Overdose of tricyclic antidepressant (TCA) presents with hypotension, neurologic depression, and anticholinergic effects. Generally TCA overdoses are the most important. Overdose of monoamine oxidase inhibitors (MAOIs) presents with hypertension, hyperthermia; the patient may have eaten tyramine-containing foods.

TCA Management:
- Manage the airway; intubate, if needed, as soon as possible.
- Start IV normal saline.
- Give bicarbonate to keep pH basic to minimize TCA cardiac effects. **This is the standard of care**.
- Get ECG and look for the wide QRS. Cardiotoxicity is the key problem in TCA overdose.
- Antiarrhythmics are not used except lidocaine and only as second-line treatment. Bicarbonate should be your Step 3 answer with a menu of therapies for TCA overdose.
- Lorazepam (Ativan) may be given for seizures.
- Get BMP, toxicology screen, and arterial blood gases.
- Calculate the anion gap because the patient may have ingested other substances. Anion gap = $[Na+] - [Cl-] - [HCO_3-]$.
- Keep K+ greater than 4.0.
- Consider dopamine or norepinephrine (Levophed) for hypotension, which is common with TCA overdose.
- Order gastric lavage with activated charcoal.
- Transfer to ICU and continue the bicarbonate drip.

MAOI Management:
- Fluids are essential.
- Use cooling blanket for hyperthermia.
- Order gastric lavage.
- Use nitroprusside for hypertension.
- Use benzodiazepines for seizures.
- Admit to ICU and observe.

Mixed, Nonspecified Drug Abuse

Presentation: anything that does not fit into the above categories.

Management:
- The history is your best tool for unkown drug use, especially if you can interview friends/family/drugmates.
- Get toxicology screen.
- Treat symptoms.

ANSWER KEY

The answer to the sample question is C.

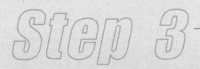

CHAPTER 8

Hematology

ANEMIA
  Pernicious anemia
  Iron-deficiency anemia
  Sickle cell anemia
  Thalassemias
  Anemia of chronic disease

GENERAL ISSUES
  Hemolysis
  Septicemia
  Agranulocytosis
  Polycythemia
  Polycythemia vera
  Enlarged spleen
  Ruptured spleen
  Viremia
  Transfusion reaction
  Coagulation disorders, hemorrhagic
  Coagulation disorders, thrombolic

Disseminated intravascular coagulation
Thrombocytopenia
Thrombocytopenic purpura/hemolytic
  uremic syndrome
Idiopathic thrombocytopenic purpura

MALIGNANCY
  Hodgkin's disease
  Multiple myeloma
  Waldenström's hypergammaglobulinemia
  Monoclonal gammopathies of undeter-
    mined significance
  Acute lymphocytic leukemia
  Acute myelogenous leukemia
  Chronic myelogenous leukemia
  Chronic lymphocytic leukemia
  Hairy cell leukemia
  Myelodysplastic syndrome
  Burkitt lymphoma

ANEMIA

Pernicious Anemia

Presentation: classic triad of symptoms: weakness, sore tongue, and paresthesias. Patient may be a vegetarian. Caused by impaired absorption of vitamin B12 due to lack of intrinsic factor or poor intake.

Management:

- Look for beefy red tongue.
- Ask about diarrhea and other GI symptoms.
- Do a thorough neurologic exam; look for gait problems and paresthesias.
- Get CBC with smear and look for classic macrocytic anemia with mean corpuscular volume (MCV) >200, oval macrocytosis, and 6-lobed polymorphonuclear neutrophils (PMNs).
- Do a Schilling test to see if absorption is the problem.
- Give cyanocobalamin injections if needed for treatment.
- Be alert to concurrent folic acid deficiency.
- Advise patient to eat meat/dairy products, which are rich in vitamin B12.

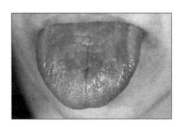

Figure 1. Pernicious anemia. (From Howard MR, Hamilton PJ: Haematology, An Illustrated Colour Text, 2e. Philadelphia, Churchill Livingstone, 2002, p 27.)

Iron-deficiency Anemia

Presentation: classically a woman or a man who has a slow GI bleed.

Management:

- Ask about pica: craving/eating dirt, ice, feces, talcum powder, or paint.
- Look for Plummer-Vinson esophageal web with dysphagia and glossitis.
- Look for spoon nails.
- Get menstrual history in women.
- Check heme status.
- Get CBC. MCV should be low in classic microcytic anemia (< 80).
- Get iron, ferritin, total iron-binding capacity (TIBC) levels.
- Supplement with ferrous sulfate.
- Consider colonoscopy to rule out colon cancer.

Sickle Cell Anemia

Presentation: African American with fatigue, joint pain, chest pain, priapism.

Management:

- Get CBC; hemoglobin will be decreased.
- Get peripheral smear to look for sickle cells.
- Look for casts in urine.
- Expect high bilirubin on CMP.
- Do hemoglobin electrophoresis for definitive diagnosis.
- Sickledex can detect trait as well as full-blown disease.
- Use pseudoephedrine to treat priapism chronically in men; untreated, it can lead to impotence.
- Consider exchange transfusions. Remove blood via central line and then give new blood.
- Put patient on chronic penicillin for infection.
- Give patient folic acid supplements.
- Be alert to acute chest syndrome.

Thalassemias

Presentation: Mediterranean heritage, beta thalassemia presents in infancy, alpha thalassemia presents at birth.

Management:

- Get CBC
- Get iron levels, which should be normal or even high.
- Get peripheral smear to look for anisocytosis, poikilocytosis, target cells, ovalocytes, basophilic stippling, polychromasia, macrocytes, nucleated red blood cells (RBCs).
- Treat with transfusions in combination with iron chelation to avoid iron overload.

Anemia of Chronic Disease

Presentation: patient with kidney failure is typical.

Management:

- Get CBC.
- Measure reticulocyte count for signs of activity.
- Transfuse as needed if hemoglobin is < 10, although chronic patients may adapt and accept lower hemoglobin than normal person. Definitely transfuse for comorbidities such as heart trouble.
- Give weekly erythropoietin (Epogen) injections.

GENERAL ISSUES

Hemolysis

Presentation:

Etiology	Presentation
Autoimmune	Lupus
Medication	Methyldopa, antibiotics.
Trauma	Artificial valves, soldiers marching. Look for bite cells.
G6PD deficiency	Person of African-American heritage after malaria or sulfa drugs. Look for Heinz bodies.
Spherocytosis	Person of northern European heritage with jaundice

Management:
- Get CBC.
- Look for high bilirubin on CMP.
- Transfuse if needed.
- Measure reticulocyte count, which should be high.
- Stop offending medications.
- Consider spleen removal in spherocytosis.

Septicemia

Presentation: fever, chills, tachycardia (rapid heart beat), and tachypnea (rapid respirations) are common acute symptoms of septicemia.

Management:
- Treat the cause, but until you know, start ceftriaxone and IV fluids.
- Get cultures of urine and blood and chest x-ray.

Agranulocytosis

Presentation: likely in sepsis with fever, chills, hypotension after starting new drug. Defined as absolute neutrophil count (ANC) < 100. ANC = total white blood cells (WBCs) × (segmented neutrophils + bands).

Management:
- Admit septic patients to ICU.
- Start fluids for hypotension.
- Start empirical antibiotics such as cefepime. Add vancomycin if fever persists after 48 hours.
- Look in mouth for sores. Give hydrogen peroxide rinse.
- Look for obvious skin lesions/infections.
- Institute neutopenic precautions: no fresh fruit or plants, aggressive hand-washing.
- Ask about propylthiouracil, chloramphenicol, sulfa drugs, clozapine—the classic players. Patient may also be undergoing chemotherapy.
- Get CBC with differential. Calculate the ANC (see under presentation).
- Order panculture of blood, sputum, urine.
- Get chest x-ray to look for pneumonia.
- Bone marrow biopsy gives the most information.
- Consider filgrastim (Neupogen) to stimulate production WBCs.

Polycythemia

Presentation: red cell mass > 36 ml/kg for men or > 32 ml/kg for women. Secondary polycythemia is seen with smoking, high altitude, and lung disease as adaptive change to hypoxia. Primary causes are usually myeloproliferative disorder; polycythemia vera is the most common primary cause. See below for management.

Polycythemia Vera

Presentation: pruritus after showers, gout, fatigue; more men than women are affected.

Management:

- Feel the spleen; it is likely to be big.
- Get CBC. In most cases, you will note high hemoglobin, high WBCs, high platelets.
- Erythropoietin levels are low.
- Hydroxyurea can be used to treat the disease.
- Phlebotomy is treatment of choice, however.

Enlarged Spleen

Presentation: can be caused by infections (including Epstein-Barr virus), malignancies (including lymphomas/ leukemias), and liver disorders such as cirrhosis (pressure back-up).

Management:

- Ask about left shoulder pain (referred).
- Get lab tests, including CBC with differential, peripheral smear, and lactate dehydrogenase (LDH) level to rule out hemolysis. These routine tests can also find sickle cell disease and thalassemias. Look for malaria on peripheral smear.
- Consider Monospot to rule out Epstein-Barr virus, mononucleosis.
- Get chest x-ray to look for tuberculosis.
- Get CT of spleen and include liver to look for liver disease.
- Treat the underlying disease.
- Advise patient to avoid rugby, ultimate fighting, wrestling, and other contact sports until spleen is of normal size.
- Call surgeon to remove spleen if severe anemia is developing as a result of splenic destruction.
- If elective spleen removal is going to be pursued, vaccinations for encapsulated organisms such as pneumococci (Pneumovax) are given ahead of time to help develop immunity before removal. Obviously in trauma there is no time for this precaution.
- Give antibiotics such as penicillin after spleen removal.
- Expect platelets to increase after removal, and be careful of deep venous thrombosis risk.

Ruptured Spleen

Presentation: can be caused by trauma following enlargement (classic cause is Epstein-Barr virus/mononculeosis) or motor vehicle accident or other trauma.

Management:

- Attend to ABCs, give fluids and blood.
- If spleen rupture is suspected, **go directly to the OR!** In situations of abdominal trauma and shock, this is the right answer. Delay for diagnostic tests is completely inappropriate.
- Otherwise diagnostic peritoneal lavage and CT of the abdomen are good choices to rule out a damaged spleen. Again, go to the OR for repair or removal of the spleen in this case.

SAMPLE CCS INPUT: Splenic Trauma

PE focused on cardiovascular system, lungs, abdomen

IV access

Blood pressure monitor

NSS 0.9%

CBC, CMP, LFTs, UA, coagulation studies, type and cross-match blood

PRBCs, transfusion (if hemodynamics are unstable)

Consult Surgery, General → POPUP: Enter reason: probable splenic rupture

Laparotomy, emergent (if rupture); otherwise continue with below:

Blood ethanol, urine drug screen

Chest x-rays (portable)

Kidney-ureter-bladder (KUB) study

Ultrasound or CT of abdomen STAT

Change location to ICU

Check vital signs every hour

Viremia

Presentation: presence of viruses in the bloodstream.

Management:

- Obviously important because viruses spread throughout body via the blood stream but also has relevance in measuring effectiveness of HIV therapies.
- Detectable viremia (over 50 copies) indicates active virus replication/therapy failure and risk for rebound.

Transfusion Reaction

Presentation: fever, chills, joint pain, back pain with ABO incompatibility, or simple antibodies to platelets/WBCs

Management:

- Minor febrile reactions are common and do not necessarily indicate ABO incompatibility. They can be avoided by premedicating with diphenhydramine (Benadryl) and acetaminophen (Tylenol).
- If the patient is anaphylactic, treat appropriately from the ABCs to intubation. Consider racemic epinephrine breathing treatment with wheezing/stridor. Consider epinephrine drip.
- Give diphenhydramine (Benadryl) for itching/rash. Also give an H1 blocker such as ranitidine (Pepcid) for even more antihistamine action.
- Give acetaminophen for fever/pain.
- Give prednisone to reduce immune response.
- Give IV fluids for hypotension and renal protection. Add furosemide (Lasix) and be more aggressive with fluids in hemolytic situations to flush kidneys and prevent renal failure.
- Monitor CBCs (look at platelets, RBCs) and CMPs (look at bilirubin and creatinine) for disseminated intravascular coagulation, anemia, and renal failure.

Coagulation Disorders, Hemorrhagic

Presentation: patient who bleeds excessively; von Willebrand disease, hemophilia.

Management:

- Get CBC. Make sure that patient is stable and has not lost excessive blood.
- Get prothrombin time (PT), partial thromboplastin time (PTT).

- Hemophilia A or B is suspected if only PTT is abnormal. 50% of males get the disease and 50% of females carry the trait as X-linked and recessive. Check factor 8 and factor 9 to confirm the diagnosis. Replace these factors as needed.
- von Willebrand disease should be suspected with high PT. Also expect a family history because inheritance is autosomal dominant. Treatment includes cryoprecipitate and factor 8.

Coagulation Disorders, Thrombolic

Presentation: frequent clots, deep vein thromboses (DVTs), pulmonary embolisms (PEs).

Management:
- Check antinuclear antibody for lupus. A rapid plasma reagin syphilis test will also be positive.
- Consider checking for antithrombin III, protein C, and protein S deficiencies as well as Leyden factor V mutation.
- Consider long-term anticoagulant use; life-long use of warfarin (Coumadin) may be required.

Disseminated Intravascular Coagulation (DIC)

Presentation: malignancy, sepsis, and septic abortion with amniotic fluid in the bloodstream are classic. Combination of hemorrhage and thrombosis consumes all of the factors/platelets in the blood while increasing fibrin.

Management:
- Get CBC. Expect platelets to decrease. Give packed red blood cells (PRBCs) if needed.
- Get D-dimer level; expect it to be elevated.
- Assess antithrombin III; expect it to be elevated.
- Get PT, PTT; expect both to be elevated.
- Assess fibrin degradation products (FDPs); expect increased levels.
- If you measure factors, expect to find decreased levels of factors V, VIII, X, and XIII as well as protein C.
- The standard answer in DIC is to correct underlying cause.
- If the underlying cause is unknown, consider giving fresh frozen plasma (FFP) to induce clotting.
- Consider giving platelets if the patient's condition is severe.
- Consider heparin for thrombosis.
- Antithrombin III is given when FFP fails.
- Aminocaproic acid is considered a last resort medication or is used with DIC in the context of promyelocytic leukemia.

Thrombocytopenia

Presentation: decreased platelets.

Management:
- Can be drug-induced; heparin is the most common cause.
- Autoimmune thrombocytopenia is classically lupus; check a Coombs' test.

Thrombotic Thrombocytopenic Purpura (TTP)/Hemolytic Uremic Syndrome (HUS)

Presentation: von Willebrand factors bind to platelets, causing hemolysis and thrombosis; the clinical picture much like DIC. The classic pentad of thrombocytopenia consists of fever, renal failure, neurologic deficit, mental status changes, and hemolytic anemia. HUS is likely in children with kidney involvement. HUS is usually preceded by GI infection with diarrhea. TTP is more likely in adults, especially in the context of pregnancy, cancer, HIV infection, or other infections.

Management:
- Get CBC; expect low platelets and low hemoglobin.
- Get CMP; expect blood urea nitrogen (BUN) to be elevated. Uremia can cause the mental status changes.

- Get a smear; look for schistocytes and burr cells as evidence of hemolysis.
- LDH is elevated due to hemolysis
- Get a D-dimer level; expect it to be normal, which helps rule out DIC.
- Urinalysis shows blood as well as casts.
- Admit patient and initiate plasma exchange/plasmapheresis. This is a very serious illness.
- Give steroids.
- Insert a Foley catheter, and treat renal failure with dialysis.
- Order splenectomy if the patient does not respond to plasmapheresis.
- Resist the temptation to give platelets (unlike DIC).

Idiopathic Thrombocytopenic Purpura (ITP)

Presentation: platelets destroyed in autoimmune process.

Management:

- Get CBC.
- Give IV immunoglobulin and steroids to arrest the process of platelet destruction.
- Give platelets if the count is extremely low. The standard of care is to intervene if platelets are under 20,000; you may give platelet transfusions below this level.
- ITP resolves in 80% of patients without intervention.
- Consider removing the spleen, depending on cause.

CCS SAMPLE INPUT 2004 TIMED BLOCK 1:

5-year-old with nosebleed and petechiae. Note history, giving history of preceding URI. The differential diagnosis should immediately include Henoch-Schönlein purpura (HSP), HUS, ITP, TTP. Vital signs appear stable.

1. Click on Interval Hx or PE button.
2. Check the Interval History, HEENT/Neck Exam. The child is still actively bleeding.
3. Click Write Orders or Review Chart.
4. On Order Sheet, click Order button. We need some immediate orders.
5. Apply pressure to nose. (Computer will automatically add phenylephrine for you!)
6. Click on Interval Hx or PE button.
7. Check the Interval History, HEENT/Neck Exam. You fixed him!
8. CBC, CMP, coagulation profile, urinalysis, antiplatelet antibodies (these lab tests give a look at patient's hemoglobin, kidney function).
9. If platelet count is low, get reticulocyte count.
10. While waiting on these lab results, do a real exam—a complete exam will run the clock.
11. Click Interval and Complete Exam. Complete exam is generally a good idea in routine office scenarios. Note the rectal exam for occult blood and petechiae on the skin.
12. Click Obtain Results or See Patient Later. Click With Next Available Result. Look at all these lab results! Note the platelet count and the blood in urine. Note that creatinine is normal. The mother is upset about the rash.
13. Move patient to ward. Platelet counts are very low, and the child needs some TLC. He may become hemodynamically unstable.
14. Continue to advance the clock. Note the antiplatelet antibody that finally pops up. Voilá—ITP.
15. Counsel patient to avoid aspirin (affects platelets).
16. Order CBC every 24 hours. Keep advancing the clock, and note that platelets are improving. Otherwise we would have to consult surgery and remove the spleen.
17. The case will end in 5 minutes and "real time" will pop up. Click OK.
18. Click on Interval Hx or PE button.
19. Enter your diagnosis: ITP

MALIGNANCY

Hodgkin's Disease

Presentation: 15- to 34-year-old patient with night sweats. From least aggressive to most aggressive form: lymphocyte-predominant, nodular sclerosis with mixed cellularity, lymphocyte depletion.

Management:

- CBC with manual differential.
- Biopsy of lymph node allows definitive diagnosis. Look for Reed-Steinberg ("owl's eye") cells.
- Order chest x-ray for staging.
- Order CT for staging.
- Initiate radiotherapy.
- Initiate chemotherapy with stem cell support (reimplant stem cells after chemotherapy).

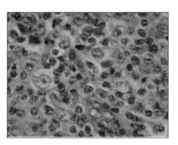

Figure 2. Reed-Sternberg cells in a lymph node biopsy. (From Howard MR, Hamilton PJ: Haematology, An Illustrated Colour Text, 2e. Philadelphia, Churchill Livingstone, 2002, p 58.)

Multiple Myeloma

Presentation: look for middle-aged person older than 40 years with back pain. Multiple myeloma affects plasma cells, proliferation of B cells. The current prognosis is survival for about 3 years.

Management:

- Order bone survey to look for classic osteolytic punched-out lesions.
- Get CBC to look for anemia.
- Check calcium on CMP.
- Get urine protein electrophoresis to look for Bence-Jones protein.
- Order plasma electrophoresis with immunoglobulin levels. Look for IgG and IgA spikes—usually IgG.
- Initiate chemotherapy.
- Initiate localized radiation.
- Be aware of impending fractures. Multiple myeloma can leave a person paralyzed.

Waldenström's Hypergammaglobulinemia

Presentation: older person presents with weakness and Raynaud's symptoms. It is similar to multiple myeloma but has an IgM spike and no excessive plasma cells.

Management:

- Cold agglutinins cause the Raynaud's symptoms.
- Get CBC with differential. The classic finding is "rouleaux" or "stacked-coin" appearance.
- Get CMP, LDH, and alkaline phosphastase.
- Get uric acid levels.
- Order serum protein electrophoresis followed by immunoelectrophoresis.
- Bone marrow biopsy is required for definitive diagnosis.
- Plasmapheresis may be needed emergently for hyperviscosity.
- Chemotherapy consists of chlorambucil and prednisone to treat the disease itself.
- Stable patients may not require any treatment at all.
- Splenectomy should be considered.

Monoclonal Gammopathies of Undetermined Significance

Management:

- Not treated but followed closely to watch for emergence of diseases such as multiple myeloma or Waldenström's hypergammaglobulinemia.

Acute Lymphocytic Leukemia (ALL)

Presentation: Look for child with fever, anemia, and pain. The prognosis depends on age and WBC count. Younger is better, and with regard to WBCs, the lower the better.

Management:

- Get CBC and look for neutropenia.
- Look for blasts on blood smear.
- Check DIC panel; DIC is common with this type of lymphoma. Check PT, fibrinogen, FDPs.
- Check uric acid level, which is elevated frequently in ALL.
- Bone marrow aspiration with biopsy is definitive method of diagnosis.
- Chemotherapy consists of hyper-CVAD.
- Replace blood with PRBCs if the patient is anemic.
- Treat infections with IV antibiotics such as cefepime and neuropenic precautions.
- Give colony-stimulating factor such as filgrastim (Neupogen) to replenish WBCs after chemotherapy.

Acute Myelogenous Leukemia (AML)

Presentation: age > 30 with fatigue, pancytopenia + Auer rods + DIC.

Management:

- Get CBC, and be sure to include absolute neutrophil count.
- Look for blasts and Auer rods on peripheral smear.
- Get DIC panel; DIC is common in M3 subtype of AML.
- Bone marrow biopsy with flow cytometry and cytogenetics is the most important study because the subtypes affect treatment.
- Initiate chemotherapy.
- Use neutropenic precautions and antibiotics.
- Replace packed red blood cells as needed.

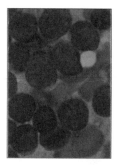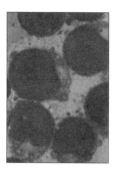

Figure 3. ALL (left). AML (right). (From Wood ME, Philips GK: Hematology/Oncology Secrets, 3e. Philadelphia, Hanley & Belfus, 2003, color plate section)

Chronic Myelogenous Leukemia (CML)

Presentation: patient aged around 40 with fatigue; usually found by accident on a routine CBC. The prognosis depends on stage. CML can be controlled if caught early; follows pattern of chronic → transitional → blast crisis phases.

Management:

- Feel for big spleen on exam.
- Get CBC with differential. Expect WBC count > 40,000; more eosinophils indicate progression toward a blast crisis.
- Get bone marrow biopsy, and look for Philadelphia chromosome on cytogenetics.
- Imatinib (Gleevec) has revolutionized the treatment of CML and led to complete remission in recent years.

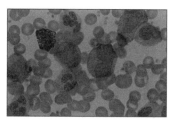

Figure 4. CML. (From Wood ME, Philips GK: Hematology/Oncology Secrets, 3e. Philadelphia, Hanley & Belfus, 2003, color plate section)

- Myelosuppressive chemotherapy is disappearing as treatment for CML.
- Interferons are still used.
- Leukapheresis to remove excess WBCs is also a possibility with very high WBC counts acutely (i.e., blast crisis).

Chronic Lymphocytic Leukemia (CLL)

Presentation: males over age 50; usually found on CBC on routine exam.

Management:

- Get CBC with differential. Look for plentiful lymphocytes and smudge cells.
- Peripheral blood flow cytometry is definitive method of diagnosis.
- Measure Ig levels and consider supplementation with IgM because patients are prone to infections.
- Bone marrow biopsy and lymph node biopsy are not always done with CLL.
- Chemotherapy is not always used unless CLL has progressed. In this case, prednisolone is used alone or with fludarabine or chlorambucil.
- Be alert to neutropenia, and admit for patient infections. Start IV antibiotics if needed.
- Give IgG to patients who keep getting infections.
- Give PRBCs, as needed, for anemia.

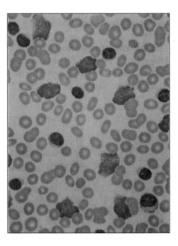

Figure 5. CLL. (From Howard MR, Hamilton PJ: Haematology, An Illustrated Colour Text, 2e. Philadelphia, Churchill Livingstone, 2002, p 46.)

Hairy Cell Leukemia

Presentation: adult men; look for easy bleeding and fatigue.

Management:

- Feel for big spleen on physical exam.
- Look for pancytopenia on CBC and hairlike projections on lymphocytes.
- Tartrate-resistant acid phosphatase staining makes the diagnosis.
- 2-Chlorodeoxyadenosine is the chemotherapy agent of choice.
- IV fluids and allopurinol are used to offset hyperuricemia during chemotherapy.
- Neutropenic precautions are advised.
- Give filgrastim (Neupogen) after chemotherapy to restore WBCs.

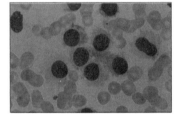

Figure 6. Hairy cell leukemia. (From Wood ME, Philips GK: Hematology/ Oncology Secrets, 3e. Philadelphia, Hanley & Belfus, 2003, color plate section)

Myelodysplastic Syndrome

Presentation: elderly patient with fatigue, bleeding, cytopenia on routine CBC.

Management:

- CBC with differential; look for anemia, thrombocytopenia, neutropenia, or any combination of the three.
- Order bone marrow biopsy and get cytogenetic studies.
- Give blood products as needed.
- Give erythropoietin (Epogen), as needed, to stimulate RBC production.
- Give filgrastim (Neupogen), as needed, to stimulate WBC production.
- For low platelets, treat bleeding with aminocaproic acid.
- Get bone marrow transplantation with suitable donor, especially in younger patients.

Burkitt Lymphoma

Presentation: occurs in children. Look for large growth mandible (African form) or large neck nodes. Non-African form affects the abdominal region. B-cell lymphoma is classically associated with EBV as well as AIDS. The disease is rapidly proliferative.

Management:
- Get CBC.
- Definitive diagnosis requires lymph node biopsy. Look for starry sky.
- Get chest x-ray for staging,
- Get CT for staging.
- Get PET for staging.
- Get a bone marrow biopsy.
- CHOP is classic chemotherapy regimen: cyclophosphamide, hydroxydaunomycin, vincristine (Oncovin), and prednisone.
- **Beware of tumor lysis!** Give generous IV fluids with bicarbonate and allopurinol.
- The outcome is good if the disease is caught early and treatment is aggressive.

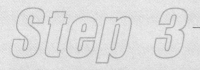

CHAPTER 9

Infectious Disease

GENERAL INFECTIONS
Local skin infection
Acute and chronic osteomyelitis
Streptococcal sore throat
Proteus infection
Pseudomonas infection
Streptococcal infection
Staphylococcal infection
Pneumococcal infection
Escherichia coli infection
Hemophilus influenzae infection
Dermatophytosis (tinea)
Candidiasis
Mycoses
Toxoplasmosis
Infections of the kidney
Acute cystitis/urinary tract infection
Infection of genitourinary tract during
    pregnancy
Other infections complicating pregnancy
Cellulitis and abscess
Enteric infections
Pertussis
West Nile virus/fever
Rickettsiosis
Malaria
Rocky Mountain spotted fever
Lyme disease
Trachoma
Diseases of conjunctiva
Cat-scratch disease

PEDIATRIC INFECTIOUS DISEASES
Impetigo
Chickenpox (varicella)
Measles (rubeola)

Rubella (German measles)
Roseola (exanthem subitum)
Erythema infectiosum (fifth disease)
Kawasaki syndrome (mucocutaneous
    lymph node syndrome)

SEXUALLY TRANSMITTED DISEASES AND HIV
AIDS, HIV infection, AIDS-related complex
Pneumocystosis (*Pneumocystis carinii*)
Kaposi's sarcoma
Syphilis
Gonococcal infections
Genital herpes
Trichomoniasis

VIRAL INFECTIONS
Hepatitis
Coxsackievirus
Adenovirus
Rhinovirus
Human papillomavirus
Retrovirus
Respiratory syncytial virus
Mumps
Herpangina
Infectious mononucleosis
Molluscum contagiosum
Foot and mouth disease-coxsackie
    viruses
Cytomegalic inclusion disease
Echovirus
Herpes zoster without complications
Herpes simplex
Herpes zoster with herpes simplex
Herpes simplex fever blisters

GENERAL INFECTIONS

Local Skin Infection

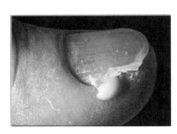

Figure 1. Acute paronychia. (From Habif, TP (ed): Clinical Dermatology, A Color Guide to Diagnosis and Therapy, 4th ed., St. Louis, Mosby, 2004, p 871.)

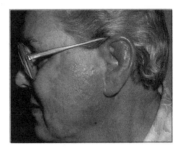

Figure 2. Erysipelas. (From Fitzpatrick, JE: Bacterial infections. In Fitzpatrick JE, Aeling JL (eds): Dermatology Secrets in Color, 2nd ed. Philadelphia, Hanley & Belfus, 2001, p 191.)

	Presentation	Management
Erysipelas	Skin cut followed by rash, blisters, lymph node enlargement (also called St Anthony's fire)	Penicillin Erythromycin
Erythrasma	Intertriginous zones with pink patches turning into brown scales	Penicillin Antibacterial soap
Paronychia	Infection around an ingrown nail; painful and full of pus	Warm water soaks Nail resection and drainage of abscess Cephalexin (Keflex)

Acute and Chronic Osteomyelitis

Presentation:

	Presentation
Acute	Sudden fever, fatigue, swelling, pain
Chronic	Patients with nonhealing open ulcers and draining sinus tracts

Management:
- Get CBC; expect left shift.
- C-reactive protein, alkaline phosphatase, and erythrocyte sedimentation rate (ESR) are elevated.
- X-ray usually shows soft tissue swelling; only much later does it show lytic lesions.
- Three-phase bone scan is initial test to evaluate for osteomyelitis.
- MRI is considered superior to other diagnostic tests.
- Nafcillin is combined with ceftriaxone to treat most cases of osteomyelitis.
- Sickle cell osteomyelitis is usually due to *Salmonella* sp.; use ciprofloxacin.
- *Pseudomonas* infections require cefepime instead of ceftriaxone.

Streptococcal Sore Throat

Presentation: red throat, fever, tender anterior cervical nodes, and no symptoms of viral upper respiratory infection.

Management:

- Inspect the posterior pharynx.
- Swab tonsils and get rapid streptococcal antigen test now.
- Send for cultures, which may take 1–2 days for incubation and interpretation.
- You have 7–9 days after symptoms appear to treat for prevention of rheumatic fever.
- Antibiotic decision time: during epidemic of streptococcal throat, do not wait for cultures. Definitely look for this judgment question on Step 3.
- Start oral penicillin VK for 10 days. Consider IM route for noncompliance: benzathine penicillin G.
- If the patient has an allergy to penicillin, use erythromycin, 250 mg 4 times/day.
- Do not give antibiotics if the cause is clearly not bacterial.
- Recurrent infections merit a cephalosporin.
- To rule out mononucleosis, you can get CBC with differential for atypical lymphocytes or order a Monospot. If you give amoxicillin to a patient with mononucleosis, there is a high likelihood that a rash will develop, and you have your diagnosis.
- Symptom relief with NSAIDs or anesthetic mouthwash, lozenges.

Proteus Infection

Presentation: symptoms of urinary tract infection may progress to back/flank pain.

Management:

- Is the patient septic? Adjust management accordingly with attention to ABCs.
- Get urinalysis. Expect high pH due to urease secretion.
- Trimethoprim/sulfamethoxazole (TMP/SMX) or levofloxacin (Levaquin) is an excellent choice due to high resistance to many antibiotics.
- Struvite renal calculi can develop with *Proteus* infection. Frequent fliers should get ultrasound or CT of kidneys to rule them out.
- Get surgical intervention for calculi.
- Prevent them by removing catheters as soon as possible and changing them frequently.

Pseudomonas Infection

Presentation	Infection	Treatment
Septic, MICU patient	Meningitis	Cefepime; add gentamicin
Septic, MICU patient	Pneumonia	Classic combination: ampicillin and gentamicin
Inpatient with catheter	Urinary tract infection	Levofloxacin (Levaquin) is a good choice
IV drug users	Bone infections	Give piperacillin/tazobactam (Zosyn)
IV drug users	Endocarditis	Give piperacillin/tazobactam (Zosyn)
Swimmers	Outer ear/ malignant otitis externa	Give ciprofloxacin ear drops for outer ear infection or ampicillin/gentamicin for malignant otitis externa
Contact lens (improperly cleaned)	Corneal erosions	Fluorescein stain with slit-lamp exam and gentamicin eye drops
Burn victims	Wound infections	Give piperacillin/tazobactam (Zosyn) with silver sulfadiazine cream topically

Management:

- Treat septic patient appropriately with ICU admission and concern for the ABCs.
- *Pseudomonas* has a distinctive "sweet" odor and green/blue color in skin infections.
- *Pseudomonas* is highly resistant to antibiotics, and two-drug combination is needed for nearly all serious infections.
- Simple infections can become disseminated systemic infections.
- Get CBC, chest x-ray, blood cultures, urinalysis for patients with suspected *Pseudomonas* infection.
- See table above for specific treatments.

Streptococcal Infection

Presentation	Infection	Treatment
Dark urine several weeks after streptococcal infection: throat/skin	Acute glomerulonephritis	Treat for renal failure, watch for electrolyte abnormalities
Hot, red skin	Cellulitis	Cephalexin
Fever and uterine pain after childbirth	Endometritis	Ampicillin
Crusty, honey-colored lesions	Impetigo	Cephalexin or dicloxacillin
Extreme pain after cut out of proportion to injury; may look like simple cellulitis	Necrotizing fasciitis	Surgical debridement and antibiotics
Fever, cough, infiltrate on chest x-ray	Pneumonia	Azithromycin
Mitral murmur after sore throat	Rheumatic fever	Penicillin, aspirin; steroids may need to treat congestive heart failure
Rash with sore throat	Scarlet fever	Penicillin
Hypotension, organ failure	Streptococcal toxic shock syndrome	Nafcillin, MICU/supportive care; find source

Staphylococcal Infection

Presentation	Infection	Treatment
IV drug user with murmur	Endocarditis	Vancomycin
Vomiting *and* diarrhea	Gastroenteritis	Fluids and supportive care
Pain in the breast	Mastitis	Continue breast feeding and ampicillin
Infection along ingrown nail	Paronychia	Augmentin and nail resection
Started as impetigo; now skin is peeling off	Scalded skin syndrome	Nafcillin or cephalexin
Hypotension, fever, rash (associated with tampons)	Toxic shock syndrome	Nafcillin, MICU/supportive care; find source

Pneumococcal Infection

Presentation	Infection	Treatment
Fever unknown origin	Bacteremia	Penicillin; consider vancomycin for sepsis
Stiff neck, lethargy, fever	Meningitis	Ceftriaxone + vancomycin if resistant
Child with bulging tympanic membrane and earache	Otitis media	Amoxicillin
Cough, weakness, chills, pain	Pneumonia	Azithromycin or ampicillin
Headache, sinus tenderness	Sinus infection	Amoxicillin

Escherichia coli Infection

Presentation	Infection	Treatment
Burning, urgency, flank pain	Urinary tract infection	TMP/SMX or levofloxacin (Levaquin)
Traveler's diarrhea	Gastroenteritis	TMP/SMX
Neonate fever and lethargy	Meningitis	Ceftriaxone
Urinary tract infection followed by shortness of breath	Pneumonia	Ceftriaxone or levofloxacin (Levaquin)
Fever, pain, jaundice	Cholangitis	Ultrasound and ceftriaxone + metronidazole (Flagyl)

Hemophilus influenzae Infection

Presentation	Infection	Treatment
Sore throat, drooling, shortness of breath	Epiglottitis	Intubate and then give ceftriaxone
Upper respiratory infection (URI), then stiff neck, fever	Meningitis	Ceftriaxone and dexamethasone
URI, then bulging tympanic membrane and earache	Otitis media	Amoxicillin
Cough, weakness, chills, pain with insidious onset, especially in smokers	Pneumonia	TMP/SMX or ceftriaxone + doxycycline
URI, then single joint pain	Septic arthritis	Ceftriaxone acutely; then oral penicillin

Dermatophytosis (Tinea)

Presentation: fungus on scalp, body, groin, feet. Patient complains of itching.

Management:

- Scrape the skin and apply potassium hydroxide (KOH).
- Look under a microscope.
- Illuminate with Woods lamp; not all will illuminate.
- Ketoconazole cream is applied.
- Also can give terbinafine orally. This is treatment of choice for nail infections.
- Treat secondary bacterial infections that frequently coexist with fungal infections because the skin is compromised.

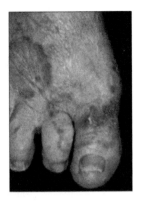

Figure 3. Tinea incognito. (From Habif, TP (ed): Clinical Dermatology, A Color Guide to Diagnosis and Therapy, 4th ed., St. Louis, Mosby, 2004, p 426.)

Candidiasis

Presentation: ranges from thrush (in mouth) or simple vaginal "yeast" infection to massive disseminated disease in the blood, which may present as fever and sepsis that do not respond to antibiotics.

Management:

- Assess risk factors in patient history, including antibiotic use, HIV/immunocompromised state, steroid use. Diabetes is a definite risk factor.
- Look at skin for cutaneous manifestations, especially in the groin area, under the breasts, and in the axilla.
- Look at the nails for signs of candidal infection. Scrape and do KOH prep.
- Look in the mouth for white plaques or simple redness at the corners of the mouth.

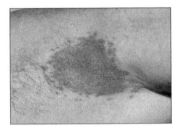

Figure 4. Cutaneous candidiasis. (From Keller, RA: Superficial fungal infections. In Fitzpatrick JE, Aeling JL (eds): Dermatology Secrets in Color, 2nd ed. Philadelphia, Hanley & Belfus, 2001, p 223.)

- Thrush in a young adult is AIDS until proved otherwise. Thrush is extremely rare in normal immune state.
- If you see the mouth lesions, be sure to ask about trouble with swallowing or reflux-type symptoms to rule out esophageal candidiasis. Do endoscopy of the upper GI tract.
- The respiratory tract can become colonized. If the patient has shortness of breath or respiratory distress, pursue a chest x-ray and then bronchoscopy.
- Do a pelvic exam; examine the vulva for redness and the vagina for white, curd-like discharge.
- Get cultures of sputum and urine to find yeast in these organ systems. Consider culturing blood for yeast as well.
- For candidal infection limited to mouth, use nystatin swish-and-swallow. Add oral fluconazole if the patient is immunocomprised or does not respond.
- Treat simple skin infections with topical antifungals.
- Treat nail infections with itraconazole.
- Treat vaginal infections with single dose of fluconazole.
- For systemic disease, IV fluconazole should be tried first; then consider amphotericin-B if the patient does not respond. Do not wait too long to start amphotericin-B, especially with a positive blood culture with yeast if you are not getting a response. Although toxic, "ampho-terrible" was formerly the initial drug of choice for disseminated canididal infection.
- Advise patient to eat live yogurt cultures to colonize the GI tract with beneficial bacteria. Some even use plain yogurt in the vagina to colonize with good bacteria in chronic infections, although this is considered a folk remedy.

Mycoses

Presentation: generally present only in immunocompromised conditions.

	Presentation
Blastomycosis	Southern United States; man who works outdoors and comes into contact with soil presents with "flu" and shortness of breath. Blasto = broad-based buds.
Histoplasmosis	Midwestern United States; associated with bird droppings/decaying leaves. Small, oval yeast cells that can be found in macrophages.
Coccidioidomycosis	Southwest United States; dust exposure.

Management:

- Get travel/exposure history.
- Get chest x-ray.
- Get a CT to follow up chest x-ray results.
- Can get serology for histoplasmosis.
- Can also get serology for coccidioidomycosis.
- Needle biopsy is the definitive diagnostic tool.
- Oral itraconazole is currently the initial treatment of choice, even for meningitis.
- Start amphotericin-B if itraconazole fails or if patient has disseminated illness.

Toxoplasmosis

Presentation: congenital infection with chorioretinitis or hydrocephalus; intracranial calcifications in an immunocompromised patient. Cats are the definitive hosts.

Management:

- Toxoplasmosis is usually asymptomatic and not treated.
- Look in patient's eyes for retinitis. Always treat retinitis if present.
- Pyrimethamine is the drug of choice. Give it with folic acid.
- Can get serum test for toxoplasmosis.
- Treat pregnant women who become infected; the risks of not treating it outweigh drug risks to fetus.
- Give dapsone with pyrimethamine to prevent toxoplasmosis in AIDS patients with low CD4 counts (< 200).

Infections of the Kidney

Presentation: symptoms of urinary tract infection (UTI) with flank pain, nausea, fever, chills.

Management:

- Ask about frequency and urgency of urination, dysuria, flank pain, nausea, fever, chills.
- Feel for tenderness at costovertebral angle over the kidneys.
- Get urinalysis with cultures and sensitivities. White casts suggest pyelonephritis.
- If the patient appears to have urosepsis:
  - Admit to ward.
  - Insert Foley catheter.
  - Start fluids.
  - Give IV antibiotics. Ceftriaxone and levofloxacin are good choices.

- If the patient is not septic and stable:
    □ Give one dose of ceftriaxone (IV/IM).
    □ Discharge with prescription for TMP/SMX.
- Schedule follow-up soon.

Acute Cystitis/Urinary Tract Infection

Presentation: UTIs presents with urinary frequency/urgency, burning, and suprapubic pain Common in women and rare in men.

Management:
- Ask about the above symptoms.
- Push on the suprapubic region to check for tenderness.
- Get a urinalysis. Look for nitrites, WBCs, or bacteria.
- In simple UTIs, urinalysis is often not done.
- Give TMP/SMX for 3 days, typically in females. Extend 7 days for male patients with catheters in place.
- Alternative drug choice is one of the fluoroquinolones.
- Phenazopyridine eliminates the burning symptoms. Counsel patients that it will make urine orange.
- Counsel women regarding hygiene: wipe from front to back after urination.
- Counsel regarding possible antibiotics after intercourse in women who have repeated infections.

Infection of Genitourinary Tract During Pregnancy

TORCH	Presentation
Toxoplasmosis	Retinitis, miscarriage
Other (syphilis, hepatitis B, coxsackie, EBV, varicella zoster virus, and human parvovirus)	Syphilis causes saber shins, teeth defects, sniffles, corneal and skin lesions
Rubella	Associated with cardiovascular defects, deafness, cataracts, small eyes. First-trimester disease is most serious.
Cytomegalovirus	Deafness is most common; small eyes, cerebral calcifications/retardation
Herpes virus	Skin lesions followed by dissemination

Other Infections Complicating Pregnancy

Presentation: green vaginal discharge (bacterial vaginosis).

Management:
- Bacterial vaginosis has been found to increase miscarriages. Women at risk for preterm labor should be treated.
- Treat with metronidazole (Flagyl).

Cellulitis and Abscess

Presentation: Cellulitis is usually due to trauma with a break in the skin followed by warmth, redness, and tenderness in the area around the injury. An abscess is a walled-off infection that is full of pus.

Management:

- Mild cases are treated with an outpatient regimen of cephalexin (Keflex).
- Serious cases should be admitted to the hospital; start IV antibiotics.
- Consult surgery for gangrenous/necrotic disease.
- Generally incision and drainage, followed by antibiotics, are required for an abscess. Cephalexin (Keflex) is a good choice, as is dicloxacillin.

Enteric Infections

Etiology	Presentation/Management
Botulism	Improperly canned foods. Causes descending paralysis. Support ventilation because patient may not be able to breathe, and give botulism antitoxin.
Cholera	Presents in underdeveloped countries as epidemic. Toxin binds in intestine and leads to osmotic diarrhea, which can be quite deadly. Requires rice-based oral rehydration therpy and IV fluids if available. Antibiotics are appropriate. Give TMP/SMX.
Escherichia coli O157:H7	Presents with bloody diarrhea after patient eats raw hamburger. Give TMP/SMX.
Enterotoxigenic *E. coli* (ETEC)	Traveler's diarrhea. Replace fluids and give TMP/SMX or tetracycline. These drugs also can be given as prophylaxis before trip.
Pseudomembranous colitis	Hospitalized patients on antibiotics. Clindamycin is classic cause, but all antibiotics cause overgrowth. Get cultures. Treat with metronidazole or vancomycin.
Salmonella infection	Raw eggs are the classic cause. Look for mucus and blood in stools. Replace fluids. If fever is present, use antibiotics. TMP/SMX or amoxicillin can be used.
Shigella infection	Children with nausea, fever, bloody stools. Replace fluids and give antibiotics such as TMP/SMX or ampicillin.
Staphylococcal food poisoning	Most common overall cause. Give fluids. No antibiotics.
Viral gastroenteritis	Rotavirus in children, Norwalk virus in cruise ship passengers. Most common cause of enteritis. Treat with rehydration. No antibiotics needed.

Pertussis

Presentation: pediatric patient with "whooping" sound to cough.

Management:

- Assess the patient's stability. Place patient in oxygen tent if needed.
- Consider steroids and breathing treatments with albuterol.
- Swab the throat and run culture for *Bordetella* sp. Culture is needed for definitive diagnosis.
- Erythromycin is appropriate and can shorten course of illness as well as decrease spread of the disease.
- Prevent it with appropriate immunization: diphtheria-tetanus-pertussis (DTP) vaccine at 2, 4, 6, 8, and 16 months and 5 years of age.
- The cough can persist long after the illness is treated.

West Nile Virus/Fever

Presentation: fever, chills, muscle weakness, headache, and photophobia. The West Nile virus (WNV) is mosquito-borne.

Management:

- Suspect in WNV endemic area—which is now most of the U.S. Dead birds and horses are monitored for the virus.
- The usual patient has transient symptoms that resolve.
- The elderly are prone to severe illness.
- Supportive care for the ABCs is all that can be done currently once illness strikes:
  - Intubation and ventilation may be needed.
  - IV fluids should be given.
- Get a lumbar puncture (LP), and send a sample of the cerebrospinal fluid (CSF) for viral cultures.
- You can get a serum test as well.
- CNS damage can be permanent.
- A new vaccine is being tested that appears to be effective.
- Advise patients to cover up and use repellant for most effective prophylaxis.

Sample question 1:

An 80-year-old woman woman is brought to the ED by her daughter. The daughter states that her mother is an avid gardener and bird watcher and spent a great deal of the summer in her rose garden. She is extremely lethargic and reports weakness in her hands. She reports that several days ago she began to feel "achy" and progressively more tired. On physical exam she has a temperature of 38°C and finds the bright lights in the ED to be extremely uncomfortable. A routine CMP shows serum sodium to be 127, and CBC shows mild leukocytosis. What is the most likely method of confirming the diagnosis for this illness?

A. CT of the head without contrast
B. Serum DNA polymerase chain reaction (PCR) or viral cultures of CSF
C. Bacterial culture of CSF
D. Blood in CSF
E. High opening pressure on LP

The correct answer is found at the end of the chapter.

Rickettsiosis

Presentation: fever 5 days after tick bite, rash, eschar.

Management:
- Give doxycycline. For many tick-borne illnesses doxycyline is a good choice even if you are not sure which exact organism is involved.
- Rickettsiosis usually resolves without problems.

Malaria

Presentation: traveler to endemic region of South America, Africa. Malaria is caused by protozoa, including *Plasmodium ovale*, *P. vivax*, *P. malariae*, *P. falciparum*. *P. falciparum* is the worst.

Management:
- Take a travel history.
- Ask about fever preceded by shaking chills and sweats. This is classic presentation of initial infection.

- Does the patient have fevers that spike throughout the day?
- Feel the spleen. An enlarged spleen is common in malaria.
- Get a CBC with peripheral smear.
- Check a special malarial Giemsa stain: thick-and-thin peripheral blood smear. If you suspect malaria, this is the test of choice. It will give you species information as well as simple positive or negative result for malaria.
- Repeat this special smear if the first one is negative.
- *P. falciparum* can affect CNS as well; consider CT with suspicious symptoms. Treat seizures if need be.
- Get chest x-ray for respiratory symptoms. Look for pulmonary edema.
- Check CMP for blood urea nitrogen, creatinine to see renal function is affected. Dark-colored urine is a sign of renal involvement.
- Look at serum glucose. Hypoglycemia is common in malaria.
- Check lactic acid level. The higher it is, the worse the prognosis.
- Give chloroquine to treat *P. falciparum*. Use with caution in patients with G6PD deficiency.
- Give primaquine to treat nonfalciparum malaria.
- Mefloquine or doxycycline can be used for prophylaxis prior to travel for *P. falciparum*. Ask patients where they are traveling to tailor therapy.

Rocky Mountain Spotted Fever

Presentation: patient gets bitten by tick (may not know it) and several weeks later presents with fever, myalgia, headache, petechiae.

Management:
- Ask about travel. Many patients do not recall a bite but have traveled to an area of exposure.
- A CBC may show decreased platelets.
- A CMP may show low sodium.
- Is the patient stable? If not, prepare for intubation, fluids.
- Give platelets and blood products as needed.
- Give tetracycline to treat infection. This should be your first choice.
- Give chloramphenicol to children to avoid staining the teeth.

Lyme Disease

Presentation: patient again presents after a tick bite that may have gone unnoticed. First stage: the "bulls-eye" rash; second stage: disseminated disease. Later (within 1 year) the third stage appears: autoimmune arthritic symptoms.

Management:
- Ask about travel to endemic areas. Lyme disease is caused by the spirochete *Borrelia burgdorferi*, which carried by the deer tick.
- Look for cranial nerve palsies on exam. They are quite common.
- Look for symptoms of meningitis on exam.
- Get a Lyme disease titer to confirm the diagnosis.
- Get an ECG if the patient presents with syncope. An intermittent/fluctuant AV block can occur with Lyme disease in the disseminated stage.
- Be prepared to pace the patient transcutaneously with AV block.
- Treat patient at first stage (rash) with doxycycline for 1 month. Consider treating any tick bite even without Lyme symptoms for simple prevention with a single dose of doxycycline.
- Any symptoms of the second stage (disseminated infection) merit doxycycline for 1 month.

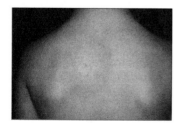

Figure 5. Lyme disease. (From Fitzpatrick, JE: Bacterial infections. In Fitzpatrick JE, Aeling JL (eds): Dermatology Secrets in Color, 2nd ed. Philadelphia, Hanley & Belfus, 2001, p 192.)

- At second stage with symptoms of meningitis, encephalitis, or AV block, give ceftriaxone IV for 1 month.
- Arthritic and fibromyalgia symptoms may persist chronically even with adequate treatment, which is the best argument for prophylactic doxycycline after any tick bite.

Trachoma

Presentation: entroprion (eyelashes that turn inward) caused by scarring of the tarsal plate results in corneal abrasion. It looks like conjunctivitis on initial exam. Trachoma is a disease of poverty and is caused by *Chlamydia trachomatis*. It is one of the leading causes of blindness in the world.

Management:
- Treat the whole family with azithromycin.
- Consider eyelid surgery to prevent blindness: incision of lid with rotation sutures.

Diseases of Conjunctiva

	Presentation	Management
Allergic	Itchy, watery, red swollen eyelids	Topical antihistamines; consider allergy testing
Viral	Adenovirus (pink eye)—endemic	Artificial tears, isolation, cool compresses, vasoconstrictors; give as prophylactic antibiotic the combination of polymyxin B and trimethoprim (Polytrim)
Viral	Herpes—usually accompanied with vesicular lesions on eyelids	Artificial tears, oral acyclovir, no steroids!
Bacterial	Purulent discharge immediately after birth	Topical erythromycin in neonate for presumed gonococcal infection. Erythromycin 0.5% ointment is also used for prophylaxis.
Bacterial	Conjunctivitis about 1 week after birth	Systemic erythyromycin for presumed chlamydial infection. Erythromycin 0.5% ointment is also used for prophylaxis.
Bacterial	"Beefy" red eye	Sodium sulfacetamide or gentamicin. Use IM/IV ceftriazone for inpatients.

Cat-scratch Disease

Presentation: Look for scratch on face/hand and swollen node in neck/arm. Caused by *Bartonella henselae*.

Management:
- Take history and ask about/be alert to possible cat/kitten exposures.
- Treat with oral erythromycin, TMP/SMX, or doxycycline.

> **Sample question 2:**
>
> An 11-year-old girl presents in your clinic with a single enlarged tender lymph node in her neck and a small red pustule on her cheek. What animal is most likely responsible?
>
> A. Tick
> B. Rabbit
> C. Cat
> D. Dog
> E. Chigger
>
> *The correct answer is found at the end of the chapter.*

PEDIATRIC INFECTIOUS DISEASES

Impetigo

Presentation: child with yellow-brown lesions on face. Impetigo can be caused by staphylococci or streptococci.

Management:

- Soap and water 3 times/day followed by antibiotic.
- Mupirocin ointment (Bactroban) is tried first.
- If it fails, add oral antiobiotic:
  - □ Streptococci respond best to erythromycin or penicillin.
  - □ Staphylococci respond best to dicloxacillin.

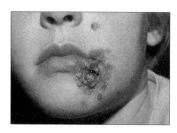

Figure 6. Streptococcal impetigo. (From Fitzpatrick, JE: Bacterial infections. In Fitzpatrick JE, Aeling JL (eds): Dermatology Secrets in Color, 2nd ed. Philadelphia, Hanley & Belfus, 2001, p 190.)

Chickenpox (Varicella)

Presentation: fever, malaise, and rash with vesicles that crust.

Management:

- In children not much needs to be done except treat secondary bacterial infections.
- Avoid aspirin in chickenpox because of association with Reye syndrome.
- Illness in adults is much more severe; acyclovir should be considered.
- Pneumonia is a complication in adults.
- Varicella-zoster immune globulin should be given to immunocompromised patients.
- Chickenpox is part of TORCH syndrome and can lead to serious birth defects. Mother should avoid exposure and ideally be vaccinated before pregnancy.
- The vaccine should be considered for adults who may be exposed for the first time.

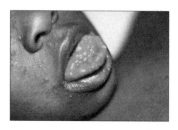

Figure 7. Chickenpox. (From English III, JC, Vaughan, TK: Fever with dermatitis. In Gates, RH (ed): Infectious Disease Secrets, 2nd ed. Philadelphia, Hanley & Belfus, 2003, p 367.)

Measles (Rubeola)

Presentation: cough, coryza, and conjunctivitis at first; then spots appear on the inside of mouth (Koplik spots). Later, the rash spreads from the head downward.

Management:

- Supportive care is the general rule.
- Give immunoglobulin to immunocompromised patients or pregnant women if they are living with a patient with measles.
- Watch for encephalitis, including subacute sclerosing panencephalitis.
- Treat superinfections, such as otitis media and pneumonia.
- Prevent measles with proper immunizations.

Rubella (German Measles)

Presentation: rubella presents much like rubeola, although it may be slightly milder.

Management:

- Treat symptoms with acetaminophen (Tylenol) and diphenhydramine (Benadryl).
- Pregnant women should avoid exposure due to TORCH syndrome.

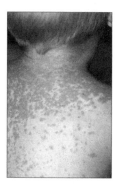

Figure 8. Rubeola. (From English III, JC, Vaughan, TK: Fever with dermatitis. In Gates, RH (ed): Infectious Disease Secrets, 2nd ed. Philadelphia, Hanley & Belfus, 2003, p 365.)

- Hearing loss is most common manifestation in newborn, along with visual problems and heart malformations.
- Get chest x-ray and echocardiogram in child that was exposed prior to birth.
- Surgical intervention may be needed.
- Immunize women before pregnancy.

Roseola (Exanthem Subitum)

Presentation: roseola prevents with fever and faint rose-pink rash. Considered the sixth exanthem of children and is caused by herpes simplex virus subtype 6.

Management:
- The general approach is to treat symptoms.
- Watch for very rare cases of encephalitis.

Erythema Infectiosum (Fifth Disease)

Presentation: classic slapped cheeks and reticulated lacy eruption on trunk. Caused by human papillomavirus B19.

Management:
- Generally nothing is done.
- Erythema infectiosum induces aplastic crisis in patients with sickle cell disease.
- Once rash appears, the patient is no longer infectious. The rash is a good prognostic indicator for recovery.
- Pregnant women should avoid exposure to fifth disease.

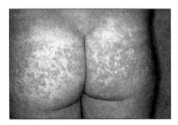

Figure 9. Erythema. (From English III, JC, Vaughan, TK: Fever with dermatitis. In Gates, RH (ed): Infectious Disease Secrets, 2nd ed. Philadelphia, Hanley & Belfus, 2003, p 366.)

Kawasaki Disease (Mucocutaneous Lymph Node Syndrome)

Presentation: fever over 5 days in duration, bulbar conjunctiva congestion, strawberry tongue, truncal rash (especially in perineal area), desquamation of skin, arthralgias. Ominous signs are tachycardia and gallops. Kawasaki disease is a systemic vasculitis with coronary aneurysms.

Management:
- Give aspirin.
- Give immunoglobulin.
- Get ECG to look for left ventricular hypertrophy, nonspecific ST changes.
- Get echocardiogram during illness and at follow-up after several weeks.
- With proper treatment (aspirin, IVIG) aneurysms usually regress.

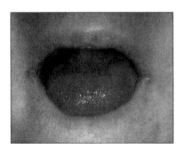

Figure 10. Kawasaki disease. Courtesy of Robert Hartman, M.D. (From Mancini AJ, Shani-Adir A: Other viral diseases. In Bolognia, JL, Jorizzo, JL, Rapini, RP (eds): Dermatology, St. Louis, Mosby, 2003, p 1267.)

SEXUALLY TRANSMITTED DISEASES AND HIV

AIDS, HIV infection, AIDS-related Complex (ARC)

Presentation: viral prodrome with fever, malaise that resolves spontaneously. More likely to present with opportunistic/associated infection such as thrush/yeast infections, Pneumocystis carinii pneumonia (PCP), herpes zoster, cryptococcal meningitis, tuberculosis, Kaposi's sarcoma. Step 3 presents these in the CCS as well as MCQ portions of the exam.

Management:

- Ask about sexual history, especially anal intercourse and unprotected sex, IV drug use/needlesticks, receipt of blood products.
- Get enzyme-linked immunosorbent assay (ELISA) for intial test, then Western blot for confirmation
- Get CD4 count, viral load.
- With AIDS you must diagnose and treat various opportunistic infections, and the CD4 count is an indicator of risk. A count below 200 is like a walking petri dish, especially for PCP, Mycobacterium avium complex (MAC).
- Examine the eyes for cytomegalovirus (CMV).
  - □ Treat CMV with ganciclovir.
  - □ CMV retinitis requires ophthalmology consultation.
- Look in the mouth for thrush, candidal infection.
  - □ Start clotrimazole for thrush.
  - □ Prescribe nystatin swish-and-swallow.
- Get chest x-ray to rule out PCP, MAC, and TB.
  - □ Give TMP/SMX (Bactrim) for PCP. Pentamidine is alternative choice. You may need to intubate patients with severe PCP. Steroids are also given in severe PCP.
  - □ TB can become disseminated in HIV/AIDS. Skin testing may give low yield due to anergy.
  - □ Give azithromycin for MAC.
- Get CT of head and lumbar puncture with cultures for suspected Cryptosporidium infection or toxoplasmosis. Look for ring-enhancing lesions on CT in toxoplasmosis. Look for positive India ink stain for Cryptosporidium infection.
  - □ Give amphotericin B to treat Cryptosporidium infection.
  - □ Give pyrimethamine to treat toxoplasmosis.
- Start treatment with zidovudine (AZT) in pregnant women because it greatly reduces vertical transmission.
- Commence antivirals, protease inhibitors when CD4 count is under 500.
  - □ Antiretrovirals: abacavir + lamivudine + zidovudine (triple drug regimen)
  - □ Protease inhibitors: lopinavir + ritonavir (double therapy)
- Patient should be followed every 6 months with CD4 count and viral load.

Pneumocystosis (Pneumocystis carinii)

Presentation: cough, fever, dyspnea on exertion in a patient with HIV (or at risk of HIV). Look for other symptoms, including thrush. Case scenario may indicate high-risk sex, needle use. This is generally an opportunistic infection when CD4 count is below 200.

Management:

- Is the patient stable? Give oxygen.
- Get arterial blood gases.
- Assess lactate dehydrogenase, and expect elevated level in PCP infections.
- Get chest x-ray to look for interstitial infiltrates.
- Get sputum samples.

- Pursue bronchoscopy with bronchoalveolar lavage and/or biopsy if sputum does not yield an answer.
- TMP/SMX is the antibiotic to give. Dapsone may be used if the patient is allergic to TMP/SMX.
- Pentamidine is second-line drug and can be inhaled and used for prophylaxis. Give adjuvant prednisone if PO_2 is <70.

Kaposi's Sarcoma

Presentation: red vascular nodules on skin that enlarge. Formerly seen in elderly men of Jewish/Mediterranen heritage; now seen mostly in gay men with AIDS and coinfection with human herpes virus 8.

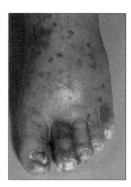

Management:

- Ascertain HIV or immunosuppressed status.
- Biopsy skin and lymph nodes to cinch the diagnosis with hemangioma-like histology.
- Kaposi's sarcoma can affect any organ system, and CT scans may be useful to stage disease.
- Chemotherapy with alkaloid agents should be instituted.
- Radiotherapy can be used for treatment in localized disease.
- Surgical excision is occasionally used as well.
- Make sure that you treat associated infections and underlying immunosuppression.

Figure 11. Kaposi's sarcoma. (From Bolognia, JL, Jorizzo, JL, Rapini, RP (eds): Dermatology, St. Louis, Mosby, 2003, p 2193.)

Syphilis (Treponema pallidum)

Presentation: first-stage symptom is a painless chancre on genitals; second stage has classic rash on palms/soles, general feeling of malaise, fever. The patient can relapse in and out of second stage. 33% of patients eventually develop tertiary syphilis.

Management:
- Take a sexual history.
- Use gloves because you can get syphilis from the lesions.
- Get rapid plasma reagin (RPR) and fluorescent treponemal antibody, absorbed (FTA-ABS) tests for confirmation. This is usually automatic, but Step 3 may make you order them sequentially.
- Positive darkfield microscopic examination is gold standard, but serologic tests are the mainstay of diagnosis.
- Treat with depot penicillin.
- Patient comes in weekly for Venereal Disease Research Laboratory (VDRL) test and another penicillin shot until negative.
- Watch for Jarisch-Herxheimer reaction in early treatment with chills, pain, intense malaise. Advise patient of this possibility.
- For neurosyphilis give IV penicillin.
- Give penicillin as your first choice in syphilis, but you can use doxycycline or erythromycin in penicillin-allergic patients. Rarely does Step 3 get this sophisticated.
- Tertiary syphilis can affect the CNS as well as the aorta. Also gummas can form in many organs of the body.
- Other STDs may occur in conjunction with syphilis, which makes one more likely to contract HIV because the tissues are compromised. Test for them as well.

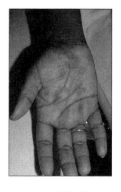

Figure 12. Secondary syphilis. (From Fitzpatrick, JE: Syphilis. In Fitzpatrick JE, Aeling JL (eds): Dermatology Secrets in Color, 2nd ed. Philadelphia, Hanley & Belfus, 2001, p 197.)

Gonococcal Infections

Presentation:

	Presentation
Males	Urethritis, prostatitis or epididymitis.
Females	Cervicitis, pelvic infection.
Either sex	Pain with urination and a discharge. Depending on site of infection, patients with alternative sexual practices may also have sore throat or rectal pain.

Management:
- Obtain a sexual history.
- Do a pelvic exam and look for "chandelier sign" when moving the cervix.
- Swab discharge from throat, urethra, cervix, or anus and send specimen for Gram stain. Use Thayer-Martin medium, which incubates soon.
- Rule out pregnancy in women.
- Treat gonorrhea with "butt and gut":
  □ "Butt" is ceftriaxone IM in the buttocks. You can also use oral ciprofloxacin instead of IM ceftriaxone if patient will be compliant.
  □ "Gut" is doxycycline by mouth. This is to treat chlamydial infection, which coexists in 50% of gonococcal infections. You can also use azithromycin.
- Treat sexual partners.
- Consider testing for other STDs.
- Counsel patient about safe sex (i.e., condoms/abstinence). Input the order on the CCS Step 3 for easy points.
- Untreated gonorrhea can lead to scarring/infertility in the female.

Genital Herpes

Presentation: painful, red vesicles that ulcerate. Herpes simplex virus (HSV) 1—lips; HSV2—genitals. However, oral sex can switch typical sites of infection.

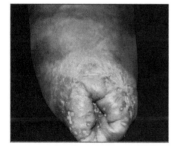

Management:
- Women with active genital herpes infection should not deliver vaginally.
- Eczema predisposes to eczema herpeticum, which can become disseminated easily. Give IV acyclovir as soon as possible to treat disseminated HSV.
- Sticking your finger in a lesion can lead to herpes whitlow infection (localized).
- A Tzanck smear may be useful for a quick diagnosis of herpes virus but is not specific.
- Culture active vesicles to get subtype of virus.
- Serum tests are available to detect latent illness.
- Valacyclovir and foscarnet can be given to shorten outbreaks and as prophylaxis.
- Recommend barrier contraceptives to avoid transmission to partners.

Figure 13. Primary genital herpes. (From Stalkup JR, et al: Human herpesviruses. In Bolognia, JL, Jorizzo, JL, Rapini, RP (eds): Dermatology, St. Louis, Mosby, 2003, p 1237.)

Trichomoniasis

Presentation: smelly, itchy, frothy green discharge in women. Men may have pain with urination.

Management:
- Do a pelvic exam and swab the vagina.
- Add KOH to the discharge. A fishy odor will fill the clinic if trichomoniasis is present.
- Do a wet mount. Put a slide under the microscope and look for pear-shaped protozoa.
- Treat with metronidazole.
- Screen for other STDs.

VIRAL INFECTIONS

Hepatitis

Presentation: ranges from jaundice, dark urine, clay stools to fulminant liver failure.

Type	Route of Infection	Prognosis	Treatment	Vaccine Available?
A	Fecal/oral (i.e., food)	Good	IVIG acute	Yes
B	Blood or sex	Can become chronic	IVIG acute Interferon alpha-2b for chronic infection	Yes
C	Blood or sex	Can become chronic carrier and develop cirrhosis or carcinoma	Interferon alpha-2b for chronic infection	No
D	Blood or sex (requires prior infection with hepatitis B)			No, but there is vaccine for hepatitis B
E	Fecal/oral (i.e., food)	Can kill pregnant women		No

Management:
- Get hepatitis panel.
- Get liver enzymes.
- Measure cholesterol, international normalized ratio (INR) and prothrombin time (PT), and ammonia if you are concerned about liver deterioration.
- Recheck panel. Hepatitis B surface antibody indicates immunity and is a good sign.
- Advise patient to avoid alcohol, acetaminophen (Tylenol), and other hepatotoxic medications.
- Advise high protein diet to enhance recovery.

Coxsackievirus

Disease	Presentation	Virus Subtype
Meningitis/encephalitis	Stiff neck, fever, lethargy	B
Myocarditis	Heart failure	B
Hand, foot, and mouth disease	Painful red oral blisters, palms, soles	A
Herpangina	Red blisters/ulcers on throat/tonsils	A
Pleurodynia	Spasms in muscles of the chest, associated with testicular pain	B
Conjunctivitis	Eye pain, red/watery eyes, photophobia	

Management:
- Supportive care is the general approach.
- Keep pregnant women away for exposure; coxsackievirus can cause abortion.

Adenovirus

	Presentation
Respiratory	Range from fever, runny nose, sore throat to pneumonia
Conjunctivitis	Large groups may be infected at a time, very contagious. Starts with one red eye then spread to both.
GI	Diarrhea in infants

Management:
- Supportive care is all that can be done.
- Treat bacterial superinfection.
- Do not miss another treatable infectious agent; be sure to culture and treat other infections.

Rhinovirus

Presentation: common cold.

Management:
- Rest
- Fluids
- Tell patient to wash hands frequently to avoid spread.
- Decongestants
- Ibuprofen for fever

Human Papillomavirus (HPV)

	Presentation	Management
Common warts	Commonly found on hands. Rough papules with thrombosed capillaries; can be spread	Salicylic acid or trichloroacetic acid, cryotherapy
Condylomata acuminata	Genital warts; cauliflower-like lesions	Podophyllin, cryotherapy
Cervical disease	Abnormal Pap smear	LEEP, laser, conization

LEEP = loop electrosurgical excision procedure.

Retrovirus

Presentation: person from Japan or Caribbean presents in similar fashion to HIV infection. Genome consists of RNA, not DNA, and uses reverse transcriptase to copy information backward. HIV is most important example (see section on HIV/AIDS). Human T-cell lymphotropic virus (HTLV) deserves special mention at this time.

Management:
- CBC may show marked leukocytosis.
- HTLV serology can confirm the diagnosis.
- Treat the same opportunistic infections as with HIV infection.
- Chemotherapy can induce remission in some cases.
- Anti-AIDS medications (antiretrovirals) are also used.
- Advise women not to breast-feed because HTLV is spread through milk.
- Also spread via IV needles, sex.

Respiratory Syncytial Virus

Presentation: child with simple cold that progresses to cough, wheezing/rales, fever.

Management:
- Supportive care is generally the main approach.
- Get arterial blood gas analysis if clinically indicated.
- Chest x-ray usually shows only hyperinflated lungs with increased interstitial markings.
- Admission with oxygen tent, ventilator, and IV fluids can be indicated in some situations.
- Ribavirin can be given in severe disease.

Mumps

Presentation: malaise, fever/chills, and sore throat followed by parotitis and swollen testes/ovaries. Usually caused by paramyxovirus.

Management:
- Labs test generally not done, but expect amylase to be elevated as well as leukocytes on CBC.
- Infertility can result from mumps.
- Hearing loss can also result.
- Meningitis/encephalitis can occur.
- Supportive care is generally the main approach.
- Apply icepack to testicles and recommend athletic supporter.
- Prevent mumps with proper vaccination.

Herpangina

Presentation: fever, malaise, sore throat, anorexia, oropharyngeal exanthem. Caused by coxsackievirus A.

Management:

- Herpangina is a clinical diagnosis, but you can swab the throat and culture the virus.
- Supportive care is the general approach.

Infectious Mononucleosis

Presentation: fatigue, swollen lymph nodes, sore throat; caused by Epstein-Barr virus (EBV).

Management:

- Look in the patient's mouth; note enlarged tonsils.
- Feel the spleen; it may be enlarged.
- Get CBC, and expect leukocytosis, which should be monitored for resolution over several weeks.
- Get a Monospot test to confirm the diagnosis.
- If you give amoxicillin thinking that the problem is streptococcal infection, do not be surprised by a rash that breaks out in 80% of patients with EBV virus.
- If spleen is large, advise patients to avoid contact sports and trauma.
- Chronic fatigue syndrome is rare and may follow EBV infection.

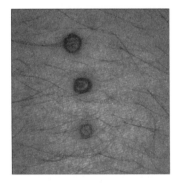

Molluscum Contagiosum

Presentation: small, flesh-colored, dome-shaped growths with dent in center. Caused by virus.

Management:

- Infection can be spread in pools and by fomites such as towels and sex.
- Atopic dermatitis and HIV are risk factors for extensive spreading of disease.
- Shaving can spread the virus.
- Treatment may involve cryotherapy (as with warts).
- Alternatively, trichloroacetic acid can also be applied in office.
- Tretinoin cream can be used on outpatient basis.
- Advise patients about risk of infecting others.

Figure 14. Molluscum contagiosum. (From Mancini AJ, Shani-Adir A: Other viral diseases. In Bolognia, JL, Jorizzo, JL, Rapini, RP (eds): Dermatology, St. Louis, Mosby, 2003, p 1266.)

Foot and Mouth Disease (Coxsackieviruses)

Presentation: viral prodrome followed first by sore mouth, then by lesions on hands and soles of feet.

Management:

- Generally no lab tests are needed.
- Diphenhydramine (Benadryl) and sucralfate swish-and-spit is used for mouth sores.
- Counsel patient about washing hands to avoid infecting others.

Cytomegalic Inclusion Disease

Presentation: fever, hepatitis, pneumonitis, retinitis, and/or a mononucleosis-like illness.

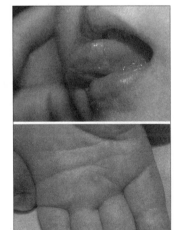

Figure 15. Hand-foot-and-mouth disease. (From Brice, SL: Bullous viral eruptions. In Fitzpatrick JE, Aeling JL (eds): Dermatology Secrets in Color, 2nd ed. Philadelphia, Hanley & Belfus, 2001, p 180.)

Management:

- Cytomegalovirus (CMV) is exchanged through body fluids, such as blood, urine, saliva, breast milk, semen, and cervical secretions.
- In immunocompromised individuals, particularly those with AIDS, CMV infection can cause encephalitis.
- CMV is a major concern in organ transplants.
- CMV retinitis occurs in 50% of HIV-infected patients.
- CMV is part of TORCH and can lead to congenital deafness and small eyes.
- Get viral cultures. Results take many weeks.
- Get CT of head in suspected congenital CMV infection. This is used to look for the cerebral calcifications that may appear.
- Ganciclovir is mainstay of CMV treatments.
- IVIG also may be given.
- Advise pregnant women to stay away from situations in which CMV can be contracted.

Echovirus

Presentation: an amazing number of presentations; see table below.

Presentation	Management
Aseptic encephalitis/meningitis	Supportive
Pericarditis/myocarditis	IVIG; steroids are controversial
Common cold	Supportive
Conjunctivitis	Supportive
Diarrhea in infants	Rehydration, supportive
Acute febrile respiratory illnesses	Supportive

Management:

- It is obvious that echovirus can imitate various other illnesses that are treatable. Do not miss them!
- You can get serum PCR for echovirus, but this test takes a long time.
- Antibiotics given empirically for meningitis are certainly not out of the question while awaiting lab results.
- Supportive care is the main approach for most manifestations, but IVIG can be given.

Herpes Zoster Virus without Complications

Presentation: infections begin as pain; then herpetiform vesicles appear in a dermatome distribution. Varicella-zoster (chickenpox) virus hides in ganglions and emerges at later date.

Management:

- Make sure that the patient is not immunosuppressed. Herpes zoster in a young or middle-aged person can herald HIV (like thrush).
- Make sure that the eye is not involved; herpes zoster ophthalmicus can lead to blindness.

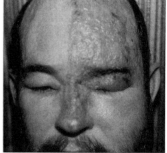

Figure 16. Herpes zoster. (From Brice, SL: Bullous viral eruptions. In Fitzpatrick JE, Aeling JL (eds): Dermatology Secrets in Color, 2nd ed. Philadelphia, Hanley & Belfus, 2001, p 178.)

- Treat the extreme pain with topical capsaicin (hot pepper extract), tricyclic antidepressants.
- Give acyclovir
- Give HZV immunoglobulin to immunocompromised patients.
- Steroids can also relieve some of the pain.

Herpes Simplex Virus (HSV)

Presentation: Painful, red vesicles that later ulcerate. Generally HSV1 infects lips, whereas HSV2 infects genitals. Oral sex can switch this pattern, however. (See Genital Herpes.)

Herpes Zoster with Herpes Simplex

Presentation: coinfection can lead to dissemination and usually presents in immunocompromised patient. One case has been documented in a patient undergoing chemotherapy with thalidomide for multiple myeloma.

Management:
- Aggressive treatment with IV acyclovir is warranted.

Herpes Simplex Fever Blisters

Presentation: vesicles on face/lips.

Management:
- Herpes simplex fever blisters are contagious.
- They reappear in the same place, generally under times of stress.
- They can be spread to genitals; oral sex should be avoided during active outbreak.
- Shaving can spread them in a wider distribution.
- Acyclovir can shorten course.

Correct answers to the sample questions:

Sample question 1: B. The diagnosis is West Nile virus encephalitis.

Sample question 2: C.

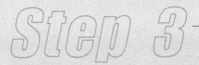

CHAPTER 10

Medical Law and Ethics

Informed consent
Patient autonomy
Treatment of minors with/without notification of parent
Guidelines for confidentiality of medical records
Opportunities for cost containment
Guidelines for physician-patient relationship
Assessment of quality-of-life decisions
Priorities in decisions to allocate transplant organs and/or other scarce resources
Use of unorthodox/experimental or folk/alternative therapies
Physician error vs. negligence
Good Samaritan laws
Guidelines for reporting findings to proper authorities
Degree of disclosure to terminally ill patients
Definitions of competence and sanity
Guidelines for commitment
Recognition of impaired physician
Appropriate prescription practices
Definition of and legal issues regarding brain death

Informed Consent

- Get signature from patient.
- Consent must contain the following elements:
  - Diagnosis
  - Nature of proposed treatment
  - Name of the procedure without abbreviations
  - Description in layman's terms
  - Risks associated with that treatment
  - Alternatives/associated risks
  - Risk of doing nothing

Patient Autonomy

- Recognize that the patient has a right to refuse treatment or testing.
- You must respect "self-governance."
- Autonomy works hand in hand with informed consent.

Treatment of Minors with/without Notification of Parent

- Urgent/emergent condition care should *never* be delayed because of problems with obtaining consent.
- Get consent from parents whenever possible.
- Emancipated minors need no consent; they are married, in the armed forces, financially independent, living on their own.
- Minors need no parental consent when pregnant, for treatment of STD, for abortions, or for drug/alcohol treatment.
- Any adult standing in *loco parentis*, whether serving formally or not, may give consent for minor charge in case of emergency. An example is an adult babysitter who takes the minor to the ED.
- Any guardian can give consent for his/her ward.
- During the absence of a parent any adult can give consent for a minor brother or sister.
- During the absence of a parent any grandparent can give consent for a minor grandchild.

Guidelines for Confidentiality of Medical Records

- Release information to third parties only with patient consent.
- Suspected child abuse **must** be reported.
- Patient statement that he or she is going to harm another **must** be reported.
- Certain diseases **must** be reported.

Opportunities for Cost Containment

- Do not order unneeded tests.
- Give a treatment time to work before trying a more expensive option.
- Convert IV medications to oral form as soon as possible.
- Move to lower acuity settings as soon as possible (i.e., from ICU to ward).
- Use outpatient services as much as possible.

Guidelines for Physician-Patient Relationship

- No sex/dating with current or former patients.
- No inappropriate touching during exam; no voyeurism or inappropriate comments during exam.
- Physicians cannot proselytize patient, but no one can require physcians to do something against their personal ethics (e.g., perform abortion).
- Maintain confidentiality.
- Maintain the bond of trust between patient and physician.

Assessment of Quality-of-life Decisions

- This is a subjective, nonmedical assessment of patients' satisfaction with their present circumstances.
- Honor patients wishes with the following caveats: Be certain that a patient is not suicidal before withholding care and determine whether the patient is clinically depressed. Depression must be treated before letting a patient die.

Priorities in Decisions to Allocate Transplant Organs and/or Other Scarce Resources

- Blood and tissue typing
- Medical urgency
- Time on the waiting list
- Geographical location
- Patient compliance/lifestyle is a big issue. If a liver transplant is likely to fail because the patient is alcoholic, he/she will be passed over for transplant.

Use of Unorthodox/Experimental or Folk/Alternative Therapies

- Folk therapy is a lay person's use of household and traditional remedies. A board classic is "coining" or "cupping," in which certain Asian cultures rub coins/place cups on the back of a child to drive out sickness. Bruises can appear to be child abuse.
- Alternative therapies include but are not limited to folk medicine, ayurveda/yoga, massage therapy, aromatherapy, mind/body interventions, diet/nutrition/herbals, manual healing/chiropractic, energy healing, chelation, ozone, DHEA, colloidal silver, asparagus extract, acupuncture, homeopathy, naturopathy.
- Ask patients *specifically* about their use of alternative therapies.
- Advise patients that little evidence confirms the safety/efficacy of alternative therapies in general. Many of the studies are poorly designed.
- The following "alternative" therapies have shown some promise:
  - St. John's wort for depression
  - Garlic to reduce cholesterol
  - Ginkgo for dementia and claudication.
  - Saw palmetto for benign prostatic hypertrophy
  - Intercessory prayer has been associated with improved outcomes. Religious commitment and prayer have been positively correlated with physical health in general.

Physician Error vs. Negligence

- Physician errors are failed processes that may/may not have caused adverse outcomes. An example is amputating the wrong leg.
- Negligence is the failure to exercise the care that would be used by a reasonably prudent physician in the same situation. An example is not getting an ECG in a patient with chest pain.

Good Samaritan Laws

- A person who renders emergency care at or near the scene of or during an emergency, gratuitously and in good faith, is not liable for any civil damages or penalties as a result of any act or omission by the person rendering the emergency care unless the person is grossly negligent or caused the emergency.

Guidelines for Reporting Findings to Proper Authorities

- Report child abuse and elder abuse.
- Report dangers to others, including threats as well as impaired drivers (e.g., poor vision, seizures).
- Certain diseases are reportable.

Degree of Disclosure to Terminally Ill Patients

- Ascertain what the patient knows.
- What does he/she want to know? Would he/she rather you talked with someone else?
- Family may not want the patient to be told. If the patient gives informed consent not to be told, it is acceptable to withhold information.
- Parents may not want a child to be told. In this case an ethics consultation may be warranted.

Definitions of Competence and Sanity

- A competent person understands the nature and seriousness of the medical condition, the purpose of the recommended medical treatment, and the risks and benefits of consenting to or refusing the recommended treatment. A competent adult is able to answer questions about his or her condition or treatment and demonstrates a rational thought process.
- Sanity is soundness of mind, emotions, and behavior—a sound degree of mental health.

Guidelines for Commitment

- *One Flew Over the Cuckoo's Nest* is a thing of the past.
- Patients who pose danger to self or others can be hospitalized against their will.
- But after about 72 hours a review is mandated; otherwise patients can leave if they wish.
- Continually review need for commitment.

Recognition of Impaired Physician

- An impaired physician is defined as "one who is unable to practice medicine with reasonable skill or safety to patients because of mental illness or deficiency, physical illness, including but not limited to deterioration through the aging process or loss of motor skills and/or excessive use or abuse of drugs including alcohol."
- Report first to in-house impaired physician office, if available; go to chief of staff if not available.
- If the physician has no privileges at a hospital, then report him/her to impaired physician program.
- State Medical Board is the next step if other options are not available.

Appropriate Prescription Practices

Guidelines vary from state to state but generally the following apply:

- Doctor-patient relationship is required, with visit every 6 months or so.
- You need to do history and physical before giving medications.
- Dispensing of controlled substances without a prescription (i.e., samples) is illegal in some states.
- Physicians may not self-prescribe schedule II, III, or IV controlled substances.
- Schedule II substances should not be prescribed to immediate family members except in emergency.
- Schedule III-IV drugs should be prescribed to family members only when history and physical exam and other elements of a doctor-patient relationship are present.

Definition of and Legal Issues Regarding Brain Death

- Brain death is defined as irreversible cessation of all brain function, including brainstem.
- You must exclude other causes before declaring brain death: metabolic derangement, intoxication, shock, hypothermia. Always warm the patient and exclude any possibility of recovery.
- Ensure that brainstem function is absent on exam: pupils fixed and dilated (penlight), corneal reflex (Q-Tip), oculocephalic/oculovestibular reflex ("doll's eyes" turn with head from side to side), gag reflex, apnea.
- Anoxic brain injury requires 24 hours' observation. Confirmatory test such as EEG can shorten observation.
- Alternatively, check cerebral blood flow with intracranial 4-vessel cerebral angiography.
- For all practical purposes, the patient who meets these criteria is dead, and you can harvest organs (with consent).

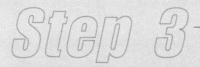

CHAPTER 11

Men's Health

Malignant neoplasm of male breast
Malignant neoplasm of prostate
Malignant neoplasm of male reproductive system
Disorders of prostate
Torsion of testes
Hydroceles/spermatoceles

Varicoceles
Inquinal hernias
Orchitis/epididymitis
Male infertility
Other disorders of male genitalia

Malignant Neoplasm of Male Breast

Presentation: mass in nipple area (different from women, in whom the classic presentation is an upper-outer mass).

Management:

- Look in history for risk factors such as Klinefelter syndrome or other hyperestrogenic state and positive family history.
- Breast cancer is rare in men (1% of cases), but tumors much more likely to be malignant.
- Mammogram may show calcifications.
- Proceed with fine-needle aspiration for diagnosis. Pick this answer if given the choice.
- Grade the disease; look for metastases to bone.
- Treatment includes surgery (mastectomy with lymph node removal), radiation, and chemotherapy (including tamoxifen).

Malignant Neoplasm of Prostate

Presentation: found in older men on routine digital rectal exam (DRE).

Management:

- Glove up and insert a finger in the anus for the DRE. A firm, hard/rocky, asymmetrical prostate definitely should cause concern.
- Get a prostate-specific antigen (PSA) level and correlate with age, since PSA rises with age as the prostate enlarges.
- Look for **low** level of free PSA in the malignant prostate.
- A sudden rise in PSA, even within the age-expected range, is also concerning.
- Get a biopsy with use of transrectal ultrasound.
- CT abdomen and pelvis for finding mets
- Consider bone scan for finding metastases.
- If the patient is old and sickly, consider watchful waiting without intervention.
- Radical prostatectomy is the most common treatment.

- External radiation therapy or brachytherapy/implants may be used.
- Antiandrogens are implanted commonly.
- Treat impotence, which frequently occurs after surgery.

Malignant Neoplasm of Male Reproductive System

	Presentation
Prostate adenocarcinoma	Discussed above
Adenomatoid tumor	Typically appears in men in their 30s. Basically a benign mesothelioma; often starts in the epididymis and is surgically removed.
Testicular tumor	Appears in young white men in their 20s and 30s.

Presentation: hard, painless, swollen testicle (classic presentation).

Management:
- Assess levels of human chorionic gonadotropin, alpha-fetoprotein (AFP), and lactate dehydrogenase.
- AFP elevation indicates seminoma.
- Get ultrasound of scrotum.
- Order a chest x-ray to detect metastases.
- Order CT of the abdomen and pelvis to detect metastases.
- Orchiectomy (removal of the testicle) is common treatment.
- Follow up with chemotherapy. Usually the regimen is platinum-based; a classic example is bleomycin, etoposide, and platinum.
- Watch for recurrence.

Disorders of the Prostate

	Presentation	Management
Prostatitis	Chills, obstructive symptoms. Usually bacterial in young men.	Treat like epididymitis below.
Cancer	See above	See above
Benign prostatic hypertrophy	Men over 50 who get up and go to bathroom many times during the night, with poor stream; can lead to urinary tract infections.	Treat with finasteride to shrink prostate hormonally or alpha blocker such as terazosin to relax prostate. Transurethral resection of the prostate (TURP) is surgical procedure of choice when medications fail. Saw palmetto may help in a manner similar to finasteride to shrink prostate.

Torsion of Testes

Presentation: young men with **severe** pain.

Management:
- Testicular torsion is a urologic emergency! Surgery is needed.
- Lift the scrotom and rotate testicle outward and laterally (when viewing from patients feet) to attempt manual detorsion.

Hydroceles/Spermatoceles

Presentation: soft and full scrotum, which should not be painful. These disorders are fluid collections.

Management:

- Transillumination of scrotum with bright light. A solid mass will not illuminate behind light. Hydroceles and spermatoceles are not solid.
- Look for hernia, which sometimes can cause hydroceles, usually idiopathic.
- Get testicular ultrasound for definitive diagnosis.
- Usually nothing is done, but if the fluid collection is large, there are two options: surgical excision of the tunica vaginalis or scrotal aspiration and sclerotherapy with doxycycline.

Varicoceles

Presentation: white men; most common on left side; feels like "bag of worms" classically. Varicocele is a dilatation of the pampiniform plexus.

Management:

- Does the mass get smaller after patient has been standing? This finding points to varicocele.
- Get an ultrasound.
- Varicocele may cause fertility problems.
- Treat with embolization or occlusion of internal spermatic vein.

Inguinal Hernias

Presentation: painful bulge in scrotum

Management:

- Have the patient cough and feel for a bulge in the scrotum.
- Is the varicocele reducible? If not, surgery is needed soon.
- Laparoscopic surgery is the cure.

Orchitis/Epididymitis

Presentation: scrotal pain that radiates to abdomen or back

Management:

- Ask if the patient has had prostate problems and surgery in the past.
- Ask about sexual history.
- Ask about symptoms of urinary tract infection.
- Rule out testicular torsion immediately.
- Glove up, insert a finger in the anus, and feel for a boggy prostate.
- Get Doppler ultrasound, which is the highest-yield diagnostic test.
- Culture the urine and/or urethra.
- Treat men under 35 with "gut-and-butt" regimen of doxycycline PO and ceftriaxone (Rocephin) IM (presumed gonorrhea/chlamydial infection).
- Treat men over 35 with ciprofloxacin (presumed gram-negative organism).

Male Infertility

Presentation: inability to impregnate after one year of unprotected intercourse. A male factor is completely or partially at fault in 50% of infertility cases

Management:

- Ask patient about intercourse frequency. Some couples complain of infertility and have sex only once a month.

- Ask about history of testicular trauma, undescended testes. Does the patient have Klinefelter syndrome, a history of chromosomal problems, or hemochromatosis? Has the patient ever had orchitis?
- Is the patient taking drugs such as testosterone or anabolic steroids? What about antiandrogens such as cimetidine? Does the patient smoke marijunana or drink alcohol heavily? Does the patient have renal failure?
- Does the patient wear tight underwear? Sperm need a cooler environment. They prefer boxers to briefs.
- Does the patient have erectile function and ejaculate properly?
- Look for gynecomastia on exam and see if both testicles are descended and of the proper size. Check the prolactin level, especially if patient has gynecomastia.
- Check for varicocele, a common cause of infertility in men. Get ultrasound and fix the varicocele surgically.
- **Semen analyis** is an excellent choice; choose it if given the option. Look at volume, motility, and morphology of sperm. This test gives the most information and can rule out many problems.
- Check levels of luteinizing hormone (LH), follicle-stimulating hormone (FSH), and testosterone if semen does not show adequate sperm.
- For secondary hypogonadism, consider LH therapy to stimulate testosterone production, followed after several months by FSH to stimulate sperm production.
- Is the patient insensitive to testosterone? This finding requires biopsy of genital skin tissue with T receptors. Testosterone levels may be high; there is no cure for this condition.
- Artificial insemination is best for low sperm volume but otherwise adequate morphology.
- Otherwise consider in-vitro fertilization.

Other Disorders of Male Genitalia

	Presentation/Management
Balanitis	Inflammation of the glans penis
Redundant prepuce	Overhanging foreskin
Phimosis	Narrowness of foreskin, which cannot be drawn back over the glans. Corrected with circumcision.
Peyronie's disease	Curvature of penis
Hypospadias	Urethra opens on the underside of the penis rather than at the tip of glans. Repair with foreskin material.

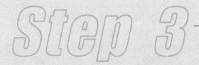

CHAPTER 12

Musculoskeletal System

GENERAL ISSUES

Diffuse diseases of connective tissue
Rheumatoid arthritis
Internal derangement of knee
Effusion of joint
Afflictions of shoulder region
Enthesopathy
Ganglion and cyst of synovium/tendon/
    bursa
Synovitis/tenosynovitis
Bursitis
Myalgia/myositis
Myositis ossificans
Osteogenesis imperfecta
Relapsing polychondritis
Achondroplasia
Abnormal head shape
Congenital musculoskeletal deformities
Spinal enthesopathy
Spondylosis/intravertebral disc disorders
Spinal stenosis
Kyphoscoliosis and scoliosis
Secondary malignant neoplasm of bone/
    marrow
Pathologic fracture

Temporomandibular joint disorders
Rotator cuff syndrome
Infective arthritis
Osteoarthritis
Monoarthritis
Arthropathy
Polyarthritis
Pain in joint/stiffness of joint
Pain in thoracic spine
Pain in limb/other musculoskeletal
    symptoms in limbs

TRAUMA

Various sprains and strains
Various contusions
Closed fracture of mandible/facial bones
Fracture of vertebral column
Fracture of ribs
Closed fracture, upper extremity
Fracture of femur
Various closed fractures of lower extremity
Dislocations/separations
Lumbosacral sprain
Sprain of sacroiliac region/back
Cauliflower ear

GENERAL ISSUES

Diffuse Diseases of Connective Tissue

	Presentation	Diagnosis	Management
Behçet's syndrome	Young man with ulcers in mouth and on penis, uveitis, retinitis	No specific test, but expect anticardiolipin antibodies, elevated ESR	Colchicine, steroids, consider MRI to rule out involvement of central nervous system

continued

Diffuse Diseases of Connective Tissue (continued)

	Presentation	Diagnosis	Management
CREST Syndrome	**C**alcinosis, **R**aynaud's syndrome, **e**sophageal dysmotility, **s**clerodactyly, **t**elangiectasias	Anticentromere anibody	Steroids
Dermatomyositis/ polymyositis	Middle-aged women with proximal muscle pain	Creatine phosphokinase (CPK), muscle biopsy, EMG studies	Steroids, azathioprine, cyclophosphamide
Mixed connective tissue disease	Similar to lupus, dermato-myositis/polymyositis	CPK, ESR	Steroids, cyclosporine, plasma-pheresis, NSAIDs
Polyarteritis nodosa/ vasculitis small/ medium	Fever, abdominal pain, and weight loss. Later hyper-tension, renal failure.	Selective arteriography has replaced biopsy	Steroids, cyclophosphamide
Polymyalgia rheumatica	Woman over 50 with pain in muscles of chest, neck, pelvis	ESR elevated	Steroids, watch for temporal arteritis
Scleroderma	Erythematous patches change to hypopigmented plaques with purple borders. Step 3 classic is picture of hands with red, "tight"-looking skin.	Autoimmune antitopoisomerase	Steroids
Sjögren's syndrome	Dry eyes, mouth	Schirmer test strips to check for tears; expect ESR elevated as well as Rh Factor	Artifical tears, salivary subsititutes, chewing gum
Systemic lupus erythematosus	Can affect every organ system, but Step 3 classic is malar rash. Look for fatigue, fever, arthralgia/ myalgia, renal failure, pleurisy, perdicarditis usually female patient	Antinuclear antibody (ANA) is highly sensitive; then anti-ds-DNA and anti-Smith antibodies, antiphospho-lipid antibodies; renal biopsy may be useful if kidney is involved.	Hydroxychloroquine, cyclopho-phamide, NSAIDs, steroids
Temporal arteritis	Patient with polymyalgia rheumatica	ESR elevated, temporal artery biopsy is diagnostic	Admit to hospital and give IV steroids as soon as possible
Wegener's granulomatosis	Dyspnea/hemoptysis, hematuria/renal failure/ nosebleeds	c-ANCA, urinalysis, renal biopsy	Cyclophosphamide, prednisone

ESR = erythrocyte sedimentation rate, c-ANCA = cytoplasmic antineutrophilic cytoplasmic antibody.

Rheumatoid Arthritis (RA)

Presentation: predominantly in females; morning stiffness, symmetric joint pain.

Management:

- The life-threatening complication is atlantoaxial instability (unstable cervical spine).
- Other systemic manifestations include vasculitis, pericarditis, pleural effusions, and diffuse interstitial fibrosis.
- Felty's syndrome presents as RA with splenomegaly and neutropenia. These patients need antibiotics.
- Ask patient about morning stiffness.
- Look for characteristic RA changes in the hands, especially in the proximal interphalangeal (PIP) and metacarpophalangeal (MCP) joints, sparing the distal interphalangeal (DIP) joints. Other changes include swan-neck deformities, boutonnière deformity, and ulnar deviation.
- On x-rays look for loss of articular bone mass, narrowing, erosions.
- Check erythrocyte sedimentation rate, rheumatoid factor.
- NSAIDs: give GI protection with chronic use. Be alert to GI bleeds in patients with RA who may swallow lots of aspirin and other NSAIDs.
- Other treatments include auranofin, hydroxychloroquine, methotrexate, D-penicillamine, and prednisone.

Internal Derangement of Knee

Presentation: athlete tackled from side, skier who twists knee.

Management:

- Check the anterior cruciate ligament (ACL) with anterior drawer sign. Flex knee to 90° and pull forward. The test is positive with 6 mm or more of movement.
- Check the posterior cruciate ligament (PCL) with posterior drawer sign. Flex to 90° and attempt to push backward. The test is positive with 6 mm or more of movement.
- Check medial collateral ligament (MCL) abduction/valgus of 30°. Place one hand on lateral knee, grasp medial ankle with other hand. The knee is abducted. Pain or laxity = MCL tear.
- Check lateral collateral ligament (LCL). Place one hand on medial knee and grasp the lateral ankle with the other hand. The knee is adducted. Pain or laxity = LCL tear.
- Check meniscus in patients with a twisting injury. McMurray test: apply a valgus force, externally rotate the tibia, and extend the knee. A pop indicates meniscal tear.
- MRI is the diagnostic tool of choice for all of the above-knee injuries.
- Treat initially with NSAIDs, knee brace, ice, and elevation.
- Then use arthroscopic surgery followed by aggressive physical therapy.

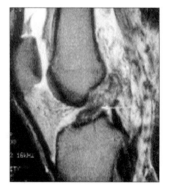

Figure 1. MRI image of torn ACL (arrow). Note irregularity in the ligament as well as no visible attachment of proximal ACL at the femur. (From Walsh WM, Helzer-Julin MJ: Office management of knee injuries. In Mellion MB (ed): Office Sports Medicine, 2nd ed. Philadelphia, Hanley & Belfus, 1996, p 264.)

Effusion of Joint

Presentation: increased amount of synovial fluid in the joint with pain and stiffness.

Management:

- Effusion can be autoimmune, infectious, or degenerative in origin.
- Fever or external wound points towards infection.
- Get CBC; look for leukocytosis or left shift.
- Arthrocentesis is likely to give the most information.
- X-ray may show osteoarthritis.
- Give antibiotics for infectious effusion.

Afflictions of Shoulder Region

	Presentation	Diagnosis	Management
Acromioclavicular (AC) arthritis	Pain, swelling	X-ray may show joint narrowing, spurs	NSAIDs, ice, steroid injection; drastic solution is to cut off end of distal clavicle
Calcific tendinitis	Severe, acute pain, especially of greater tuberosity	Calcium deposits on x-ray	NSAIDs, physical therapy, steroid injection, surgical decompression
Cervical radiculopathy	Pain that radiates in arm, neck pain; patient may show numbness in arm/shoulder	Get x-rays to look at neck; get MRI if you really want to see it	NSAIDs, physical therapy, surgery
Frozen shoulder	Pain with motion/no motion; patient may have worn sling due to injury	Physical exam	NSAIDs, physical therapy; drastic solution is putting patient under anesthesia and moving shoulder
Gout	Usually in men; big toe may hurt also	Serum uric acid, crystals in joint fluid	Colchicine, NSAIDs, allopurinol, fluids
Impingement	Pain with motion, night pain, under age 40	Inject with lidocaine; relief suggests the diagnosis	NSAIDs, physical therapy, steroid injection, surgical decompression
Lupus	Look for other lupus signs/symptoms	Antinuclear antibody (ANA), elevated erythrocyte sedimentation rate (ESR)	NSAIDs, methotrexate
Milwaukee shoulder	Elderly women, blue tint to skin	Calcium hydroxyapatite in synovial fluid	Colchicine, NSAIDs
Pseudogout	Similar to gout	Calcium pyrophosphate dihydrate crystals in joint fluid	Colchicine, NSAIDs
Rheumatoid arthritis	Bilateral, multi joint disease	X-ray shows joint narrowing, serum test positive for rheumatoid factor, ANA	NSAIDs, steroid injection, DMARDs
Rotator cuff tear	Weakness, atrophy; patient may have fallen on outstretched arm, over age 40	MRI may show tears	Physical therapy, surgery
Rotator cuff tendinitis	Weakness, atrophy, over age 40	MRI	Physical therapy; eliminate aggravating factors
Septic arthritis	Pain, fever, chills	Aspirate the joint; x-ray classically normal at first, then joint erodes	IV antibiotics, surgery
Thoracic outlet syndrome	Weak/no pulses and numbness/pain	Angiography	Surgery

Management:

- Do not miss other symptoms that masquerade as shoulder pain (e.g., cardiac pain that radiates to the shoulder).
- Try conservative treatments before surgery.

Enthesopathy

Presentation: disease at site of insertion of tendons and ligaments into bones or joint capsules. Frequently accompanied by ankylosing spondylitis, Reiter's syndrome, and psoriatic arthritis.

Management:

- Steroids are used frequently.

Ganglion and Cyst of Synovium/Tendon/Bursa

Presentation: rubbery swelling from tendon, usually at wrist.

Management:

- This condition is generally benign, unless painful.
- Cyst is fluid-filled.
- You can order surgical excision or even attempt drainage in the office with a needle.
- Recurrences are common.

Synovitis/Tenosynovitis

Presentation: synovitis is inflammation of the lining of the joints.

Management:

- You need to rule out pigmented villonodular synovitis, which is a slow-growing, benign, and locally invasive tumor of the synovium. It usually presents as a monoarticular hemarthrosis.
- Get MRI.
- Arthroscopic synovectomy may be needed.

Bursitis

Presentation: pressure/irritation of bursa; frequent sites are olecranon (elbow), subdeltoid (shoulder), and prepatellar (knee). Usually caused by overuse or infection.

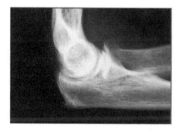

Management:

- Rest and NSAIDs for simple inflammation due to too much activity. Steroids can also be injected.
- Ask patients about risk factors for infection.
- If the bursa is infected, likely organisms are *Staphylococcus aureus* or streptococci A.
  - Treatment requires bursal drainage and antibiotics.
  - Remember to get Gram stain and rule out gout.

Figure 2. Chronic olecranon bursitis of elbow. (From Shubert S, Cassidy C: Olecranon bursitis. In Frontera WR, Silver JK (eds): Essentials of Physical Medicine and Rehabilitation. Philadelphia, Hanley & Belfus, 2002, p 128.)

Myalgia/Myositis

	Presentation	Diagnosis	Management
Dermatomyositis/ polymyositis	Middle-aged women with proximal muscle pain	CPK, muscle biopsy, EMG studies	Steroids, azathioprine, cyclo-phosphamide
Fibromyalgia	Young women with fatigue, pain	Check pressure points	NSAIDs, antidepressants
Medication-related disease can progress to rhabdomyolysis	Simvastatin combined with clofibrate classic	CPK	Stop medication, IV fluids in frank rhabdomyolysis
Mixed connective tissue disease	Similar to lupus, dermato-myositis/polymyositis	CPK, ESR	Steroids, cyclosporine, plasmapheresis, NSAIDs
Polymyalgia rheumatica	Woman over 50 with pain in muscles of chest, neck, pelvis	ESR elevated	Steroids; watch for temporal arteritis
Trichinosis	Raw meat	High eosinophil count on CBC, CPK elevated, muscle biopsy	NSAIDs for pain, albendazole for intestinal worms

CPK = creatine phosphokinase, ESR = erythrocyte sedimentation rate.

Myositis Ossificans

Presentation: abnormal formation of bone within muscle in response to soft tissue injury or autosomal dominant genetic disorder with complete penetrance.

Management:
- Look for bone formation in muscle 6 weeks after injury.
- Get x-rays.
- Biopsy shows lamellar bone.
- For the traumatic variety, surgery can be attempted.

Osteogenesis Imperfecta (OI)

Presentation: fragile bones, hearing loss, and blue sclerae.

Management:
- Get x-rays.
- Collagen studies on skin punch biopsy are diagnostic.
- Offer genetic counseling since OI is inheritable disease.
- Rods can be placed in bones to increase strength.
- OI is frequently misinterpreted as child abuse.

Relapsing Polychondritis

Presentation: saddle nose deformity, joint pain. This is an autoimmune disorder of cartilage.

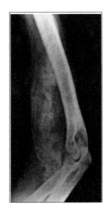

Figure 3. Myositis ossificans. (From Math KR, Cushner FD: Extremity trauma. In Katz DS, Math KR, Groskin SA (eds): Radiology Secrets. Phila-elphia, Hanley & Belfus, 1998, p 451.)

Management:

- Rule out other autoimmune disorders with antinuclear antibody test, erythrocyte sedimentation rate.
- Biopsy of cartilage is most definitive method of diagnosis.
- Steroids are the treatment of choice.
- Methotrexate may also be helpful.

Achondroplasia

Presentation: short upper arms/thighs, normal back length, large head and depressed nasal bridge, small nose and large forehead.

Management:

- Achnondroplasia is carried in a single gene and is inherited in dominant fashion.

Abnormal Head Shape

Presentation: in patients with craniosynostosis, sutures close prematurely; alternatively, positional deformity may reveal as posterior flattening due to sleep position.

Management:

- Physical exam should focus on sutures. Are they closed?
- The more sutures that close prematurely, the earlier surgery is required.
- Perform surgery.
- Molding cap is used for positional deformity.

Congenital Musculoskeletal Deformities

	Presentation	Management
Hip dysplasia	Barlow/Ortolani signs	Pavlik harness, open reduction
Slipped capital femoral epiphysis	Frog leg on x-ray	Pin fixation, osteotomy
Legg-Calvé-Perthes disease	Avascular necrosis	Brace
Osgood-Schlatter disease	Prominent tibial tuberosity	Activity restriction with casting for 6 weeks

Spinal Enthesopathy

Presentation: paraspinal ligaments degenerate and then ossify, usually by attrition.

Management:

- Diagnose with x-rays; look for osteophytes on one side of spine.
- Get MRI if neurologic symptoms are present.
- Really not much can be done.

Spondylosis/Intravertebral Disc Disorders

Presentation: starts with disc degeneration and then leads to pain and neurologic symptoms.

Management:

- NSAIDs and lifestyle modifications are mainstays of therapy.
- Surgery may be needed, especially if cervical radiculopathy presents with a lot of pain.

Spinal Stenosis

Presentation: narrowing of spinal canal causes compression of nerve roots.

Management:
- Full neurologic exam, not just weakness or atrophy.
- Ask about changes with bladder, other neurologic functions.
- Get x-rays.
- Order an MRI.
- Order EMG studies.
- Give NSAIDs.
- Give steroid injections.
- Surgery may be needed to correct severe stenosis.

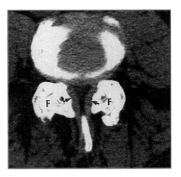

Figure 4. Spinal stenosis. The combination of facet hypertrophy (F), ligamentum flavum buckling and hypertrophy (*arrows*) and a posteriorly bulging disc result in significant degenerative spinal stenosis. (From Barckhausen RR, Math KR: Lumbar spine diseases. In Katz DS, Math KR, Groskin SA (eds): Radiology Secrets. Philadelphia, Hanley & Belfus, 1998, p 329.)

Kyphoscoliosis and Scoliosis

Presentation: kyphosis = posterior curvature of the spine; scoliosis = lateral curvature of the spine. Both are twice as common in girls.

Management:
- If the curvature is less than 25°, generally no bracing is needed.
- If curve is more then 25° but less than 30°, a back brace may be used for treatment; it will halt progression in 85% of cases.
- Stage of growth is most important in decision-making. A child with several more years of growth should be treated, but if growth has been completed, treatment should be deferred.

Pitfall:
- Failure to treat low curvatures when significant growth remains.

Secondary Malignant Neoplasm of Bone/Marrow

Presentation: patient with cancer that metastasizes to bone.

Management:
- Cancer of the breast, lung, and prostate commonly metastasize to bone; in rare cases, cancer of the thyroid, kidney, bladder, endometrium, and cervix may metastasize to bone.
- Expect serum calcium and alkaline phosphatase to be elevated.
- Skeletal survey (x-rays) helps rule out pending fractures in axial skeleton, femur, and humerus.
- X-rays may show lytic holes.
- Get bone scan. Make absolutely sure that the problem is a metastasis and not a treatable disease such as osteomyelitis.
- Chemotherapy, hormone therapy, radiotherapy, or bone surgery may be part of treatment.
- Bone marrow or stem cell transplantation is also a possibility.

Pathologic Fracture

Presentation: low-energy injury through area of bone weakness. The patient may be an elderly female with osteoporosis.

Management:
- Get lab tests, including ESR, CBC, serum calcium, alkaline phosphatase.
- Skeletal survey (x-rays) help rule out pending fractures in axial skeleton, femur, and humerus.
- Get bone scan and biopsy to rule out osteomyelitis.

Temporomandibular Joint Disorders

Presentation: clicking, headaches, pain, usually in a female patient.

Management:

- Conservative treatment such as soft foods is first approach.
- Proceed to an appliance such as a jaw guard.
- Surgery is the last resort.

Rotator Cuff Syndrome

Presentation: pain, weakness, and loss of motion of shoulder.

Management:

- Causes of impingement include acromioclavicular (AC) joint arthritis, calcific coracoacromial ligament, structural abnormalities of the acromion, and weak rotator cuff muscles, also known as SITS muscles: **s**upraspinatus, **i**nfraspinatus, **t**eres minor, and **s**ubscapularis.
- On exam note pain with supination/adduction.
- Elicit history of repetitive overhead motion.
- X-ray may show structural abnormalities.
- MRI is the diagnostic tool generally ordered.
- The next step is arthroscopy.
- Try conservative treatment initially, including rest, ice, NSAIDs, and physical therapy.
- Consider steroid injection.
- Surgery may be required.
- A sling can cause frozen shoulder.

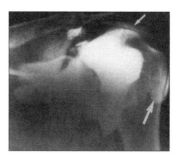

Figure 5. Rotator cuff tear with contrast extending into the subacromial (short arrow) and subdeltoid (long arrow) bursae. (From Vogelgesang S: Osteoarthritis. In West SG (ed): Rheumatology Secrets. Philadelphia, Hanley & Belfus, 1997, p 373, with permission.)

Infective Arthritis

Presentation: patient complains of a single joint that is red, edematous, hot, and painful.

Management:

- If the patient is sexually active, the infection may be gonococcal. If the patient is an IV drug user, the infection may be staphylococcal.
- On exam note any signs of trauma, infection, or skin changes.
- Get an x-ray of the joint.
- Aspirate the joint. What color is the fluid?
- Send the fluid for Gram stain, urate crystal analysis, and WBC count.
- Treat with cephalexin (Keflex) or dicloxacillin for streptococcal or staphylococcal infection.

Osteoarthritis

Presentation: older adults; frequently affects hip, knee, spine, hands.

Management:

- On exam note Bouchard nodes at the proximal interphalangeal joint and Heberden's nodes at the distal interphalangeal joint.
- Note pain, crepitus on exam.
- Get x-ray to look for osteophytes, subchondral bone sclerosis, loss of cartilage.
- Give NSAIDs, local steroid injections for relief.
- Celecoxib and rofecoxib are good choices with fewer GI side effects.
- Recommend swimming/low-impact exercise to avoid further aggravation.

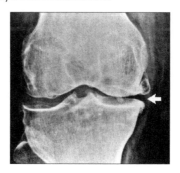

Figure 6. Osteoarthritis of knee. (From Vogelgesang S: Osteoarthritis. In West S (ed): Rheumatology Secrets, 2ed. Philadelphia, Hanley & Belfus, 2002, p 367.)

Monoarthritis

Presentation: patient complains of a single joint that is red, edematous, hot, and painful.

Management:
- In history ask about any complaint like this in the past. Does the patient have gout?
- If the patient is sexually active, the problem may be gonococcal infection. If the patient is an IV drug user, the problem may be staphylococcal infection.
- On exam note any signs of trauma, infection, skin changes.
- Get an x-ray of the joint.
- Aspirate the joint. What color is the fluid?
- Send the fluid for Gram stain, urate crystal analysis, WBC count.
- Treat most infectious cases with cephalexin (Keflex).
- Treat inflammatory disesase with NSAIDs.
- If you are uncertain of the precise cause, treat both infectious and inflammatory causes simultaneously.

Arthropathy

Presentation: be familiar with neuropathic arthropathy (Charcot's joint); presents initially as OA, then suddenly deteriorates. The joint can be destroyed in a short time.

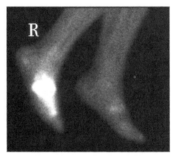

Management:
- This rapidly destructive arthropathy results from impaired pain perception/position sense.
- It is often confused with OA and should be suspected in diabetics with neuropathy.
- Get an x-ray.
- Immobilization can protect the joint.
- Replace joints surgically if needed.

Figure 7. Charcot joint. (From Silver RM, Smith EA: Rheumatology Pearls. Philadelphia, Hanley & Belfus, 1997, p 103.)

Polyarthritis

	Presentation
Gonococcal arthritis	Urethritis; ask about sexual history
Lupus	See section on Systemic lupus erythematosus
Psoriatic arthritis	Atopic disease
Reiter's syndrome	Uveitis, urethritis, arthritis: "can't see, can't pee, can't climb a tree" is the medical school mnemonic
Rheumatic fever	History of streptococcal infection
Rheumatoid arthritis	See section above on RA
Still's disease	Juvenile chronic arthritis (rheumatoid factor absent)
Viral infections	Hepatitis B or C is classic cause, but mumps, rubella, fifth disease, and human immunodeficiency virus can also be cause

Pain in Joint/Stiffness of Joint

	Helpful Tests
Osteoarthritis	Xrays
Autoimmune disease	Joint fluid aspiration with Gram stain, crystal exam, cell count and differential, and glucose assessment Sedimentation rate, Rh factor, complement levels, antinuclear antibody
Crystal arthropathies	Joint fluid aspiration with Gram stain, crystal exam, cell count and differential, and glucose Uric acid
Infectious/septic arthritis	Joint fluid aspiration with Gram stain, crystal exam, cell count and differential, and glucose assessment CBC with differential Bone scan

Pain in Thoracic Spine

	Helpful Tests
Muscular pain	Clinical exam is most useful; diagnosis may be process of exclusion
Metastasis	X-ray, bone scan
Disc degeneration	X-rays, MRI
Vertebral fracture	X-rays, MRI
Other	Rule out aortic dissection, myocardial infarction, gallbladder disease

Pain in Limb/Other Musculoskeletal Symptoms in Limbs

	Presentation
Arthritis	Joints swollen and stiff?
Fracture	History of trauma? Osteoporosis?
Growing pains	Young people may awaken with them at night
Ischemic	Risk factors for deep venous thrombosis or outlet syndrome?
Muscular	History of overuse or strain?
Neurogenic	Consider nerve impingement/compression
Phantom	Amputee

TRAUMA

Various Sprains and Strains

Presentation: sprain (ligament) commonly presents as twisted ankle; presentation of strains (muscle or tendon) can range from simple pain to complete muscle tear.

Management:
- In history note mechanism of injury.
- On exam note bruising that might result from exsanguination of blood from torn muscle. Also note popeye bulge from torn bicep or pectoralis, especially in steroid users.
- In patients with complete muscle tear, splint the body part and call an orthopedist as soon as possible.
- For simple muscle strains give NSAIDs and advise warm, moist heat.
- For sprains of grade I or II: rest, ice, compression, elevation.
- Grade III (severe tear) sprain requires surgery to prevent long-term instability.

Various Contusions

Presentation: blunt trauma to muscle, as in rugby/football player, that causes muscle bruising.

Management:
- Note tenderness on exam and look for hematoma.
- Note range of motion; reduced range of motion is a more ominous sign.
- Your main concern is to rule out a compartment syndrome.
- Consider getting a creatine phosphokinase level if rhabdomyolysis is suspected.
- Myositis ossificans may develop after about 5-6 weeks; consider x-ray at that time.
- Advise patient to keep weight off affected area initially.
- Then physical therapy and rehabilitation are warranted.

Closed Fracture of Mandible/Facial Bones

Presentation: car accident victim with breathing impairment from blockage by bone fragments, edema, blood clots, or teeth. Skin is not broken.

Management:
- Secure an airway!
- Get an x-ray
- Check for leaking CNS fluids on exam.
- Treatment consists of surgical reduction and fixation.

Fracture of Vertebral Column

Presentation: osteoporosis or trauma.

Management:
- Patient should be immobilized! Long board is the preferred method.
- Do a full neurologic exam and note any deficits. Note any incontinence.
- Get x-rays of the spine first.
- MRI is the diagnostic choice for evaluation of the spinal cord.
- High-dose steroids may protect the cord.
- Surgery may be needed to save neurologic function.
- Percutaneous vertebroplasty by interventional radiology can be used effectively to relieve pain. Polymethylmethacrylate cement is injected.

Fracture of Ribs

Presentation: patient with pain after trauma, coughing violently. Pain increases with movement, including coughing/breathing.

Management:

- Does the patient have an injury somewhere else? Evaluate patient fully.
- In examining the patient, indirect stress causes pain with a rib fracture.
- Get posteroanterior and lateral chest x-rays to rule out pneumonia or other serious pulmonary complication. The oblique view is best for finding fractures of ribs.
- X-rays do not always detect rib fractures.
- Admit the patient if arterial blood gases and pulmonary function tests are too worrisome or if the patient is elderly.
- Rib wrap can be attempted to control pain for only a few days.
- Pain control is essential.
- Pneumonia is a complication because patients hurt when they take a deep breath.

Closed Fracture, Upper Extremity

Presentation: "closed" indicates that the fracture is not open to air; caused commonly by trauma, child abuse.

Management:

- Check for pulses, nerve injury (especially of radial nerve with humerus injury and ulnar nerve with elbow injury). Look for wrist drop and claw hand, respectively.
- Get x-rays: posteroanterior and lateral.
- Note into how many pieces the bone is broken. Is it rotated? Angulated? Where is the break in the bone—in the middle or near the ends? How far is it displaced from where it should be? The more complicated the situation, the more likely you should go to the OR.
- For simple closed fractures, you can use closed reduction with traction and sling. You are trying to realign the bones to natural placement. Give anesthesia before reducing!
- Immobilize with cast and traction only after realignment is successful.
- Exceptions:
  □ Clavicle fractures generally use sling only.
  □ Distal supracondylar humerus fractures in children are perilous and difficult to reduce.
  □ Humeral head fractures require open reduction with internal fixation (ORIF); blood supply is in danger. These usually occur after direct blow to lateral shoulder.
  □ Elbow requires ORIF.
  □ Forearm requires ORIF.
  □ Colles' fractures require closed reduction
  □ Hand fractures require closed reduction with K-wire fixation.

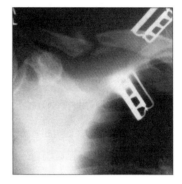

Figure 8. Clavicle fracture. (From Masih S, Bakhda R: Imaging modalities in diagnosis and management of fractures. In Mehta AJ (ed): Physical Medicine and Rehabilitation, State of the Art Reviews, Rehabilitation of Fractures Vol. 9:1, Philadelphia, Hanley & Belfus, 1995, p 225.)

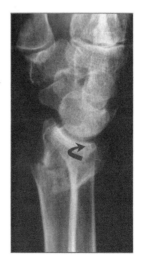

Figure 9. Typical Colles' fracture of the distal radius with the distal fracture fragment angulated in the dorsal direction (*arrow*). (From Metz VM, Gilula LA: Radiologic examination of the wrist. In Weinzweig J (ed): Hand & Wrist Surgery Secrets. Philadelphia, Hanley & Belfus, 2000, p 189.)

- Go to the OR for fractures that you cannot reduce, femur fractures, fractures that involve joints, or forearm fractures.
- Do not go to the OR for fracture in children or clavicle fractures.
- Spiral fractures are child abuse until proved otherwise. Consider skeletal survey if you suspect child abuse, and alert the authorities. Step 3 loves this topic.
- If growth plate is involved in child, the final length of extremity can be affected. Go to OR.
- Watch for complications such as nerve damage, compartment syndrome, nonhealing, ischemia, deep venous thrombosis, fat embolus.

Fracture of Femur

Presentation: direct trauma or indirect force transmitted from knee.

Management:
- ABCs → Watch for blood loss and consider pneumatic splint for this reason. Start fluids if needed. A lot of blood can hide in a thigh (> 1 liter).
- Check for pulses, nerve injury.
- Reduce to anatomic alignment with traction after pain medications are given. Use serious pain control, such as IV morphine.
- For open fracture given tetanus booster and antibiotics. Open fracture requires surgical debridement.
- Get x-rays: anteroposterior and lateral.
- Get ready to go to the OR. The standard of care is operative fixation with intramedullary nailing.
- Be aware of the risk of avascular necrosis of femoral head.
- Watch for complications such as nerve damage, compartment syndrome, nonhealing, ischemia, deep venous thrombosis, fat embolus.
- Do not forget to rule out child abuse.

Various Closed Fractures of Lower Extremity

Presentation: trauma, child abuse.

Management:
- Check for pulses, nerve injury.
- Get x-rays.
- Specific therapies/concerns:
  □ Knee: patella fracture is treated with weight restriction, crutches, knee immobilization. Peroneal nerve damage correlates with knee injury; look for foot drop.
  □ Tibia/fibula: treatment is generally nonoperative unless the fracture is displaced. Then ORIF is needed. Fractures of the tibia/fibula are frequently open fractures, in which case tetanus boosters and antibiotics should be given and the patient sent to OR for debridement by orthopedic surgeon.
  □ Ankles: anything beyond simple lateral malleolar fracture usually needs ORIF.
- Watch for complications such as nerve damage, compartment syndrome, nonhealing, ischemia, deep venous thrombosis, fat embolus.

Dislocations/Separations

Presentation:
Shoulder: blow or knock to humeral head anteriorly. Note bulge in deltopectoral groove, prominent acromion with depression below.
Elbow: fall on extended abducted arm or nursemaid elbow with child picked up by the arm
Hand: sports injury, commonly hyperextension while playing goalie.

Management:

- Check for neurovascular compromise.
- Pain control is essential.
- Get an x-ray before attempting reduction unless it is a recurring injury.
- Reduce:
  - Shoulder: flex elbow at 90°. Pull humerus inferiorly while externally rotating the forearm. Scapular manipulation is another excellent choice. Give IM/IV pain medications or inject lidocaine into the joint space.
  - Elbow: flex elbow to 90° in supine position. Then push humerus posteriorly with simultaneous pressure on the proximal forearm. Give IM/IV pain medications.
  - Fingers: pull on digit and manipulate in direction opposite to that of deformity. Do a digital block first for pain control.
- Get x-rays after reduction.
- Open dislocations always merit surgery.
- You should stop after 2 or 3 attempts at reduction and call orthopedist.

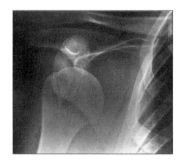

Figure 11A. Anterior shoulder dislocation.

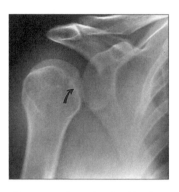

Figure 11B. Posterior shoulder dislocation. (From Math KR, Cushner FD: Extremity trauma. In Katz DS, Math KR, Groskin SA (eds): Radiology Secrets. Philadelphia, Hanley & Belfus, 1998, p 443-44.)

Lumbosacral Sprain

Presentation: generally male with weight-lifting injury at L4/L5 with lateral twisting combined with flexion.

Management:

- Get an x-ray to rule out fracture or other pathology.
- Prescribe cold for 2 days and rest.
- Refer for physical therapy.
- Give NSAIDs and muscle relaxants.

Sprain of Sacroiliac Region/Back

Presentation: similar to above.

Management:

- Similar to above.
- In this region, you need to rule out ankylosing spondylitis. Look for bamboo spine on x-ray and check erythrocyte sedimentation rate, HLA-B27.

Cauliflower Ear

Presentation: the classic patient is a wrestler.

Management:

- Trauma to pinna results in hematoma between the cartilage and perichondrium on the anterior surface of the ear. Fibroneocartilage forms, and permanent deformity may result.
- Drainage of the effusion via needle aspiration/incision and application of pressure dressing at time of injury prevents permanent deformity.

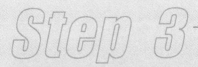

CHAPTER 13

Neurology

CENTRAL NERVOUS SYSTEM
Tetanus
Acute poliomyelitis
Creutzfeldt-Jakob disease (scrapie, kuru)
Rabies
Meningitis
Encephalitis
Brain abscess
Alzheimer's disease/cerebral atrophy
Parkinson disease
Multiple sclerosis
Amyotrophic lateral sclerosis
Seizure disorder
Brain death
Cerebral palsy
Intracranial neoplasm/malignant neoplasm
Cerebral hemorrhage
Transient cerebral ischemia

Cerebrovascular disease
Cerebral embolism and thrombosis
Reye syndrome
Migraine
Convulsions
Headache
Abnormal involuntary movement
Coma

GENERAL ISSUES
Mental retardation
Myasthenia gravis
Neuropathies/neuralgia/neuritis
Sleep disturbances
Aphasia
Psychalgia
Syncope and collapse/ataxia

CENTRAL NERVOUS SYSTEM

Tetanus

Presentation: trismus (pain on opening the mouth), dysphagia, generalized muscular rigidity, and/or spasm. The "spatula test": touch the oropharynx with a tongue blade. This should elicit a gag reflex in healthy patients, who try to expel the blade. Patients with tetanus have reflex spasm of the masseters and try to bite the spatula.

Management:
- Mind the ABCs: toxin-mediated muscle stiffness can suffocate; seriously consider admission to ICU for tracheotomy and ventilation in patients with clinical tetanus.
- Once the patient is in the ICU and the ABCs have been managed, give muscle relaxants, sedatives, and neuromuscular blocking agents, if needed.
- Penicillin G is the drug of choice in clinical tetanus; it may inhibit multiplication of *Clostridium tetani*.
- After exposure: if the patient has not received immunization in the past 5 years, give age-appropriate tetanus/diphtheria toxoid IM.

- After exposure: if the patient has never had original three tetanus immunizations, add tetanus immunoglobulin IM and age-appropriate tetanus/diphtheria toxoid IM. Do not forget to make patient come back for follow-up immunizations to complete series.
- If the patient is hypersensitive to tetanus toxoid, give immunoglobulin only. Such patients will never have passive immunity.

Pitfalls:

- Do not assume adequate immunization. Lower socioeconomic patients are the least likely to be immunized.
- Do not assume that having tetanus in the past confers immunity—it does not.
- Too frequent tetanus immunizations can cause reactions.
- Absolute contraindication: history of immediate hypersensitivity (i.e., anaphylaxis symptoms).

Sample question 1:

A 21-year-old Hispanic man is brought to your clinic after stepping on a rusty nail in an old board earlier today while working at his roofing job. He speaks mainly Spanish and came from Mexico less than 1 year ago. It is nearly impossible to elicit his past medical history, and you desperately wish you had taken Medical Spanish or that you could simply ask ¿Usted ha tenido una infección del tétanos?. You remove his work boot and find a puncture wound in his foot. After proper cleansing and debridement of the wound, what would be next most appropriate step?

A. Tetanus/diphtheria toxoid IM
B. Tetanus immunoglobulin IM
C. Tetanus/diphtheria toxoid IM and tetanus immuoglobulin IM in the same extremity
D. IV ceftriaxone (Rocephin) followed by discharge with oral ciprofloxacin.
E. Tetanus/diphtheria toxoid IM and tetanus immunoglobulin IM in opposite extremity

The correct answer is found at the end of the chapter.

Acute Poliomyelitis

Presentation: viral prodrome, sore throat, anorexia, nausea, vomiting, and muscle aches proceed to incubation period, then to paralysis stage with flaccid asymmetric weakness and muscle atrophy. Risk factors include poor sanitation, poor hygeine, and crowding. Rare in U.S. except in groups without vaccination (e.g., Amish people).

Management:

- Prevent it with immunizations. All children should receive 4 doses of inactivated polio virus (IPV) at 2, 4, and 6 months and 4 years of age. Adults get live Salk vaccine for 3 doses.
- Give immediate respiratory assistance and ICU care. Monitor vital signs carefully.
- Get CBC and lumbar puncture, along with viral studies of stool, throat, blood, and cerebrospinal fluid (CSF).
- Consider EMG, nerve conduction studies, and MRI of spinal cord.
- Give supportive care.
- Give physical therapy, occupational therapy, speech therapy, and rehabilitation.
- Prognosis: > 90% are asymptomatic when infected or have mild illness such as sore throat and/or gastroenteritis symptoms. Then the illness aborts. The mortality rate is 5%. Prognosis is good for those who recover from respiratory failure. Most recover at least 60% of muscle strength.

Pitfall:

- Do not give live Salk virus to immunocompromised patients or members of their household.

Creutzfeldt-Jakob Disease (Scrapie, Kuru)

Presentation: patient in 60s with dementia, cortical blindness, motor disorders, rigidity, myoclonus, trembling.

Management:

- It always fatal, usually within 6 months.
- It has been associated with European, particularly British, beef.
- It also has been associated with cadaver-derived pituitary hormones, corneal transplants, and other iatrogenic infections. The prion can survive autoclaves and sterilization.
- EEG is sometimes diagnostic before an invasive study. Brain biopsy is the diagnostic tool of choice.
- There is no cure.
- It is frequently misdiagnosed as Alzheimer's disease.

Rabies

Presentation: animal bite: bats, skunks, foxes, and dogs. Progresses over 7-14 days from eclipse to peripheral to central nervous system. Viral prodrome: aphasia, lack of coordination, paresis, paralysis, mental status changes, high fever, salivation, spasms with swallowing. Hyperactivity leads to hypotension, coma, disseminated intravascular coagulation, cardiac arrhythmias, cardiac arrest, and **certain death**. Step 3 is most likely to present question about decision in relation to postexposure prophylaxis rather than actual rabies.

Management:

- Start with the basics. Clean/debride wound thoroughly. Irrigate with soap and water.
- Call local health department to learn the prevalence of rabies in the area.
- Definitive diagnosis is by direct fluorescent antibody from the brain. You can also use nerves surrounding hair follicles in the nape of neck in place of brain tissue. Lumbar puncture with high CSF protein is also suggestive; you can isolate virus from saliva or CSF.
- You need to make decision about postexposure prophylaxis:
  - After bite, observe domestic animal for a week; if the animal becomes symptomatic, it can be killed and checked for rabies. You can wait for vaccine.
  - If the patient is bitten on a distal extremity by a wild animal that is captured, the animal should be killed and checked for rabies. You can wait for vaccine.
  - If the patient is bitten on the face/neck (i.e., close to brain) by a wild animal that is captured, immediately give rabies immunoglobulin and human diploid cell vaccine (HDCV). You have no time to waste because the virus travels to the CNS. Treatment can be stopped later if the test on the animal turns out to be negative. Give rabies immunoglobulin for passive protection. Begin immunization with human diploid cell vaccine and repeat 3, 7, 14, and 28 days after exposure.
  - If the patient is bitten by a wild animal, especially a bat or raccoon, that could not be captured, assume that the animal is rabid, and give a full course of rabies immunoglobulin and HDCV. Unprovoked wild animal attacks carry a high risk of rabies.

Pitfalls:

- Have a high level of suspicion if the animal is a bat. It has been suggested that exposure to bats **without** known bites can transmit virus.
- Do not give rabies vaccine for rodents/legomorphs.
- Do not neglect potential bacterial infection. Treat bites properly, and give tetanus injection if needed.
- Do not neglect to vaccinate people at high risk (e.g., veterinarians, forest rangers). Preexposure prophylaxis consists of 4 doses of HDCV.
- Do not miss another type of encephalitis. Rabies is rare. If you see it, you should write it up as a case report and present it at a national conference.

Sample question 2:

A 9-year-old girl is brought to your office after being bitten on the hand by a border collie that lives in the neighborhood. The dog is normally friendly, and the attack appears unprovoked. The owner has been contacted and can verify that vaccination status is current. The animal is now quarantined by local animal control and does not appear to be acting inappropriately. What is the most appropriate therapy?

A. Clean and debride the wound and withhold rabies prophylaxis for now.
B. Give rabies immunoglobulin and HDCV, 1 dose.
C. Give rabies immunoglobulin and full course of HDCV.
D. Give tetanus prophylaxis.
E. Request that the animal be sacrificed immediately and the brain checked with fluorescent rabies antibody.

The correct answer is found at the end of the chapter.

Meningitis

Presentation: nuchal rigidity, high fever, irritability, mental status changes, lethargy. Most patients are lethargic, listless children.

Management:

- Order emergency CT with contrast, especially for patient with focal signs.
- Perform lumbar puncture.
- Send CNS fluid for culture.
- Initial choice of antibiotic: broad-spectrum third- or fourth-generation cephalosporin such as ceftriaxone
- Once cultures come back, tailor therapy to causative organism.

	Antibiotic
Streptococci	Penicillin G
Neisseria meningitidis	Penicillin G
Hemophilus influenzae B	Ceftriaxone
Staphylococcus aureus	Oxacillin
Staphylococcus epidermidis	Vancomycin
Gram-negative organism	Cephalosporin
Listeria spp.	Ampicillin

Pitfall:

- Do not perform lumbar puncture (LP) without first getting a CT scan, especially if there are focal neurologic findings such as unilateral motor weakness. LP may result in catastrophic uncal herniation. Instead do the CT and rule out mass, bleeding, and midline shift, all of which suggest that the diagnosis is probably not meningitis.

Sample question 3:

A 59-year-old man is brought to the ED by his adult son, who found him at home very lethargic. On physical exam he has a temperature of 41°C and involuntary flexing of the hip and knee when the neck is flexed forward. Which is the most appropriate IV therapy to begin?

A. Ceftriaxone
B. Ciprofloxacin
C. Glucocorticoids
D. Acyclovir
E. Mannitol

The correct answer is found at the end of the chapter.

Encephalitis

Presentation: general viral prodrome for several days conisisting of fever, headache, nausea and vomiting, lethargy, and myalgias. Later symptoms include behavioral and personality changes, decreased level of consciousness, stiff neck, photophobia, lethargy, generalized or localized seizures, acute confusion/ amnesia, flaccid paralysis. Prognosis depends on the virus and the patient's current state of health.

Management:
- Get CT of head, with and without contrast, prior to an LP to search for evidence of elevated intra-cerebral pressure (ICP), obstructive hydrocephalus, or mass effect. It is helpful also in the differential diagnosis. MRI shows results earlier in disease course than CT.
- Order CBC with differential, serum electrolytes, serum glucose, blood urea nitrogen/creatinine, liver function tests, and coagulation profile. Also get urinary electrolytes and urine and serum toxicology screen.
- LP with CSF analysis is essential; you must get viral cultures. Brain biopsy is definitive diagnostic tool but requires neurosurgery consultation.
- Give anticonvulsants and glucocorticoids to reduce cerebral edema, sedatives to minimize restlessness, and aspirin or some other mild analgesic to relieve headache and control fever.
- Give acyclovir for suspected herpes simplex encephalitis (HSE) as soon as possible.

Pitfalls:
- Failure to give acyclovir in the ED with or without antibiotics as HSE and varicella-zoster encephalitis are treatable.
- Failure to treat hypotension/shock, hypoxemia, hyponatremia due to SIADH, which is quite common in encephalitis.
- Failure to diagnose an acute stroke or other CNS process.

Brain Abscess

Presentation: headache, low-grade fever, and a focal neurologic defect or seizure. The most likely vignette is a postdental procedure or after sinusitis; look for streptococcal infection. Immunocompromised patients may have fungal, toxoplasmosis infection. Swimmers may be infected with amebae. Vignette is likely to show CT with ring-enhancing lesions.

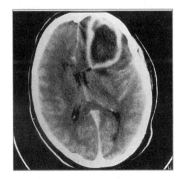

Figure 1. Brain abscess. (From Carlini ME, Harris RL: Infectious disease, including AIDS. In Rolak LA (ed): Neurology Secrets, 3e. Philadelphia, Hanley & Belfus, 2001, p 330.)

Management:
- Order CT **with contrast,** which shows ring-enhancing lesions. ESR, CBC may be useful, but CT is your best weapon.
- Give antibiotics: penicillin + choramphenicol is the classic regimen.

Cefotaxime + metronidazole is an alternative regimen. Add nafcillin or vancomycin for *Staphylococcus aureus*/methicillin-resistant *S. aureus* (MRSA).

- Dexamethasone (Decadron) is the steroid of choice for ICP reduction. Give it.
- Consult a neurosurgeon, who will probably incise, aspirate, drain, or excise the abscess. Conservative management is rare.

Pitfalls:

- Performing LP can cause CNS herniation and death.
- Do not fail to get CT in anyone with a new neurologic defect and headache.
- Do not neglect to consult neurosurgery.
- Do not forget to stabilize the patient (i.e., intubation) **before** getting diagnostic imaging. ABCs are critical.

Alzheimer's Disease/Cerebral Atrophy

Presentation: insidiously progressive memory loss leads to language and executive functional deficits, aphasia, apraxia. Lesions consist of tangles, plaques, amyloid deposits.

Management:

- Do Mini-Mental Status Exam and complete history and physical exam.
- Get CBC, vitamin B12 levels, liver function tests, ammonia and TSH levels, rapid plasma reagin test, and lumbar puncture, if indicated;
- MRI or CT shows cerebral atrophy in a patient with Alzheimer's disease. The gyri are narrowed and the sulci widened toward the frontal pole.
- Give tacrine or donepezil (Aricept) + antidepressant, antipsychotic, and/or anti-anxiety medications for symptoms.
- Estrogen and NSAIDs may offset progression,
- Recommend mentally challenging activities.
- The 1:2–1:4 lifetime risk of developing Alzheimer's disease increases with age, especially over 80 years. Patients often have low education levels.

Pitfalls:

- Failure to treat reversible delirium.
- Failure to treat depression (very high rates in Alzheimer's patients).
- Failure to consider medicolegal aspects of competency to make decisions.

Parkinson Disease

Presentation: three cardinal signs: resting tremor, rigidity, and bradykinesia; average age = 60 years with insidious onset.

Management:

- Parkinson disease (PD) may occur in young users of designer drug MPTP (synthetic heroin).
- PD is noted for loss of pigmented dopaminergic neurons in the substantia nigra and the presence of Lewy bodies.
- On exam look for cogwheeling, fenestrating gait, and glabellar reflex.
- Selegiline may be neuroprotective and should be started, especially in young patients. It is a monoamine oxidase (MAO) inhibitor.
- Symptomatic therapy: levodopa, bromocriptine, pergolide.
- Assess serum ceruloplasmin to rule out Wilson disease, especially with symptoms in patients under 40.

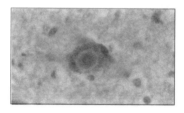

Figure 2. Parkinson's disease (classic Lewy body). (From Allen CMC, Lueck CJ: Neurological disease. In Haslett C, et al: Davidson's Principles and Practice of Medicine, 19e. Philadelphia, Churchill Livingstone, 2002, p 1174.)

Pitfall:

- Failure to treat depression.

Multiple Sclerosis (MS)

Presentation: **optic neuritis**, transverse myelitis, internuclear ophthalmoplegia, paresthesias. Patients feel worse after hot bath. Caucasians are twice as likely to present with MS; the typical patient is a 40- to 60-year-old female.

Management:

- MS is an inflammatory demyelinating disease of the CNS.
- MRI is the diagnostic tool of choice.
- Lumbar puncture shows oligoclonal bands in IgG.
- Flex the neck for Lhermitte's sign, which results in an electric shocklike feeling in the torso or extremities.
- Treat with interferon beta, glatiramer (Copaxone), steroids.

Pitfalls:

- Do not forget CBC and electrolytes to rule out other causes of neurologic findings.
- Do not fail to treat autonomic dysfunction such as incontinence, impotence.
- Do not overlook trigeminal neuralgia.
- Do not forget to treat depression.

Amyotrophic Lateral Sclerosis (ALS)

Presentation: middle-aged man with wrist drop, foot drop, and slurred speech. Initial subtle symptoms are followed by hyperreflexia, spasticity, fasciculations, dysphagia, and dysarthria.

Management:

- ALS is a slowly progressive degeneration of upper and lower motor neurons with glutamate/mitochondrial dysfunction; autoimmunity is involved. It is a fatal disease with 10% autosomal dominant inheritance, but 90% of patients have no family history.
- Give respiratory support, if needed, because muscles become weak. BiPAP is an excellent choice.
- EMG or MRI may be useful.
- Glutamate agonists such as riluzole may slow early progression.
- Give antispastic agents such as baclofen.
- Recommend living will.
- Get physical therapy, occupational therapy, and speech therapy.

Pitfalls:

- Failure to diagnose associated pneumonia, urosepsis, constipation, depression, muscle cramps, immobility-related problems.
- Do not forget that some patients may not want mechanical ventilation with such poor prognosis.

Sample question 4:

On a routine visit a healthy 32-year-old woman is concerned about the likelihood of developing ALS like her father, who was recently diagnosed. Upon further questioning she states that she knows of no other family members with the illness. Her physical exam is normal. What is the most appropriate response?

A. Without further testing it is impossible to know.
B. There is a 90% likelihood that she will develop ALS.
C. There is a 10% chance that she will develop ALS.
D. She will certainly develop ALS.
F. Until she is older, there is no way to know.

The correct answer is found at the end of the chapter.

Seizure Disorder

Presentation: symptoms range from jerking in a single extremity to movement of entire body, lip-smacking, and staring spells. Patients may become incontinent with loss of bladder and bowel control. Patients often bite their tongue.

Management:

- Get metabolic profile. Focus on electrolytes: sodium, glucose, calcium, magnesium. Hypoglycemia is a common cause.
- Get CBC with differential to rule out infection.
- Get blood urea nitrogen/creatinine to rule out renal failure.
- Get toxicology screen to rule out drugs.
- Get antinuclear antibody/erythrocyte sedimentation rate to rule out autoimmune process.
- Get CT, but be sure to stabilize the patient first. CT can rule out subarachnoid hemorrhage, stroke, and tumor.
- Get EEG in patients with new onset of tonic/clonic seizure.
- Get lumbar puncture if meningitis/encephalitis is suspected.
- Give oxygen for hypoxia, which can also cause seizures.
- Give phenytoin or carbamazepine for tonic-clonic seizures.
- If the patient is in status epilepticus (30 minutes of continuous seizure), immediately give lorazepam + thiamine + glucose + phosphenytoin, and **possibly** proceed to general anesthesia with full neuromuscular blockade. This is the most serious seizure and requires aggressive treatment.
- New seizure in a middle-aged person is caused by a brain tumor until proved otherwise.

Pitfalls:

- Never fail to treat the underlying cause.
- Do not miss eclampsia in pregnant women, which presents with hypertension.
- Do not fail to treat injuries afterward as well as complications such as aspiration pneumonia.

Brain Death

Presentation: cessation and irreversibility of all brain function, including brainstem. Watch for an ethics question requiring a decision about organ transplantation.

Management:

- You must exclude other causes before declaring brain death: metabolic derangement, intoxication, shock, hypothermia. Always warm the patient and exclude any possibility of recovery.
- Ensure that brainstem function is absent on exam: pupils fixed and dilated (penlight), corneal reflex (Q-Tip), oculocephalic/oculovestibular reflex ("doll's eyes" that turn with head from side to side), gag reflex, apnea.
- Anoxic brain injury requires 24 hours of observation. Confirmatory test such as EEG can shorten observation.
- Alternatively check cerebral blood flow with intracranial four-vessel cerebral angiography.

Cerebral Palsy (CP)

Presentation: most likely presents as gross motor development delay in first year of life. Other presentations of CP include spastic hemiplegia, spastic diplegia, dyskinesis, spastic quadriplegia.

Management:

- Damage to fetal brain can result from maternal infections, drug/alcohol abuse, anemia, and rubella. This damage leads to disorders of movement and posture.
- Initial physician tasks include detailed history of maternal exposure to toxins or infections, APGAR scores, and review of developmental milestones. Physical exam should certainly include complete neurologic exam.

- Check for mitochondrial dysfunction and order thyroid dysfunction studies. Rule out metabolic disorders with serum/urine amino acid studies. Consider DNA testing for genetic problem.
- If you must order a radiologic study, MRI will give you the most information.
- The prime responsibility is managing the complications of CP: seizures (epilepsy is quite common in CP), nutritional deficiencies due to feeding difficulties, high risk of aspiration, skin breakdown, orthopedic problems (e.g., contractures or curvature of the spine), and sensory problems (e.g., vision and hearing).
- Prescribe physical therapy, consider PEG tube, and give anticonvulsants, muscle relaxants.
- Outfit patient with communication devices, orthotics, walkers, wheelchairs, seating aids.

Pitfalls:

- Do not assume that CP is due to negligence on anyone's part; asphyxia at delivery has not been found to be the primary cause, as was thought in the past.
- Do not assume that patients with CP cannot have meaningful life. Many have normal or above normal IQ.

Intracranial Neoplasm/Malignant Neoplasm of CNS

Presentation: gliomas, meningiomas, pituitary adenoma, acoustic neuroma, and craniopharyngioma are the most common primary tumors. In adults, most primary brain tumors are above the tentorium (supratentorial); in children, most originate below the tentorium (infratentorial). Metastases include, in order of occurrence, lung, breast, melanoma, kidney, thyroid, prostate, and ovarian cancer. Primary CNS lymphomas frequently are associated with HIV. The prognosis depends on histology and location. Average life expectancy in metastatic brain cancer is 1 month without treatment. Headache is the classic presenting symptom, along with altered mental status, ataxia, nausea, vomiting, weakness, and gait disturbance. Other symptoms include focal seizures, visual changes (double vision is the classic symptom of pituitary adenoma), speech deficits, or sensory changes. Symptoms are usually insidious, but bleeding or ventricle blockage may present acutely. New seizure in older adults = tumor until proved otherwise.

Management:

- Get CBC, coagulation profile, electrolytes. Cancer patients are susceptible to hyperviscosity, hypercalcemia, and SIADH.
- CT with contrast is very useful and is the easiest modality to get at most institutions.
- MRI is better for acoustic neuroma. It should also be used if contrast is contraindicated due to allergy or renal insufficiency.
- Reduce intracranial pressure (ICP) with dexamethasone; do not give mannitol without consulting neurosurgery because it can cause rebound increases in ICP.
- If intubation is needed, do it. You can then use hyperventilation to decrease ICP as well.
- Surgery, radiation and chemotherapy are the mainstays of therapy.
- Hemorrhage and herniation are life-threatening: do not miss them, and do not cause them!

Pitfalls:

- Give prophylactic anticonvulsants for seizures in patients with newly diagnosed brain tumors unless they are actively seizing.
- Performing lumbar puncture can cause CNS herniation and death.
- Do not fail to get a CT scan in anyone with new neurologic defect and headache.
- Do not neglect to consult neurosurgery, radiation oncology, and oncology.
- Do not forget to stabilize the patient (i.e., intubation) **before** diagnostic imaging. ABCs are critical (as always).

Cerebral Hemorrhage

Presentation: "the worst headache of my life" is the classic presentation of subarachnoid hemorrhage (SAH), with focal neurological deficits and bloody lumbar puncture. Common causes include SAH, intracerebral hemorrhage, trauma, and intracranial aneurysm. Other causes include vascular malformations, tumors, and infection.

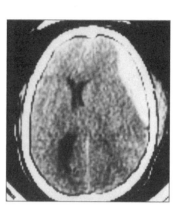

Figure 3. Acute epidural hematoma. (From Waclawik AJ, Sutula TP: Neurology Pearls. Philadelphia, Hanley & Belfus, 2000, p 101.)

Management:

- CT without contrast is the weapon of choice for imaging head bleeds.
- Lumbar puncture is generally contraindicated because it can lead to herniation and death, especially with intracerebral bleed.
- High-resolution four-vessel cerebral angiography is the best modality to show aneurysm.
- Consult neurosurgeon to clip an aneurysm or radiologist to insert coil. The neurosurgeon may elect to insert a shunt.
- *After* clipping an aneurysm, give **triple H** therapy to treat vasospasm: induced **h**ypertension, **h**emodilution to improve cerebral blood flow, and **h**ypervolemia (maintenance of high normal circulating blood volume). Hyperventilation is good for lowering ICP, but excessive amounts can precipitate vasospasm.
- Consider dexamethasone (Decadron), mannitol, furosemide (Lasix) for lowering ICP.
- Do frequent neurologic checks.
- Treat the underlying cause of the bleeding.

Pitfalls:

- Do not neglect seizure prophylaxis.
- Do not neglect SIADH, which occurs frequently.
- Do not neglect pulmonary edema, which is common after SAH (presumably neurogenic).
- Do not neglect cardiac dysfunction (also neurogenic).
- Do not neglect to watch for rebleeding, the most dreaded complication.

Transient Cerebral Ischemia

Presentation: similar to stroke, but symptoms last less than 24 hours and usually less than 10 minutes. Risk factors include hypertension, obesity, smoking, old age, diabetes, and hyperlipidemia. Oxygen is briefly cut off to the brain.

Management:

- CBC, international normalized ratio (INR), partial thromboplastin time (PTT), and BMP are basic lab tests.
- Assess proteins C and S, erythrocyte sedimentation rate if you are worried about hypercoagulability or hematologic cause.
- Chest x-ray and ECG are reasonable upon presentation in this patient population because the risk factors are similar to those for heart attacks.
- An immediate CT of the head is essential.
- Give heparin, then warfarin. Enoxaparin (Lovenox), 1 mg/kg $\times$ 12 hours, is an excellent approach until INR reaches therapeutic level.
- Start aspirin and ticlodipine for prophylaxis.
- Find the cause. Ataxia suggests the vertebrobasilar system, and carotid disease presents frequently with unilateral visual loss. Angiography or carotid Doppler ultrasounds may be helpful. Vascular surgery may be warranted.
- Consider echocardiogram if an embolus is suspected.

Pitfall:

- Do not neglect to treat risk factors; remember that hypertension is the major cause of strokes. Consider a statin, glucose control.

Cerebrovascular Disease

Presentation: stroke and transient ischemic attack constitute the spectrum of impaired blood supply to the CNS with focal neurological deficits.

Management:
- Control the risk factors.
- Risk factors are hyperlipidemia, hypertension, smoking, diabetes, advanced age, and male sex.
- Also under consideration are C-reactive protein, homocysteine, and fibrinogen.

Pitfall:
- Failure to thoroughly check the heart and renal function. If the patient has disease in the head, he or she has it in the heart and other vasculature as well.

Cerebral Embolism and Thrombosis

Presentation: can be caused by atrial fibrillation, ischemic cardiomyopathy, myocardial infarction, artificial heart valves, endocarditis, myxoma, fat emboli, or septal aneurysm.

Management:
- Mind the ABCs.
- Get CBC and other basic lab tests.
- Start anticoagulation with heparin if platelet count is high enough.
- Consider thrombolytics.
- For hypercoagulability work-up, assess proteins C and S, factor V Leyden, and antithrombin. Inform the lab that you have started heparin and/or warfarin.
- Get an ECG, which may show atrial fibrillation.
- A transthoracic echocardiogram may show vegetations or a hole in the heart and help find a cardiogenic source.
- Get D-dimer and Doppler ultrasounds of the legs to rule out deep venous thrombosis and/or ventilation/perfusion (V/Q) scan if you suspect pulmonary embolism as the cause of the embolism/thrombus.

Reye Syndrome

Presentation: child with fever after taking aspirin; usually after viral infection. Symptoms include nausea, vomiting, fever, lethargy, stupor, or coma, often followed by convulsions. Wild delirium and restlessness often are noted. Reye syndrome affects brain, liver, and kidneys.

Management:
- Liver panel: Abnormal levels of aspartate aminotransferase and alanine aminotransferase strongly suggest a diagnosis of Reye syndrome. Bilirubin is usually elevated.
- CT with contrast is important to exclude other possibilities.
- Metabolic panel: elevated blood urea nitrogen and creatinine.
- Coagulation profile: INR is usually increased because liver synthesis of factors is decreased.
- Admit to ICU and monitor carefully. Treat acidosis, electrolyte abnormalities.
- Treat elevated ICP and seizures as needed.
- Treat bleeding with fresh frozen plasma and vitamin K

Pitfalls:
- Do not overhydrate with fluids; overhydration can increase cerebral edema. Use albumin instead.
- Do not forget to order dialysis if electrolyte or ammonia levels become too high.

Migraine

Presentation: bilateral or unilateral headache, classically preceded by aura. Most patients have a positive family history; women are three times as likely as men to have migraines. Triggered by sleep, hunger.

Management:

- Prophylaxis: atenolol, amitriptyline, methysergide, cyproheptadine, valproic acid.
- Abortive therapies: clonidine, nifedipine, NSAIDs, sumatriptan with or without caffeine, meperidine, rest in dark and quiet room
- Consider giving metoclopramide (Reglan) in ED with 1 liter of normal saline to abort migraine.

Pitfall:

- Do not overlook other neurological problems, such as subarachnoid hemorrhage, meningitis.

Convulsions

Presentation: violent, involuntary contraction/spasm caused by epilepsy or sudden illness. Most common examples are benign febrile convulsions that persist for 3 months to 5 years and brief fits with jerky movements of arms and legs, lasting less than 10 minutes

Management:

- Ask about family history of febile seizures.
- Position patients on their front with neck extended.
- Cool the patient.

Headache

Presentation:

	Presentation
Tension	More common in women. Usually chronic and bilateral with neck muscle rigidity. Occurs later in day, waxes and wanes. Give NSAIDs.
Migraine	See section above devoted to migraine.
Cluster	More common in men. Unilateral headache that can last days and occurs over periods of months. Give indomethacin, prednisone or verapamil.
Other	May be associated with benign causes such as menstruation, caffeine withdrawal, or may be sign of serious illness with dreadful prognosis.

Management:

- Detailed history and physical exam are the keys to management.
- Do not overlook meningitis, tumors, temporal or giant cell arteritis, or head injury.
- Look for environmental exposure (e.g., chemicals such as carbon monoxide).

Abnormal Involuntary Movement

Presentation: dystonia, tremor, chorea, myoclonus, and tics.

	Presentation
Tardive dyskinesia	Psychiatric patient presents with orofacial tremor; the patient may be taking dopamine antagonists.
Chorea gravidarum	Pregnant Caucasian woman in early 20s presents with abrupt, brief, nonrhythmic, nonrepetitive movements of limb and facial grimaces.

Management:

- Tardive dyskinesia occurs in up to 15% of patients taking antipsychotic drugs. Changing to a new atypical agent may be warranted (e.g., clozapine, risperidone).
- Ask about what aggravates the symptoms; emotional stress and chorea gravidarum are linked. Symptoms subside with sleep. Treat with haloperidol (Haldol) or benzodiazepines. Symptoms generally subside with delivery.

Pitfalls:

- Do not recommend abortion for chorea gravidarum; it is not warranted.
- Do not make a diagnosis without ruling out other possible neurologic causes.

Coma

Presentation: patient delivered to ED with no information and loss of consciousness.

Management:
- Mind the ABCs.
- Immobilize spine, start IV line.
- Order CBC, and assess arterial blood gases, cultures, glucose, CMP, blood urea nitrogen, calcium, liver enzymes, ammonia, prothrombin time, and activated partial thromboplastin time. Order blood type/cross-match.
- Order toxicology screen.
- Give thiamine, dextrose, naloxone, and oxygen.
- Flumazenil is not recommended as empirical therapy because it may induce status epilepticus. It should be used only if the coma is clearly due to benzodiazepines.
- Now assess eyes, verbal and motor response.
- Once the patient is stabilized, get CT of head immediately.
- Dilated, unilateral, fixed pupil = high likelihood of uncal herniation. You need to lower intracranial pressure with hyperventilation, mannitol, and steroids. Uncal herniation may also be visible on CT.
- Consider lumbar puncture unless the patient has midline shift or mass lesion on CT. If meningitis is found, start broad-spectrum antibiotics immediately.
- Treat underlying cause when lab results arrive. Differential diagnosis of coma is summarized by the mnemonic **AEEIOU TIPPS**: **a**lcohol encephalopathy, **e**pilepsy, **e**lectrolytes, **i**nsulin, **o**piates, **u**remia, **t**rauma, **i**nfection, **p**oisoning, **p**sychiatric disorder, **s**yncope/stroke.

GENERAL ISSUES

Mental Retardation

Presentation: more common in boys than girls; tends to occur in poverty. Causes include congenital hypothyroidism, fetal alcohol syndrome, and genetic factors such as fragile X syndrome and Down syndrome.

Management:
- Get social support.
- Treat depression. Bupropion (Wellbutrin) is a good choice, especially with attention deficit/hyperactivity disorder (ADHD).

- Treat ADHD, which occurs frequently in mental retardation, with methylphenidate (Ritalin).
- Treat self-injury, aggression with risperidone (Risperdal), haloperidol (Haldol).
- Prevent it with education about alcohol use in pregnancy, genetic testing; check the mother's thyroid level, order screening test for phenylketonuria.

Pitfalls:

- Do not assume that patients with mental retardation cannot make decisions. They can if they are over 18.
- Do not fail to find genetic cause, which may be helpful to other family members.
- Do not assume that patients with mental retardation cannot lead a useful life. Step 3 question is likely to concern counseling to parents about the child's future.

MR	IQ	Prognosis
Mild	55 to 70	Educable
Moderate	40 to 54	Trainable
Severe	25 to 39	Nontrainable
Profound	< 25	Nontrainable

Myasthenia Gravis (MG)

Presentation: women in young adulthood and men in old age; presenting symptoms include ptosis, diplopia. Step 3 may show CT of thorax with thymus tumor and ask indirect question about MG. Antibodies against acetylcholine nicotinic receptors are usually present. MG is also associated with thymus tumors.

Management:

- Give edrophonium test. Edrophonium leads to dramatic improvement in muscle weakness in less than 1 minute. Then you have your diagnosis.
- Neostigmine or pyridostigmine is used for long-term maintenance. Both are longer-acting cholinesterase inhibitors.
- Order CT of the thorax to look for thymus tumor. Consider surgical removal of thymus.
- Consider prednisone or cyclosporine to reduce the autoimmune component of the illness.
- Plasmapheresis and immunglobulins are also effective.
- Add beta-agonist inhalers to treat the bronchospasm and respiratory distress caused by the cholinesterase inhibitors.

Pitfalls:

- Failure to maintain the airway. MG can lead to respiratory crisis due to muscle weakness.
- Watch out for sludge caused by cholinergic crisis from treatments.
- Do not miss MG effects in newborn due to vertical transmission from mother. Watch for floppy infant.

Neuropathies/Neuralgia/Neuritis

Presentation: alcoholic or diabetic patient with sensory changes in feet. Diabetics may also have impotence, swallowing difficulties. Neurogenic pain may be presenting symptom. Carpal tunnel syndrome is linked to hypothyroidism and amyloidosis.

Management:

- Do a complete history and physical exam with attention to drinking habits, neurologic exam. Glove-and-stocking pattern is consistent with diabetic neuropathy. Ask about heavy metal (arsenic, mercury, lead) and insecticide exposure. Do not forget infections: shingles, polio, tetanus, leprosy, or Guillain-Barré syndrome.

- Basic metabolic profile should include electrolyes, TSH, vitamin B12, folate levels.
- HgBA1C should also be considered for diabetics.
- Look for antinuclear antibody if you suspect autoimmune cause. Erythroycyte sedimentation rate is a marker of systemic illness.
- If you suspect porphyria, check for aminolevulinic acid synthase in urine.
- Give tricyclic antidepressants such as amytriptyline for neurogenic pain. Topical capsaicin is effective also.
- Trigeminal neuralgia or sciatica pain may require stronger medications.
- Give GI motility agents (e,g., metoclopramide) if needed.
- Give bethanechol for genitourinary problems.
- Treat the underlying cause. Dysfunction of peripheral or autonomic nerves is due most commonly to diabetes, uremia, hypo/hyperthyroidism, liver failure, vitamin B12/folate deficiencies, or nerve compression. Amyloidosis and monoclonal gammopathies should also be in your differential diagnosis.

Pitfalls:
- Do not forget to watch for asymptomatic myocardial infarction due to autonomic dysfunction.
- Do not neglect foot ulcers.
- Do not forget that folic acid may mask signs of vitamin B12 deficiency for macrocytic anemia but will not prevent nerve damage, Make sure that you supplement both together.

Sleep Disturbances

Presentation: hypersomnia and insomnia are the most common.

Management:
- The history is your best tool. Ask whether patient has difficulty with getting to sleep, waking up frequently, or staying asleep.
- Encourage good sleep hygiene: use the bed only for sex and sleep, go to bed at regular time, wake at regular time, avoid naps.
- Ask patient and spouse about snoring. If sleep apnea is suspected, recommend sleep study or overnight oximetry. You may also recommend weight loss, continuous positive airway pressure (CPAP), or ENT surgery.
- Advise patients that as we age, we get less deep sleep. This change is normal.
- Patients with fibromyalgia show changes in stage 4 sleep. Look for a graph on the test showing the stages of sleep and tertiary question.
- Primary hypersomnia or narcolepsy is treated with amphetamines or methylphenidate (Ritalin).

Pitfalls:
- Do not encourage dependency on drugs.
- Do not ignore sleep apnea; it can be deadly.
- Be sure to watch out for "narcoleptics" attempting to get stimulants.

Aphasia

Presentation: loss of the ability to communicate verbally or use written words. It is a symptom, not a diagnosis.

Management:
- Do detailed mental state examination.
- Order CT of head to look for acute changes in first 48 hours.
- Get MRI of head after 48 hours.
- Give speech therapy.

- Stroke, head injury, dementia, multiple sclerosis, and Parkinson disease should be in your differential diagnosis. Board favorites are Broca's aphasia, which is due to frontal lesions associated with right-sided weakness, and Wernicke's aphasia, which is a temporal lesion.

Psychalgia

Presentation: This is the most frequent somatoform disorder and involves only one area.

Management:
- Schedule regular appointments with a physician designated as case manager.
- Keep a positive, optimistic attitude.
- Excessive testing should be avoided.
- Avoid making promises about abolishment of symptoms.
- Avoid establishing dependency in patients.

Syncope and Collapse/Ataxia

Presentation: A transient loss of consciousness that resolves on its own.

Management:
- You need to establish the cause. First do a thorough history and physical exam. Syncope may be cardiac in origin, with a sudden drop in systemic vascular resistance; other causes include hypovolemia, CNS hemorrhage, and seizure.
- Get vital signs, check oxygen saturation, establish volume status.
- Basic lab tests may rule out simple hypoglycemia or electrolyte disturbance.
- Check the heart for regurgitation/stenosis, failure, arrhythmias, or heart block. Syncope in cardiac patients carries a poor prognosis in the Framingham study. Get chest x-ray, ECG, echocardiogram.
- Syncope can be secondary to vasomotor instability, autonomic failure, or vasodepressor/vasovagal response. Do tilt-table and orthostatic exams.
- EEG, CT, and MRI can rule out neurologic origin.

Cause	Presentation	Prognosis	Workup	Intervention
Orthostatic autonomic	Warmth, nausea, flushed	Good usually	Orthostatics, tilt-table	Dangle legs when getting up, volume expansion
Cardiovascular	Usually sudden	Poor	ECG, echocardiogram with or without carotid Doppler	Pacemaker, valve replacement
Neurologic	Seizure, transient ischemic attack	Moderate	MRI, CT, EEG	Depends
Psychiatric		Good		

Correct answers to sample questions:

Sample question 1: E is the correct answer. Immigrants, elderly people, and southern African Americans are the groups least likely to have been immunized.

Sample question 2: A is the correct answer.

Sample question 3: A is the correct answer.

Sample question 4: A is the correct answer.

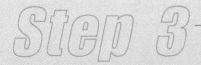
Nonspecific Symptoms

Chest pain
Fever of unknown origin
Malaise and fatigue
Abnormality of gait
Lack of normal physiological development
Septic shock/systemic inflammatory
  response syndrome/sepsis

Allergy
Chronic pain
Malignant neoplasm, unspecified site
Secondary malignant neoplasm, other sites
Palliative care
Abnormal weight gain
Abnormal weight loss

Chest Pain

Presentation: may be related to cardiac, chest wall, pleural, or reflux disorders.

Management:

- You must immediately separate life-threatening from minor causes.
- Evaluate the patient's risk factors in each organ system.
- Get a chest x-ray to look for pneumonia, pneumothorax, wide mediastium (aortic dissection).
- Rule out heart attack with ECG and cardiac enzymes.
- Consider pulmonary embolism in patients with high risk of deep venous thrombosis (DVT), and get CT chest, VQ scan, D-dimer level.
- Intramuscular ketorolac (Toradol) can relieve costochondritis/chest wall pain.
- Be aware that nitroglycerin can relieve esophageal spasm, clouding the diagnosis.
- When in doubt, do complete cardiac workup to rule out MI/ACS.

Fever of Unknown Origin

Presentation: infections account for 35% of cases, neoplasms for about 25%, collagen vascular diseases for about 20%, and other causes for about 20%.

Management:
- Get a good history, including recent travel (malaria) and exposure to humans (TB), animals, insects.
- On exam feel for lymph node enlargement.
- Order CBC with manual differential and smear.
- Panculture blood and urine; order a chest x-ray.
- Consider echocardiography to rule out vegetations in heart; you may also hear new murmur.
- Consider abdominal CT to rule out abscesses.
- Consider tagged white blood cell scan.
- Consider bone scan to rule out osteomyelitis.

Malaise and Fatigue

Presentation: Malaise is a vague feeling of illness/discomfort. Fatigue is feeling weak or tired and lacking energy. Middle-aged women are much more likely to present with chronic fatigue symptoms.

Management:
- Ask about sleep patterns, work schedules, timing of fatigue, exercise.
- Look at patient's medications; some are classic for causing tiredness.
- Evaluate for depression/sadness.
- Consider sleep apnea as cause of excessive daytime sleepiness.
- Get CBC and look for anemia.
- Check thyroid function as well as CMP for electrolytes and glucose.
- Consider autoimmune process and assess antinuclear antibody, Rh factor.
- Do not neglect to consider HIV or other infectious process.
- Consider evaluating cardiac function for congestive heart failure.

Abnormality of Gait

Presentation: can result from neurological or orthopedic problem.

Management:
- Is the abnormality acute or chronic? The patient may be having a stroke.
- Get lab tests to evaluate for electrolyte abnormality, thiamine deficiency.
- Do complete neurologic exam.
- Do complete musculoskeletal exam, focusing on the hips.
- Consider CT or MRI of head as indicated.

Lack of Normal Physiological Development

Presentation: failure to thrive; a child who is below the expected growth curve for height and weight.

Management:
- The first step is to establish that patient nutrition is adequate.
- Ask about diarrhea and vomiting to establish whether food is being absorbed and digested.
- Get routine lab tests such as CBC with differential, CMP, urinalysis.
- Consider cystic fibrosis, and get sweat chloride test if needed.
- Never forget to consider neglect as a possible reason for lack of growth.
- In an older child, consider checking growth hormone levels.
- Look at the parents to evaluate whether the patient is truly underdeveloped or simply comes from a genetically "small" family.

Septic Shock/Systemic Inflammatory Response Syndrome/Sepsis

Presentation: fever or hypothermia with temperature > 38°C or < 36°C. Tachycardia, tachypnea, white blood cell count high or low (>12,000 or <2,000), and/or left shift/bandemia. Usually caused by bacterial infection.

Management:
- Mind the ABCs.
- Give oxygen and intubate if needed.
- Start fluids and bolus in hypotensive patient.
- Get blood, urine, and sputum cultures.
- Start broad-spectrum antibiotics such as cefepime, ceftriaxone, or piperacillin/tazobactam.

- Start pressors/inotropes if the patient remains hypotensive, especially after a lot of fluid is given. Tailor to patient need. Dopamine, a mixed vasoconstrictor/inotrope, is the first choice of most house officers. Dobutamine is mostly inotropic, and norepinephrine (Levophed) is mostly vasoconstrictive.
- Have an arterial line inserted to monitor blood pressure more accurately. An arterial line facilitates easy and frequent readings of arterial blood gases.
- Order an arterial blood gas analysis.
- Consider Swan-Ganz catheter for better monitoring of wedge pressure.
- Move patient to the MICU.
- Monitor for disseminated intravascular coagulation by checking platelets, D-dimer, fibrin degradation products (FDPs), antithrombin III.
- Give blood, platelets.
- Make sure a Foley catheter is in place and monitor urine output.
- Get chest x-ray to watch for acute respiratory distress syndrome and volume overload.
- And, of course, try to locate the source of infection.

Allergy

Presentation: ranges from rash to anaphylaxis. Patients can be allergic to dyes used in radiology, bee stings, antibiotics, or even foods.

Management:
- Management depends on the severity of the reaction.
- Mind the ABCs in anaphylaxis, as usual. Bear in mind that intubation may be difficult if the airway is swollen.
- Epinephrine treats bronchospasm and hypotension in anaphylaxis.
- Breathing treatments with racemic epinephrine may be enough in a patient who is starting to react to a medication.
- Give histamine blockers such as diphenhydramine (Benadryl). Ranitidine, an H2 blocker, may also be useful because about 15% of histamine receptors may be H2 receptors outside the GI system.
- Steroids are not a bad choice at this time.
- Admit and monitor.
- You may need to continue epinephrine drip in ICU.
- Allergic skin testing or serum RAST may be useful in the future to discover cause of the reaction.
- Patients may need to carry Epi-Pen if, for example, they are found to be allergic to bee stings.
- If the patient is allergic to an antibiotic, densensitization may be possible, especially for penicillin, if it is absolutely needed in the future.

Chronic Pain

Presentation: a very broad spectrum, including somatic, visceral, neuropathic, or ischemic causes of pain.

Management:
- Take a detailed history. What work-ups have been completed in the past? What makes the pain better? What makes it worse?
- Most chronic pain is undertreated in the U.S. due to physician worries about legal implications.
- Treat the cause.
- Consider physical therapy, occupational therapy, exercise.
- Consider amitriptyline or gabapentin (Neurontin) for neurogenic pain.
- TENS electrodes can be used for arthritis.
- Consider nerve blocks.
- Consider intrethecal pain killers.
- Treatment involves pain medications that may or not be opioid in nature. Oxycodone is a long-acting opioid. Some physicians, especially surgeons, use fentanyl for their patients.

Malignant Neoplasm, Unspecified Site

Presentation: tumor that is malignant and tends to spread to other parts of the body. Presentation may be ill-defined, but keep the common causes of cancer in mind when managing the patients presented on Step 3. Look for uncommon presentations of the common.

Most common cancers in descending order of occurrence	
Men	Prostate, lung, colon/rectal, bladder, non-Hodgkin's lymphoma
Women	Breast, lung, colon/rectal, corpus/uterus, ovary

Secondary Malignant Neoplasm, Other Sites

Classic Secondary Malignant Neoplasms	
From breast	Bone, brain, GI, lung, liver
From melanoma	Small bowel, skin, brain, bone, lung, liver, eye
From lung	Bone, liver, adrenals, kidney, brain
To bone	Breast, lung, thyroid, testes, kidney, prostate
To brain	Lung, breast, skin, kidney, GI
To liver	Colon, stomach, prostate, breast, lung
To lung	Metastases from everywhere

Palliative Care

Presentation: enhanced quality of life in terminal condition. The goal is to make the patient as comfortable as possible.

Management:

- Pain control is essential. In the U.S. this aspect of palliative care is woefully neglected because physicians fear giving too many narcotics.
- Treat dyspnea with oxygen.
- Treat agitation, depression, anxiety, grief. Patient may request euthanasia, but you should seek to alleviate depression and other psychological issues.
- Treat nausea, vomiting, seizures.
- Consider hospice care so that patient can be with family.
- Treat spiritual needs of patients with visits from clergy.

Abnormal Weight Gain

Presentation: usually caused by imbalance between activity and food intake, but some medical conditions and medications can contribute.

Management:

- Rule out hypothyroidism, Cushing syndrome, other metabolic causes.
- Does the patient have ascites, congestive heart failure, kidney failure, or liver failure?
- Is the patient pregnant? Weight gain certainly should be expected, and pregnancy may be a surprise.

- Screen for depression.
- Review medications, focusing on prednisone, antidepressants, and birth control pills. Remember that megestrol (Megace) is a progesterone used to treat anorexia. Do not be too surprised by weight gain in Depo-Provera users.
- Prader-Willi syndrome and Angelman's syndrome are classic causes of hyperphagia, but their presentation is not likely to be acute.
- Polycystic ovarian syndrome frequently is associated with obesity.

Abnormal Weight Loss

Presentation: weight loss when the patient is not trying to lose weight.

Management:

- Does the patient have anorexia nervosa (AN)? This is a hot topic. Look for a young women from an affluent home. Physicians' children have the highest incidence of AN.
- Is malignancy involved? Look for other risk factors, and order the appropriate tests.
- Does the patient have tuberculosis or some other infection? An HIV/AIDs work-up may be justified.
- Is the patient a new diabetic? Get a glucose level.
- Is the patient hyperthyroid? Order a TSH level.
- Is the patient depressed? Patients can either overeat or not eat when depressed. Screen with **SIGECAPS**: **s**leep, **i**nterest, **g**uilt, **e**nergy, **c**oncentration, **a**ppetite, **p**sychomotor status, **s**uicidal ideation.
- Is the patient anxious or highly stressed? Did the patient just start residency/medical school?
- Consider drugs, especially cocaine, amphetamines, pseudoephedrine. You will never meet a fat crack addict.

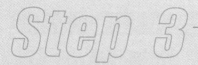

CHAPTER 15

Obstetrics

ANOMALIES
  Chromosomal anomalies
  Congenital anomalies

ISSUES RELATED TO PREGNANCY
  Adolescent pregnancy
  Abortion
  Fetal demise
  Ectopic pregnancy
  Eclampsia
  Other complications of pregnancy
  Third-trimester bleeding
  Complications of labor/delivery
  Cesarean delivery
  Multiple fetuses
  Delivery and labor with minor or no
    complications

Supervision of normal pregnancy
Single live birth before admission to
  hospital

POSTNATAL ISSUES
  Fetal growth retardation
  Post-term infant
  Birth trauma
  Respiratory problems after birth
  Hypocalcemia
  Conditions specific to the perinatal
    period
  Congenital infections
  Hemolytic disease due to Rh
    isoimmunization
  Perinatal jaundice
  Feeding problems in newborns

ANOMALIES

Chromosomal Anomalies

Anomaly	Etiology	Presentation
Aneuploidy	Monosomy X or trisomy	First-trimester loss
Down syndrome	Trisomy 21	Older mother Palmar crease Cardiac defects Early Alzheimer's disease Low-set ears, slanted eyes
Edward syndrome	Trisomy 18	Severe mitral regurgitation Small mandible Index finger overlapping third finger

continued

Chromosomal Anomalies (*continued*)

Anomaly	Etiology	Presentation
Patau syndrome	Trisomy 13	Rocker-bottom feet Severe mitral regurgitation Deafness
Turner syndrome	XO	Short with webbed neck Infertilify Amenorrhea
Cri-du-chat	Chromosone 5 deletion, short arm	Severe mitral regurgitation Catlike cry
Klinefelter syndrome	XXY	Tall Lack of secondary sex characteristics Infertility

Congenital Anomalies

Anomaly	Presentation	Management
Tracheoesophageal fistula (TEF)	Respiratory distress Excess oral secretions Air in GI tract on x-ray	Put baby in head-up prone position for sleeping and eating Repogle tube to suction Surgical division and closure of TEF and anastomosis of esophagus
Duodenal atresia	Emesis after feeding Double bubble on x-ray	Surgery
Congenital diaphragmatic hernia	Respiratory distress Shift of heart sounds and loss of breath sounds on one side Scaphoid abdomen	Intubate and ventilate Extracorporeal membrane oxygenation for pulmonary hypertension Repogle tube to decrease GI distention Muscle relaxants Surgical repair
Omphalocele	Abdominal viscera herniates through umbilical wall into sac	C-section to prevent rupture Usually requires staged surgical repair
Gastroschisis	Polyhydramniosis	Nasogastric tube to suction Cover with gauze Surgery
Cleft lip and/or palate	Persistent labial groove Maldevelopment of palate	Surgical repair at birth for lip At 12–24 months for palate

Management:

- Cardiac abnormalities and neural tube defects are the most common congenital defects.
- Caudal regression syndrome/sacral agenesis is mostly related to maternal diabetes.
- Also watch for shoulder dystocia from brachial plexus injury in macrosomia.
- See Congenital Anomalies of the Heart and Congenital Musculoskeletal Disorders.

ISSUES RELATED TO PREGNANCY

Adolescent pregnancy

Presentation: patient under 19 years old.

Management:

- Adolescents have a much higher risk of having serious medical complications such as toxemia, pregnancy-induced hypertension, significant anemia, premature delivery, and/or placenta previa compared with women in their 20s.
- Infants born to teens are much more likely to have low birth weight due not only to prematurity but also to intrauterine growth retardation during pregnancy.
- Counsel about lifestyle choices: smoking, alcohol, and drugs should be strongly discouraged. Good nutrition should be encouraged.

Abortion

Presentation	Cause	Management
First trimester	Usually fetal cause: abnormal karyotype	D&C if product of conception not passed
Second trimester	Usually maternal cause: uterine duplication/septum, cervical incompetence, gestational diabetes, sepsis (pyelonephritis), no prenatal care	Resection of uterus Cervical cerclage
Septic abortion	Botched abortion	IV gentamicin and clindamycin, then D&C

Fetal Demise

Demise	Presentation
Early	Lack of growth of fundus
Late	Lack of movement

Management:

- Fetal demise can be caused by gestational diabetes mellitus, anomalies, pregnancy-induced hypertension, cord problems, uteroplacental problems (insufficiency secondary to intrauterine growth retardation is common), antiphospholipid syndrome, trauma.
- Frequently cause is not known but may be undiagnosed sepsis. Watch for sepsis (i.e., pyelonephritis, urinary tract infection) and get culture with sensitivity. Also get CMP with liver enzymes.
- Get panel for disseminated intravascular coagulation, which may occur after fetal demise.
- Proceed with
  - □ D&C in first trimester
  - □ D&E in second trimester or possibly labor management with oxytocin (see below)
  - □ Labor management with oxytocin or prostaglandin E2 in third trimester, depending on mother's health

Ectopic Pregnancy

Presentation: amenorrhea, abdominal pain, and (sometimes) vaginal bleeding.

Management:

- Major risk factors include prior history of ectopic pregnancy and pelvic inflammatory disease.
- Get both urine and serum beta human chorionic gonadotropin (bHCG), urinalysis, complete blood count.
- Is the patient stable?
- Rupture may require IV fluids, blood. Get to the OR!
- Get a transvaginal ultrasound, and expect not to find a gestational sac.
- Surgery is done by laparoscopy or laparotomy. On the CCS section of Step 3 make sure you order this procedure specifically. Consult obstetrician, and also order the procedure.
- Methotrexate can be used in **early** ectopic pregnancy.
- RhoGAM should be given if the mother is Rh-negative.
- Follow up with serial bHCG levels.

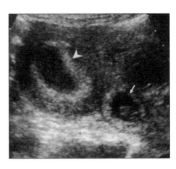

Figure 1. Ectopic pregnancy. (From Paspulati RM, McElro TM: Ectopic pregnancy. In Dogra V, Rubens DJ (eds): Ultrasound Secrets. Philadelphia, Hanley & Belfus, 2004, p 77.)

Eclampsia

Presentation	
Preeclampsia	Hypertension, 1+ proteinuria Also may present as HELLP syndrome: hemolysis, elevated liver enzymes, and low platelets
Eclampsia	Hypertension, proteinuria, edema, *and* convulsions

Management:

- Obtain pregnancy history; most likely to present in first pregnancy.
- Does the patient have chronic hypertension, renal problems, or diabetes? These conditions predispose patient to preeclampsia/eclampsia.
- Observe as outpatient only for mild chronic hypertension:
  - Bed rest on left side
  - Frequent follow-up
- Observe as inpatient in more severe cases
  - Do ultrasound, nonstress test, biophysical profile, basic lab tests.
  - Then give hydralazine or labetalol for hypertension. Atenolol can be continued on outpatient basis.
  - Bed rest on left side
- After 36 weeks, move to prompt delivery!
  - Give magnesium sulfate to prevent convulsions.
  - Give hydralazine or labetalol for hypertension.
  - Try to induce labor with prostaglandin 2 or oxytocin. The newest drug is misoprostol (Cytotec) per rectum.
  - Move to C-section, especially if the mother's condition is deteriorating.
- Hypertension related to preeclampsia/eclampsia will resolve with pregnancy, although chronic hypertension will persist.

Other Complications of Pregnancy

Complication	Presentation	Management
Anemia	Hemoglobin <10	Iron and folate
Cholestasis	Itching from build-up of bile salts	Cholestyramine Avoid fatty foods
Deep venous thrombosis	Tenderness in legs Usually postpartum	Heparin only *No warfarin* (birth defects)
Gestational diabetes	Fasting blood sugar over 90 at 28 weeks	Insulin only *No oral agents*
Urinary tract infections	Urgency, frequency, burning Can be asymptomatic in pregnancy	Simple: nitrofurantoin Pyelonephritis: admit and start cephalosporin IV

Third-trimester Bleeding

Cause	Presentation	Management
Placenta previa (most common cause)	Placenta implants over the cervical os; presents with painless third-trimester bleeding	Get ultrasound to diagnose C-section (depending on presentation)
Bloody show	Bloody mucus plug ejected from cervix before labor begins	Continue with delivery
Abruptio placentae	Premature separation of a normally implanted placenta from the uterus; presents with third trimester bleeding, pain, and hyperactive contractions	Diagnose with ultrasound Watch for disseminated intravascular coagulation Induce delivery as soon as possible
Vasa previa	Fetal vessels cross the membranes over cervix; presents with fetal bleeding with fetal tachy- cardia followed by bradycardia as fetal vascular volume is depleted	Get Apt test to figure out whether the blood is fetal or maternal C-section

Management:

- Mind the ABCs for patient stability.
- **Never** do pelvic exam with fingers or speculum until you do ultrasound. You do not want to cause severe hemorrhage.
- Do Apt test to figure out if blood is fetal or maternal. This test is **not** in the CCS accepted orders but may be encountered in the MCQs.
    □ Pink = fetal hemoglobin
    □ Yellow/brown = adult hemoglobin

Complications of Labor/Delivery

Complication	Presentation	Outcome	Management
Premature rupture of membranes (PROM)	Amniotic fluid leaks and turns nitrazine paper blue with ferning pattern under microscope	1. Sepsis 2. Preterm 3. Respiratory distress in fetus 4. Fetal death 5. Retinopathy	> 36 weeks: induce delivery or do a C-section Preterm 24–35 weeks: bed rest, ampicillin, steroids < 24 weeks: induce labor for safety of mother
Preterm delivery	<37 weeks Contractions Cervical dilation	1. Prematurity 2. Respiratory distress in fetus 3. Fetal death 4. Retinopathy	Slow down labor with magnesium sulfate, terbutaline, nifedipine Give steroids for underdeveloped fetal lungs
Postdates	> 42 weeks	Macrosomia Placental insufficiency	Induce with oyxtocin Suction meconium generously

Cesarean Delivery

Presentation: late deceleration of fetal heart tones.

- Failure to follow normal labor curves is most common reason to perform C-section. Nonreassuring fetal heart tones (especially late deceleration) may require emergent C-section.
- Low segment transverse incision is most common.
- Latest guidelines from American College of Obstetricians and Gynecologists:
  - Vaginal birth after C-section (VBAC) is generally not recommended anymore.
  - But with transverse incision, VBAC may be attempted only when emergency care is immediately available with obstetric supervision.
  - Vertical incision VBAC is absolutely contraindicated in any case due to rupture risk.

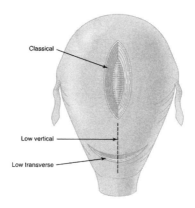

Figure 2. Incisions for cesarean delivery. (From Chmait RH, Moore TR: Obstetric procedures. In Hacker NF, Moore GJ, Gambone JC (eds): Essentials of Obstetrics and Gynecology, 4th ed. Philadelphia, Elsevier Saunders, 2004, p 254.)

Multiple Fetuses

Presentation: women receiving therapy for infertility frequently present with multiple fetuses. Otherwise twins are most common example.

Management:
- Watch for fundus to be larger than dates would indicate with very high levels of serum alpha-fetoprotein (AFP) and bHCG. Get ultrasound.
- The more fetuses, the greater the risk to the mother of eclampsia, hemorrhage, anemia, and preterm labor.
- Multiple fetuses are likely to suffer more from growth restriction, early placental separations, malpresentation, and uteroplacental insufficiency.
- Premature delivery is the most common problem in any instance of multiple fetuses.
- Watch for twin-twin transfusion in twins sharing placenta; one twin gets less blood and is smaller.

- For delivery of twins
  - ☐ Cephalic/cephalic presentation = vaginal delivery
  - ☐ Cephalic/breech presentation = C-section recommended
  - ☐ Breech/cephalic presentation = C-section mandated

Delivery and Labor with Minor or No Complications

Stages of Labor

Stage	Presentation	Friedman Rules
First latent	Regular uterine contractions and cervical dilation from 0 to 3 cm	20 hours (nulligravida) 14 hours (multigravida)
First active	3 cm to 10 cm dilation of cervix	Approximately 1 cm per hour
Second	10 cm dilation to delivery of fetus	$1/2$ hour to 3 hours (nulligravida with epidural) Under $1/2$ hour (multigravida) Add 1 hour if epidural in place
Third	Delivery of fetus to delivery of placenta	Under $1/2$ hour

Cardinal Movements of Labor

Movement	Presentation
Engagement	Fetal head to pelvic inlet plane
Descent	Fetus down birth canal
Flexion	Chin to chest
Internal rotation	Head rotates from transvere to anteroposterior (in birth canal)
Extension	Chin away from chest
External rotation	Head rotates from anteroposterior to transverse position (outside mother)
Expulsion	Body of fetus leaves mother

Management:
- Be aware of the stages of labor.
- Monitor fetal heart tones (FHTs) and uterine contraction patterns in relation to FHTs every 15 minutes until second stage.
- Get fetal scalp pH with any worrisome patterns. If pH is under 7.2, go to immediate C-section.

Presentation	Prognosis	Management
Early deceleration	Normal	No worries; indicates head compression
Variable deceleration	Can be concerning	Get fetal scalp pH; indicates cord compression

continued

Presentation	Prognosis	Management
Late deceleration	Worrisome	Change mother's position first; then C-section. May indicate utero-placental insufficiency
Loss of variation	Worrisome	Get fetal scalp pH and immediate ultrasound of head stimulation

Management:
- Oxytocin can help with weak contractions.
- Prostaglandin E2 can ripen the cervix.
- Give epidural anesthesia in most cases for pain.
- Episiotomy can be considered to avoid traumatic tears, but not always predictable.
- Use of forceps if not below +2 station (i.e., mid or high forceps) involves high risk. Vacuum assist is similar. Use only with decelerations (late) in second stage.

Supervision of Normal Pregnancy

Presentation: 9 months with normal growth pattern/weight gain.

Management:
- Initiate prenatal care:
  - Take history family, number of pregnancies, GP TPAL (gravida para, total premature abortion live-births), outcomes.
  - Get patient to stop using cigarettes, alcohol, caffeine.
  - Folate and iron supplementation (if anemic) should be started ideally before pregnancy.
  - Counsel regarding diet.
  - Screen for psychosocial issues such as domestic abuse, which can be triggered by pregnancy.
  - Check for hepatitis B surface antibody and immunize before conception or after delivery.
- First visit after conception:
  - Get a Pap smear, urinalysis, and CBC.
  - Check blood type and Rh type.
  - Check for syphilis and rubella as part of partial TORCH screen.
  - If history merits, check HIV status as well.
- At 4 months/16 weeks:
  - Triple screen/AFP: low = Down syndrome, fetal demise; high = neural tube defects.
- At 6 months/24 weeks:
  - Check for diabetes with glucose tolerance test.
- Near term (8 months/36 weeks):
  - Get group B streptococcal culture; give ampicillin if positive.
- Urinary tract infections are common in pregnancy; be aware!
- Listen for fetal heart tones using Doppler after 10 weeks' gestation.
- Measure the uterine size from the symphysis pubis to top of fundus
  - At 20 weeks fundus is at umbilicus.
  - From 20–35 weeks fundal height = weeks of gestation.
  - Do ultrasound with any discrepancy from expected pattern.
- Expect weight gain of 15–35 lbs. If the mother is obese already, she should be expected to gain a little less weight.
- Watch for postpartum hemorrhage.
  - Usually caused by uterine atony due to too much magnesium sulfate or multiple gestations. Treat with massage, oxytocin, methylergonovine maleate.
  - Other causes include lacerations, retained placenta, uterine inversion.

- Watch for postpartum fever.
  - Usually due to atelectasis, urinary tract infection.
  - Wound infections present with obvious wound signs/symptoms such as spiking fevers.
  - Endometritis presents with fever, uterine tenderness. Treat with clindamycin and gentamicin. This can become a pelvic abscess, which can be diagnosed with CT and requires surgery.
  - Septic pelvic thrombophlebitis is associated with spiking fevers and no response to antibiotics. Treat with heparin.
  - Mastitis presents with unilateral breast pain. Ampicillin is usually given with or without I&D.
- After delivery lochia is normal for a few days.
  - Rubra = red for 3 days
  - Serosa = pink for weeks 1–2
  - Alba = white after week 2
  - If lochia becomes smelly, suspect endometritis.
- Some cramping is normal after delivery. NSAID is recommended.
- Give stool softeners for constipation and hemorrhoids, which are common. Recommend sitz baths.
- Give RhoGAM within 3 days of delivery if the mother is Rh-negative and the baby is Rh-positive.
- If the mother is not immune to rubella (based on titers), now is the time to update rubella status with vaccine. Advise the mother not to become pregnant again for 3 months.
- Recommend a contraceptive. Progestin is used frequently because it does not interfere with breast milk production. Ordinary estrogen-containing oral contraceptives reduce milk production.
- Encourage breast-feeding.
- Watch for postpartum depression. Most psychiatric problems diminish during pregnancy but are accentuated in the postpartum period. Symptoms may present prior to delivery. Does the patient have a psychiatric history?

Single Live Birth Before Admission to Hospital

Presentation: women delivers baby in automobile on way to hospital.

Management:
- See postpartum issues above.
- Risk of sepsis is increased.
- Make certain that there is not a twin lurking within.
- Perineal tears may need to be repaired.
- Placenta may not have been fully delivered; consider ultrasound.
- Mother may not have gotten proper prenatal care; be especially alert for possible congenital infections such as herpes, syphilis, hepatitis B, tuberculosis.

POSTNATAL ISSUES

Fetal Growth Retardation

Presentation: size under 10th percentile.

	Cause
Maternal	Smoking
	Poor nutrition
	Adolescent
	Maternal small vessel disease in type 1 diabetes
	Lupus
Placental	Hypertension/preeclampsia
Fetal	Congenital defects
	Infections

Management:
- Make certain that dates are accurate before assuming this diagnosis.
- Use consecutive ultrasound exams to measure biparietal diameter, head circumference, abdominal circumference, and femur length.
  □ If these are symmetric (decreases in biparietal diameter, head circumference, abdomen circumference and femur length), fetal growth potential will be diminished, and the insult was probably early in pregnancy.
  □ If asymmetric (only abdomen circumference is decreased), the insult occurred later and the outcome is likely to be normal.
- Watch for oligohydramnios with too little fluid; the cause may be intrauterine growth retardation.
  □ < 5-cm pocket delivery
  □ < 7 cm biophysical profile

Post-term Infant

Presentation: delivered after 42 weeks.

Management:
- Make sure that dates are accurate.
- Watch for macrosomia with large baby that causes trauma during delivery, including damage to brachial plexus.
- Be aware that placenta can become insufficient and deprive the fetus of oxygen and lead to meconium aspiration.
- Watch for hypoglycemia.

Birth Trauma

Trauma	Injury	Presentation	Management
Shoulder dystocia	Brachial plexus injury/ Erb-Duchenne palsy, and fractured clavicle	Absent Moro reflex; cannot abduct arm, externally rotate upper arm, or supinate forearm	Supportive care generally, although nerve grafting is a possibility

continued

Birth Trauma (*continued*)

Trauma	Injury	Presentation	Management
Forceps delivery	Cephalohematoma	Subperiosteal hemorrhage	Get CT Should resolve
Vaginal birth	Caput succedaneum	Head deformation and soft tissue injury	No treatment needed
Vaginal birth	Clavicle fracture	Most common in vaginal birth due to entrapment under pubic symphysis, usually on right side	No treatment needed

Respiratory Problems After Birth

Presentation: premature infant with tachypnea, cyanosis in first 3 hours of life.

Management:
- Lecithin:sphingomyelin ratio will be under 2.0 in the amniotic fluid, and there will be no phosphatidylglycerol. Check ratio.
- Give steroids to the mother before birth to accelerate surfactant production, if possible.
- Get chest x-ray. Expect to find ground-glass pattern on air bronchograms.
- Give artificial surfactant.
- Respiratory support is the main management. Try to keep FiO_2 as low as possible because high oxygen damages the retinas and leads to chronic lung disease.

Hypocalcemia

Presentation: tetany from DiGeorge syndrome presents in this context.

Management:
- DiGeorge syndrome consists of multiple defects.
- Congenital heart defects are to be expected, and the thymus is missing.
- Hypocalcemia is due to missing parathyroids.
- See Hypocalcemia in Endocine chapter; give calcium.

Conditions Specific to the Perinatal Period

Condition	Presentation	Management
Biliary atresia	Jaundice in week 2–3; HIDA scan shows no excretion to intestine	Hepatoportoenterostomy
Hirschsprung disease	Males with abdominal distention	Surgery
Hypoglycemia	Presentation of gestational diabetes most commonly ranges from lethargy to seizures	IV dextrose Glucagon Steroids
Intussusception	Currant jelly stools, sausage mass	Barium enema

continued

Conditions Specific to the Perinatal Period (*continued*)

Condition	Presentation	Management
Meconium aspiration	Tachypnea, hypoxia, hypercapnia	Oxygen and ventilation
Meconium ileus	Cystic fibrosis	None specific
Mongolian spots	Transient macules on back	Do nothing; normal
Necrotizing entercolitis	Bilious vomiting, abdominal distention with pneumatosis intestinalis on x-ray	Orogastric tube IV antibiotics Urgent exploratory laparotomy
Neonatal sepsis	Symptoms of respiratory distress syndrome such as grunting, cyanosis; fever >100.5°F	Ampicillin and gentamicin
Respiratory distress syndrome	Premature baby with lack of surfactant	Respiratory support; artificial surfactant

Congenital Infections

Infection	Presentation	Management
Toxoplasma gondii	Hydrocephalus, retinitis, jaundice	Pyrimethamine with sulfadiazine
Rubella	IUGR, cataracts, deafness, blueberry muffin rash	
Cytomegalovirus	IUGR, retinitis, deafness, anemia	
Herpes simplex virus II	Retinitis, microcephaly	Acyclovir
Varicella-zoster virus	Retinitis microphthalmia cataracts	Acyclovir
Syphilis	Snuffles, condylomata lata, keratitis, other bone and CNS maladies	Penicillin
HIV	Failure to thrive, frequent infections	Zidovudine, IVIG, trimethoprim-sulfamethoxazole

IUGR = intrauterine growth retardation, IVIG = intravenous immunoglobulin.

Hemolytic Disease Due to Rh Isoimmunization

Presentation: mother is Rh-negative but baby (and father) are Rh-positive.

Management:
- This condition will not occur in nulliparous mother because prior sensitization is required. Abortions count as prior parity, and mother is at risk.
- If both mother and father are Rh-negative, there is no risk.
- Give Rh IgG (RhoGAM) to prevent this problem at week 28 and 3 days after delivery or after any procedure such as amniocentesis. If you fail to give RhoGAM appropriately, there is no "make-up" schedule.

- At birth immediately get umbilical cord blood and test it for ABO/Rh type, hemoglobin levels, serum bilirubin, peripheral smear, and direct Coombs' test.
- Watch infant for erythroblastosis fetalis/fetal hydrops with hemolytic anemia, cardiac failure, edema/ascites, pericardial effusion, and jaundice.
- Note on fetal monitor sinusoidal rhythm.
- Get exchange transfusion if indicated by the above tests.

Perinatal Jaundice

Presentation: ranges from mild physiologic jaundice to kernicterus with seizures.

Management:
- Measure total, direct, and indirect bilirubin.
- Normal physiologic jaundice peaks at 12–15 on the third day of life and returns to normal in 2 weeks
- Breast milk jaundice can develop; if so, the infant should be switched to formula.

Feeding Problems in Newborns

Presentation:

Cause	Presentation
Allergy	Eczema, wheezing, feeding aversion
Colitis	Anemia, bloody stools
Malabsorption	Diarrhea, abdominal distention
Colic	Inconsolable crying late in day; infant draws knees to abdomen

Management:
- Feeding intolerance can lead to food aversion; allergy/intolerance to cow milk is most common type.
- A baby should feed every 1–2 hours.
- It is normal for baby to lose 10% of birth weight over 3 days, but it will be regained by week 2.
- It is best to recommend breastfeeding only during first 6 months of life.
- A trial of soy protein should be attempted in infants with suspected milk allergy.

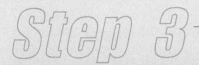
Ophthalmology

ANTERIOR
- Pterygium
- Cataract
- Glaucoma
- Acute conjunctivitis
- Disorders of eyelids/lacrimal system
- Corneal abrasion
- Orbital cellulitis

NEURO-OPHTHALMOLOGY
- Visual disturbances
- Diplopia
- Visual field defects
- Diseases of optic nerve/visual pathways
- Strabismus
- Anomalies of pupillary function
- Nystagmus

POSTERIOR
- Ophthalmologic manifectations of diabetes
- Retinal detachments
- Retinal defects and disorders
- Chorioretinitis
- Macular degeneration

ANTERIOR

Pterygium

Presentation: patient with great deal of sun exposure.

Management:
- Counsel to avoid sun exposure.
- Surgery if central cornea is invaded.
- Be aware it can induce astigmatism.

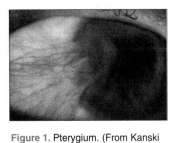

Figure 1. Pterygium. (From Kanski JJ: Clinical Ophthalmology: A Synopsis. Boston, Butterworth Heinemann, 2004, p 55.)

Cataract

Presentation: Loss of red reflex, loss of visual acuity, glare, monocular diplopia. Three possibilities: nuclear cataract, cortical cataract, or posterior subcapsular cataract. Cataracts can be congenital but usually present as senile cataracts.

Management:

- Identify risk factors: female sex, estrogen, cortisol, diabetes, and trauma. High risk after lightning strikes.
- Surgery is definitive correction. The surgery available today is elegant and the most commonly performed surgical procedure in the U.S.

Glaucoma

Presentation: blurry vision, halos around lights, pain, headache. African-Americans at highest risk.

Management:
- Can result from increased production or decreased drainage of aqueous humor.
- Open angle: primarily managed with medications, including miotics, beta-adrenergic blocking agents, and carbonic anhydrase inhibitors.
- Closed angle: generally treated with medications; laser iridectomy may be used.
- More aggressive surgical intervention includes trabeculoplasty, cyclophotocoagulation, and filtering.
- Acute angle closure is an emergency; give acetazolamide + pilocarpine + timolol immediately.

Acute Conjunctivitis

Presentation: redness and discharge.

Management:
- Nongonococcal: trimethoprim/polymyxin B, qid for 7 to 10 days.
- Neonatal gonococcal: ceftriaxone, 25 to 50 mg/kg IM.
- Neonatal chlamydial: erythromycin ethylsuccinate, 50 mg/kg/day PO.

Disorders of Eyelids/Lacrimal System

Presentation: Stye is the most common disorder seen by GP and relevant to Step 3.

Management:
- Warm compresses.
- Baby shampoo to lid margins.
- Will need ophthalmologist to drain if it does not go away in 2–3 days.

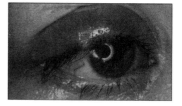

Figure 2. External hordeolum (stye). (From Kanski JJ: Clinical Ophthalmology: A Synopsis. Boston, Butterworth Heinemann, 2004, p 12.)

Corneal Abrasion

Presentation: patient working under car gets foreign body in eye. Most common eye problem that a GP or emergency physician is likely to encounter.

Management:
- Apply topical anesthetic.
- Do complete eye exam with visual acuity, funduscopy, anterior chamber.
- Do fluorescein exam with orange fluorescein dye strip. Darken room and use cobalt blue; look for scratch to fluoresce green.
- Remove foreign bodies.
- Evert the lids to look for hiding foreign body.
- Irrigate eye.
- Use erythromycin, tobramycin for antibiotic coverage.
- Small abrasion need not be covered. Large or deep abrasions should be patched with the eye taped shut.
- Use oxycodone, ibuprofen, naproxen for pain.
- Arrange ophthalmologic follow-up within 24 hours.

Orbital Cellulitis (Ophthalmic Emergency)

Presentation: swollen lids, fever, swollen conjunctiva, proptosis.

Management:

1. Hospitalize; infection can spread to brain.
2. Begin IV antibiotics immediately: nafcillin + cefotaxime + metronidazole.
3. IV antifungals possibly needed.
4. Surgical drainage if infection does not resolve with medical treatment in 48 hours.

Pitfall:

■ Dilly-dallying.

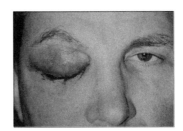

Figure 3. Orbital cellulitis. (From Gault JA: Ophthalmology Pearls. Philadelphia, Hanley & Belfus, 2003, p 67.)

NEURO-OPHTHALMOLOGY

Visual Disturbances

Presentation: can result from defects in nervous system from cornea to retina to brain.

Management:

■ History and physical exam: ask about duration of visual loss or changes, one or both eyes, trauma, prior episodes/ophthalmologic history. Review of systems: photophobia, headache, pain. Ask about hypertension, hypercholesterolemia, collagen vascular disease, hematological disorders, cancer, family history.
■ Pinhole test can rapidly establish cause as anterior: lens or cornea.
■ Ophthalmologic examination with Snellen visual acuity and visual fields.
■ Ophthalmologic consultation for dilated examination.
■ Do not miss retinal detachment.

Visual Disturbances Neurologic Etiology	Presentation
CN3	Down and out
CN4	Gaze medial; cannot look down
CN6	Cannot look lateral
CN5	Tear, blink
CN7	Closed eye

Diplopia

Presentation: double vision, ghosting

Management:

■ If it resolves when one eye is covered, the cause is probably neurological.
■ If it persists in one eye when the other is covered, the cornea is probably at fault; consider getting corneal topography.
■ Ask about history of refractive surgery; may be induced astigmatism.

Visual Field Defects

Defect	Location	Cause	Imaging	Management
Monocular	Retina, optic nerve	Optic neuritis, tumor, vascular	MRI, carotid Dopplers	Steroids, surgery
Bitemporal	Chiasma	Pituitary tumors	MRI or CT	Bromocriptine, surgery
Homonymous hemianopia	Optic tract Lateral geniculate Optic radiations Occipital cortex	Vascular, tumor Vascular Stroke PCA stroke	MRI MRI MRI MRI	Surgery if tumor Anticoagulation if stroke
Homonymous quadrantanopia, disconjugate	Optic radiations	MCA stroke	MRI	Anticoagulation
Homonymous quadrantanopia, conjugate	Occipital cortex	PCA stroke	MRI	Anticoagulation
Sudden bilateral blindness	Occipital cortex	Psychiatric	MRI to rule out organic cause	Psych consult

Diseases of Optic Nerve/Visual Pathways

Presentation: Optic neuritis is associated with multiple sclerosis. Compressive optic neuropathy is another possibility that is usually caused by tumors. Sarcoidosis is also possible.

Management:

- Look for ethambutol, isoniazid, and amiodarone in history—all can cause toxic optic neuropathy.
- Angiotension-converting enzyme is elevated in sarcoid.
- TSH to rule out thyroid ophthalmopathy.
- MRI is essential to figure out what is really going on.
- Orbital ultrasound may be useful, but MRI is still needed.
- Steroids are the first choice generally for most causes of compression, but treat the underlying cause.
- Surgical decompression is definitive but not without its risks.

Strabismus

Presentation: Deviation of the alignment of one eye in relation to the other. More common in pediatric patients. In adults look for diabetes, stroke, brain injury, Guillain-Barre syndrome, botulism.

Management:

- Pediatric ophthalmologist should correct strabismus because it can lead to amblyopia, which is permanent vision loss. This is the most serious outcome of not intervening.
- Glasses, eye muscle exercises may be prescribed.
- Amblyopia requires patching of the "good" eye to force the child to use the amblyopic eye.
- Surgery may be required to realign eye muscles.

Anomalies of Pupillary Function

Presentation: physiologic anisocoria, Horner syndrome, oculomotor (CN III) nerve palsy, tonic pupil, iris damage

Management:

- Rule out serious underlying cause. For example, uncal herniation indicates CNIII palsy, Horner syndrome may herald carotid dissection. Do not miss vision-threatening iritis.
- Miosis, anhydrosis, and ptosis are classic signs of Horner syndrome. Cocaine will not dilate affected side.
- CNIII palsy presents with blown Hutchinson pupil. Look for other global neurological defects.
- Physiologic anisocoria is a diagnosis of exclusion, present in up to 20% of population. Look for less than 1 mm difference in light and dark, with no other associated problems.

Nystagmus

Presentation: periodic rhythmic ocular oscillation of the eyes. Causes include Ménière disease, drug/alcohol toxicity.

Management:

- Neuroimaging (MRI) if you cannot attribute nystagmus to the above or if other neurologic focal deficit is present.
- Warm water in the same ear produces a horizontal nystagmus directed to the same side as the water. The mnemonic is **COWS**: **c**old—**o**pposite, **w**arm—**s**ame. If this sign is not present, there is a vestibular defect.
- You can use muscle relaxants, anticonvulsants, even botox for treating nystagmus.

Pitfalls:

- Missing a tumor causing the nystagmus.

POSTERIOR

Ophthalmologic Manifestations of Diabetes

Presentation: microaneurysm proceeds to dot-and-blot hemorrhages, neovasculization, and macular edema. These signs tend to manifest after 15 years of diabetes.

Management:

- Ophthalmologist must be seen yearly.
- Fluorescein angiography is invaluable for better imaging of the retina.
- Lifestyle modifications: glucose control, control of hypertension, smoking cessation.
- Laser treatment can prevent further visual loss.

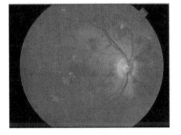

Figure 4. Neovascularization of disc and elsewhere, dot-and-blot hemorrhages, and hard exudates. (From Gault JA: Ophthalmology Pearls. Philadelphia, Hanley & Belfus, 2003, p 121.)

Retinal Detachments

Presentation: floaters, flashes, "curtain"; most common in high myopes, over 50 years old, patients with history of injury or positive family history. Three categories: rhegmatogenous, exudative, and tractional.

Management:

- Prompt surgical intervention is needed. Options include scleral buckle, pneumatic retinopexy, and vitrectomy.

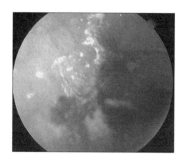

Figure 5. Tractional retinal detachment. (From Borne MJ: Retinal detachment. In Vander JF, Gault JA (eds): Ophthalmology Secrets, 2e. Philadelphia, Hanley & Belfus, 2002, p 362.)

Retinal Defects and Disorders

Disorder	Presentation
Central retinal artery occlusion	Usually emboli
Central retinal vein occlusion	Associated with hypertension, diabetes, and glaucoma, "blood and thunder fundus"
Retinitis pigmentosa	Gradual degeneration of the rods and cones. Usually begins with night blindness and progresses to loss of peripheral vision

Chorioretinitis

Presentation: Exudative inflammatory process. For Step 3, think of HIV/AIDs with viral or protozoan origin.

Management:
- If the cause is cytomegalovirus, ophthalmologist may perform surgical implant of ganciclovir.
- Consult infectious disease specialist and treat underlying illness.
- TB or toxin also may be the cause, in which case you should use antibiotics and steroids.

Macular Degeneration

Presentation: lines looking bent, blind spots, decreased central vision.

Management:
- Eliminate controllable risk factors, encourage healthy lifestyle choices. Risk factors are age, white race, smoking, hypertension, vascular disease, fatty diet, being hyperopic, UV light.
- Use Amlser grid to diagnose macular degeneration.
- Ophthalmologist may elect to utilize fluorescein or indocyanine green angiography.
- For wet macular degeneration, photodynamic therapy is used. Give IV light-activated verteporfin (Visudyne), then laser the abnormal vessels.

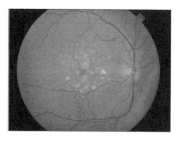

Figure 6. Nonexudative ("dry") macular degeneration. (From Gault JA: Ophthalmology Pearls. Philadelphia, Hanley & Belfus, 2003, p 219.)

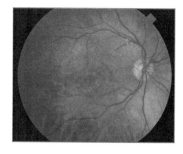

Figure 7. Exudative ("wet") macular degeneration. (From Gault JA: Ophthalmology Pearls. Philadelphia, Hanley & Belfus, 2003, p 137.)

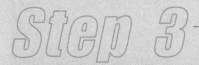

CHAPTER 17

Otolaryngology

ISSUES RELATED TO THE EARS
  Diseases of ear and mastoid process
  Otitis media
  Otitis externa/disorders of tympanic
    membrane
  Vertiginous syndromes
  Otalgia
  Hearing loss

ISSUES RELATED TO THE NOSE, SINUSES,
AND THROAT
  Streptcoccal sore throat
  Acute upper respiratory tract infection
  Chronic rhinitis
  Allergic rhinitis
  Peritonsillar abscess
  Diseases of the nasal cavity
  Acute sinusitis
  Chronic sinusitis

ISSSUES RELATED TO THE ORAL CAVITY
  Herpetic gingivostomatitis
  Disorders of the teeth and jaw

MALIGNANCY
  Malignant neoplasm of larynx
  Malignant neoplasm of lip, oral cavity,
    pharynx

ISSUES RELATED TO THE EARS

Diseases of Ear and Mastoid Process

Presentation: acute otitis media untreated with antibiotics, pain behind the ear. Inflammatory process of the mastoid air cells in the temporal bone.

Management:
- Give IV antibiotics such as ceftriaxone to improve condition; then perform myringotomy.
- If myringotomy fails, perform mastoidectomy.
- Check for hearing loss.
- Watch for CNS spread.

Pitfall:
- Failure to manage complications such as meningitis.

Otitis Media

Presentation: pain, nausea, vomiting, bulging tympanic membrane (TM). Typically caused by streptococci, *Hemophilus influenzae* B, or *Moraxella* sp.

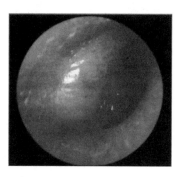

Figure 1. Acute otitis media. (From Yellon RF, McBride TP, Davis HW: Otolaryngology. In Zitelli BJ, Davis HW (eds): Atlas of Pediatric Physical Diagnosis, 4e. Philadelphia, Mosby, 2002, p 829.)

Management:

- Give amoxicillin (or trimethoprim-sulfamethoxazole) as front-line antibiotic.
- Then give high-dose amoxicillin.
- The second-line antibiotic is ceftriaxone (Rocephin).
- Give analgesics.
- If eardrum perforates, do not panic; this complication is common. Add ciprofloxacin or gentamicin eardrops. Instruct patent to wear earplug and keep out water. Follow-up needs to be more aggressive.
- ENT specialist must perform tympanocentesis if antibiotics fail.

Pitfalls:

- Failure to diagnose meningitis.
- Failure to diagnose mastoiditis.

Otitis Externa/Disorders of Tympanic Membrane

Presentation: ear pain, exposure to water. Most commonly caused by *Pseudomonas aeruginosa*.

Management:

- Examine the ear. Otitis externa is very painful. Patient may resist examination/manipulation of ear.
- Remove exudate from the ear; this is the medium for bacterial growth.
- Send for cultures if you suspect a fungal etiology.
- Insert ear wick.
- Use acetic acid solution on the wick (e.g., VoSol)
- Advise patient to keep ear from getting wet while swimming,
- If the patient is diabetic, he or she may have malignant otitis externa, which can spread to bone. In this case, admit patient to hospital and start IV antibiotics. Use ceftazidime + piperacillin.
- You can switch to ciprofloxacin once symptoms abate. Generally in Step 3 you will be quizzed on the initial choice.

Pitfalls:

- Failure to diagnose malignant otitis externa in diabetics.
- Wiskott-Aldrich syndrome should be suspected in males with recurrent otitis, eczema, and thrombocytopenia.
- Seborrheic dermatitis can masquerade as otitis externa due to scaling in the ear canals.

Vertiginous Syndromes

Presentation: tinnitus, hearing loss, nausea, vomiting. Typically the cause is Ménière's disease, but other causes include multiple sclerosis, cardiovascular and CNS disease.

Management:

- Check for positive Romberg sign. The patient falls over when standing with feet together and both eyes closed.
- Check with Dix-Hallpike maneuver: Move patient from sitting to lying position with head turned to left. Then sit patient up rapidly and move patient to lying position with head turned to right. Watch for nystagmus and vertigo.

- Use Weber or Rinne test to check for associated hearing loss. This finding points to Ménière's disease, acoustic neuroma, drug-induced ototoxicitiy, labyrinthitis.
  - Weber test: apply tuning fork to forehead; ask the patient if it sounds loudest on the right or left. It will sound loudest on side with conductive loss or quietest on side with neurologic loss.
  - Rinne test: apply tuning fork to mastoid and close to external meatus. In normal patient, tuning fork is loudest on external meatus.
- Order lab tests to check for systemic problems: TSH, erythrocyte sedimentation rate, antinuclear antibody, CBC, electrolytes.
- Diuretics, low salt diet, and steroids can reduce endolymphatic pressure.
- Aminoglycosides are ototoxic and can be used for bilateral vestibular disease. This is a last-resort effort to cure intolerable disease that is recalcitrant to therapy.
- Meclizine is the standard vestibulosuppressant.
- Consider MRI for working up other causes.

Pitfall:
- Failure to find a brain tumor or other serious cause of vertigo.

Otalgia

Presentation:

Presentation	Causes
Primary otalgia	Otitis media, mastoiditis, and auricular infections.
Referred otalgia	Dental problem is number-one cause, but consider herpes zoster oticus (Ramsay Hunt syndrome).

Management:
- Look in the mouth; dental problem is prime culprit. Get x-rays of teeth.
- Apply lidocaine to nose, larynx, ear canal, or even inject it into muscles to find trigger points.
- Treat infections with antibiotics; ampicillin is a good choice initially for the usual suspects.

Pitfalls:
- Stopping the pain without finding the cause.
- Do not miss malignancy causing the pain.

Hearing Loss

Presentation: generally conductive or neural.

Management:
- Inspect the ear for blockages (e.g., earwax); ask about objects inserted in ear.
- Ask about associated vertigo.
- Check for hearing loss with the Weber or Rinne test. This points to Ménière's disease, acoustic neuroma, drug-induced ototoxicitiy, labyrinthitis.
  - Weber test: apply tuning fork to forehead; ask patient if it sounds loudest on the right or on the left. It sounds loudest on side with conductive loss or quietest on side with neurologic loss.
  - Rinne test: apply tuning fork to mastoid and close to external meatus. In normal exam it sounds loudest at the external meatus.
  - Audiometry is best diagnostic tool for bilateral loss.

- Look for infection and treat it.
- Ask about exposure to ototoxic drugs.
- Ask about firearms, loud music.
- Consider hearing aid.
- Consider cochlear implant.

ISSUES RELATED TO THE NOSE, SINUSES, AND THROAT

Streptococcal Sore Throat

Presentation: red throat, fever, tender anterior cervical nodes, and no symptoms of viral upper respiratory infection.

Management:
- Inspect the posterior pharynx.
- Swab tonsils and get rapid streptococcal test at least.
- Send for cultures, which may take 1–2 days for incubation and interpretation.
- You have 7–9 days after symptoms appear for prevention of rheumatic fever.
- Antibiotic decision time: if there is an epidemic of streptococcal throat, do not wait for cultures. Definitely look for this judgment question on Step 3.
- Start oral penicillin/amoxicillin. Consider IM ceftriaxone (Rocephin) for noncompliant patients.
- If the patient has an allergy to penicillin, use erythromycin.
- Do not give antibiotics if the cause is not clearly bacterial.
- Recurrent infections merit a cephalosporin.
- To rule out mononucleosis, you can get CBC with differential to look for atypical lymphocytes or order a Monospot test. If you give amoxicillin to a patient with mononucleosis, there is a high likelihood that a rash will develop—and you have your diagnosis.
- Offer symptomatic relief with NSAIDs or anesthetic mouthwash, lozenges.

Pitfall:
- Failure to diagnose epiglottitis, abscesses, gonococcal pharyngitis, myocarditis, or diphtheria, all of which may present as sore throat.

Acute Upper Respiratory Tract Infection

Presentation: runny nose, cough, sore throat.

Management:
- Fever, headache, and myalgia merit acetaminophen and/or ibuprofen. You can alternate doses.
- Decongest with oxymetazoline (Afrin) nose drops for 2–3 days and add systemic pseudoephedrine.
- You may add antihistamines for runny nose.
- For cough suppression, add dextromethorphan or codeine.
- Consider inhaled bronchodilators such as albuterol and inhaled steroids such as beclomethasone.

Pitfall:
- Giving antibiotics for viral illness.
- Failure to diagnose life-threatening epiglottitis. Watch for inspiratory stridor, sitting in the "tripod" position leaning forward.

Chronic Rhinitis

Presentation: unresolved acute sinusitis with nasal stuffiness, postnasal drip, facial fullness, and malaise.

Management:
- X-rays are okay, but CT is the diagnostic tool of choice.
- Functional endoscopic sinus surgery is the curative weapon of choice except in children.
- Medical care is an adjunct to surgery.

Pitfall:
- Do not miss invasive fungal sinusitis (e.g., *Aspergillus, Mucor,* and *Rhizopus* spp.) in immunosuppressed/ diabetic patients. Fungal sinusitis requires a very aggressive and urgent approach.

Allergic Rhinitis

Presentation: polyps, sneezing, allergic shiners, and nasal crease (from wiping nose constantly).

Management:
- Order skin test, RAST to identify allergens.
- Look for high IGE levels on serum protein electrophoresis (SPEP) and eosinophils on CBC with differential.
- Prescribe antihistamines, nasal steroids.
- Attempt desensitization.

Peritonsillar Abscess

Presentation: severe pain with swallowing, fever, holding head tilted toward abscess, and trismus. The tonsil is displaced medially and often displaces the uvula. The soft palate is erythematous and swollen. Also known as quinsy, this is an acute infection located between the tonsil and the superior pharyngeal constrictor muscle.

Management:
- Order CT of neck. A CT is not always needed with classic quinsy. However, you can proceed directly to ENT drainage.
- Definitive treatment is incision and drainage by ENT specialist.

Sample question:

An 18-year-old Caucasian male comes to the ED with persistent tonsillitis after being treated with ampicillin the week before by a physician's assistant at a walk-in clinic. After getting no relief, he paid a second visit to the clinic, where a resident physician who recently passed his Step 3 and was moonlighting at the clinic gave him a third-generation cephalosporin. He now presents at the ED, stating he has no relief from the pain. His temperature is 102°F. He now has difficulty opening his mouth (trismus). and his left tonsil appears enlarged. What is the next most appropriate step?

A. CT of the neck
B. Immediate needle aspiration
C. Admit to hospital and begin IV antibiotics
D. Rapid streptococcal test
E. Monospot test

The correct answer is found at the end of the chapter.

Diseases of the Nasal Cavity

Presentation: swelling nasal septum, drainage of pus.

Management:

- Use incision and drainage for abscess.
- Watch out for osteomyelitis.
- Watch out for deformity of nose since the cartilage is destroyed.
- Watch out for orbital cellulitis, which can occur with swelling and redness around the eyes.

Acute Sinusitis

Presentation: pain in face, bad breath, low-grade fever, tenderness on palpation, purulent discharge from the nose. Often described by the patient as "a cold that won't go away."

Management:

- Help open nasal passages with phenylephrine/oxymetazoline nose drops.
- On physicial exam look for drainage.
- Give systemic decongestant pseudoephedrine.
- If the cause appears to be bacterial, give amoxicillin (or trimethoprim-sulfamethoxazole for penicillin-allergic patients).
- If this is a recurrence, use cephalosporin or Augmentin (amoxicillin/clavulanic acid).
- Give NSAIDs or oxycodone for pain relief.
- Try vapor inhalation.
- Get x-ray and ask for Water's view. Look for air-fluid level and/or opacification.
- Give treatment straightaway *without imaging* if symptoms are classic.

Chronic Sinusitis

Presentation: nasal stuffiness/fullness, postnasal drip, bad breath, and general malaise. Subtle compared with acute sinusitis.

Management:

- Give maximal medical therapy.
- X-ray is okay, but contrast-enhanced CT scan is the standard of care before surgical intervention.
- Bear in mind that neoplasms can present as sinusitis.
- ENT specialist will probably examine the patient endoscopically after CT and get cultures/biopsies.
- Functional endoscopic sinus surgery is the curative weapon of choice except in children.

Pitfalls:

- Do not miss invasive fungal sinusitis in immunosuppressed/diabetic patients (i.e., *Aspergillus, Mucor,* and *Rhizopus* species). This requires a very aggressive and urgent approach.

ISSUES RELATED TO THE ORAL CAVITY

Herpetic Gingivostomatitis

Presentation: fever, general malaise, lymphadenopathy. Oral mucosa red with blisters that burst and then leave ulcers behind.

Management:

- Herpes simplex fever blisters are spread in crowded conditions such as dormitories and prisons and among the urban poor.
- Antivirals are not helpful for the simple disease, but they may help prevent complications.
- Tell patient that blister will last about 1 week no matter what you do.
- Herpes simplex virus can hide in ganglion and reappear with stress—warn the patient.

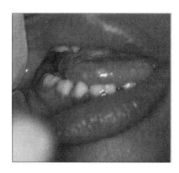

Figure 2. Herpetic gingivostomatitis. (From Davis HW, Michaels MG: Infectious disease. In Zitelli BJ, Davis HW (eds): Atlas of Pediatric Physical Diagnosis, 4e. Philadelphia, Mosby, 2002, p 405.)

Disorders of the Teeth and Jaw

Presentation:

Disorder	Presentation
Caries	Presents as pain generally
Temporomandibular joint (TMJ) disorder	Clicking, headaches, pain, usually in a female patient

Management:

- Prevent caries with oral hygiene, diet, fluoride, sealants, and antibacterial therapy.
- Fix the cavities before infection spreads and requires root canal.
- Recommend orthodontia for crooked teeth.
- For TMJ disorder, conservative treatment begins with soft food, then use of appliance like jaw guard. Surgery is the last resort.

MALIGNANCY

Malignant Neoplasm of Larynx

Presentation: hoarseness, dyspnea, breathy voice, aspiration, dysphagia, pain, otalgia, hemoptysis.

Management:

- Specifically ask about the above symptoms.
- CT is most helpful. It is important for establishing borders.
- Laryngoscopy is essential.
- Radiation therapy is the mainstay of treatment.
- Watch out for cartilage necrosis after radiation.

Malignant Neoplasm of Lip, Oral Cavity, Pharynx

Presentation: look for white spots on gums in someone who smokes or uses snuff.

Management:

- Diagnosis is made with biopsy. Squamous cell carcinoma is the most common malignancy.
- Direct laryngoscopy + bronchoscopy + esophagoscopy are the classic ENT triple play to exclude further neoplasm.
- Treatment is radiation therapy, not chemotherapy. Good prognosis if only the lip is involved.
- Surgery is used for pharynx and can progress to radical resection, jaw removal, and even radical neck dissection—all this for a 5-year survival rate of only 50%.

Pitfall:

- Failure to use triple play (direct laryngoscopy + bronchoscopy + esophagoscopy) to seek out further neoplasm.

Answer to sample question:

The correct answer is A because the patient ended up in ED.

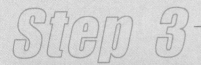

CHAPTER 18

Psychiatry

BEHAVIORAL DISORDERS AND SUBSTANCE ABUSE
- Abuse of other person
- Sexual dysfunction
- Conduct disturbance
- Attention deficit/hyperactivity disorder
- Autistic disorder
- Phobic disorders
- Obsessive-compulsive disorder
- Somatoform disorders
- Eating disorders
- Alcohol-related disorders
- Chemical/drug abuse/dependence

EMOTIONAL DISORDERS
- Schizophrenia
- Paranoid states
- Anxiety disorders
- Post-traumatic stress disorder/acute stress disorder
- Bereavement
- Depressive disorders
- Bipolar disorders

GENERAL ISSUES
- Psychological factors associated with other medical condition
- Personality disorders
- Confusional states
- Postconcussion syndrome

BEHAVIORAL DISORDERS AND SUBSTANCE ABUSE

Abuse of Other Person

Presentation: victim may be elder, child, or domestic partner. Abuse may be sexual, physical, or neglect. Abuse of another person is commonly asked on Step 3.

Management:

- Suspect child sexual abuse if the child has knowledge beyond his/her years, anal/genital trauma, STDs, urinary tract infections. Most sex abusers are male and known to the child.
- Suspect child physical abuse in the presence of bruises, spiral fractures, burns, belt marks. Most physical abusers are female.
- Suspect elder abuse with signs of poor hygiene, bruises, fractures. The most likely abuser is a spouse or caretaker.
- Try to get victim away from abuser to talk in private.
- Do not confront the abuser directly.
- You have a legal obligation to report suspected child abuse but not domestic partner abuse. Also report elder abuse if the victim is mentally impaired.

SAMPLE CCS INPUT—Suspected Child Abuse

Complete exam
Urinalysis
CBC, CMP, coagulation profile
Chest x-ray
For sexual abuse
  Culture rectum, vagina, or penis
  Venereal Disease Research Laboratory (VDRL) test for syphillis (serum)
For physical abuse
  Immediate skeletal survey
  Consult, ophthalmology → retinal hemorrhages
  Change location to ward
  Child protective services consult

Sexual Dysfunction

Presentation: erectile dysfunction (ED), low desire, inability to climax, premature ejaculation.

Management:

- In all cases do a detailed history and physical exam, and ask about aspects of the relationship besides the sexual aspect.
- Ask if this is a new problem or has been lifelong.
- Be alert to other medical problems, especially diabetes in men with ED.
- Ask about all medications.
- Low desire: check hormone levels, especially testosterone in men,
- Erectile dysfunction: can give sildenafil (Viagra) or, if it fails, injectable vasodilators.
- Orgasmic disorder: you may suggest masturbation, vibrators to find effective techniques for stimulation.
- Premature ejaculation: suggest squeeze technique or sensate focus. Selective serotonin reuptake inhibitors (SSRIs) also may be helpful.

Conduct Disturbance

Presentation: Usually in boys: aggressive and cruel behavior to people and animals.

Management:

- Treat coexisting disorders: learning disabilities, attention deficit/hyperactivity disorder, drug abuse, bad environments.
- Enforce appropriate punishments.
- Teach social skills.
- Boys with conduct disturbance (CD) are at high risk to be antisocial and commit crimes as adults. CD in youth is required to give antisocial diagnosis in adult.

Attention Deficit/Hyperactivity Disorder

Presentation: usually a boy before age 7 who cannot focus, is disorganized, cannot sit still. Subtypes are inattentive, hyperactive, and combined.

Management:

- ADHD is a risk factor for future conduct/substance abuse problems.
- Psychological testing of child, parents, and teachers.
- Stimulant therapy is the mainstay of treatment, combined with behavioral treatments.

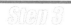

- Methylphenidate, dextroamphetamine are the stimulants of choice. Do not be afraid to use them.
- Bupropion is an emerging choice and is not a controlled substance.
- Atomoxetine (Strattera) is the newest medication and is not a controlled substance.
- Consider drug holidays, especially on summer vacation. These drugs may stunt growth.

Autistic Disorder

Presentation: poor relationships, subnormal IQ, inflexible to environment change. Affects boys more than girls except for Rett syndrome, which mostly affects girls.

Management:

- Do a thorough medical evaluation to rule out medical problems.
- Check for lead poisoning. Consider DNA testing.
- Psychological/neuropsychological testing is needed.
- Consult a speech pathologist and special education teacher.
- Epilepsy is frequent in autistic children; treat for seizure disorder, if needed.

Phobic Disorders

Presentation: fear of snakes or fear of social situation that may be embarrassing. Can be a specific phobia or generalized social phobia.

Management:

- Systematic desensitization is a mainstay of treatment.
- Benzodiazepines and beta blockers may be used for autonomic symptoms.
- MAO inhibitors and assertiveness training can be added for social phobia.
- Be aware of secondary morbidity from social dropout.

Obsessive-Compulsive Disorder

Presentation: a patient who washes hands repeatedly or repeatedly checks locks.

Management:

- Behavioral therapy (e.g., flooding) is a mainstay of treatment.
- Give SSRI or the the tricyclic antidepressent clomipramine (Anafranil).
- Look for eating disorders and depression as well.
- Obsessive-compulsive disorder is associated with Tourette syndrome in relatives.

Somatoform Disorders

Subtype	Presentation
Conversion	Manifests as sudden neurologic symptoms in stress—for example, sudden bilateral blindness
Hypochondria	Excessive worry about health
Somatization	Multiple complaints in multiple systems
Factitious disorder	Deliberately produced/falsified illness for purpose of assuming the sick role (also known as Munchausen syndrome)
Malingering	Complaints to avoid work or get money (i.e., disability checks)

Presentation: symptoms seem to be part of a medical condition, but no organic cause can be found.
Management:

- Make absolutely certain no real medical condition is present.
- Know the criteria for somatization disorder:
  - 4 pain symptoms: head, neck, back, stomach, and limbs
  - 2 GI symptoms: pain, nausea, indigestion
  - 1 sexual (or menstrual) complaint
  - 1 pseudoneurogenic complaint
- Treat underlying depression and anxiety.
- Treat frequent comorbidities of drug and alcohol use.

Eating Disorders

Disorder	Presentation	Management
Obesity	20% over ideal weight. The U.S. is a veritable flabalanche, with an obesity rate of 30%+—and it's getting worse.	Treat with sensible diet and exercise. Phentermine is still used in some cases.
Anorexia nervosa	Look for perfectionist girl from upper-middle class family, especially doctor's child.	Admit immediately if 20% below normal weight. Check for electrolyte abnormalities. Get family therapy.
Bulimia	Anorexia with binge and purge	Look at teeth and hands for signs of self-induced vomiting.

Alcohol-related Disorders

Presentation: spectrum ranges from abuse to dependence.

Management:

- Get routine lab tests. Elevated gamma-glutamyl transferase (GGT) may be a sign of drinking.
- On admission for acute intoxication, give thiamine, folate, and magnesium.
- Give benzodiazepines and diazepam for withdrawal, which can be fatal. Look for withdrawal 72 hours after admission.
- Recommend Alcoholics Anonymous for ongoing support.
- Consider disulfiram (Antabuse) to discourage drinking.

Chemical/Drug Abuse/Dependence

Presentation: abnormal use that leads to impairment of social functioning; dependence characterized by tolerance/withdrawal, compulsive use.

Drug	Management
Nicotine	Give nicotine patch and consider bupropion (Wellbutrin) for helping with cessation.
Marijuana	Benzodiazepines for acute agitation.
Barbituates/benzodiazepines	Flumazenil is an antidote for overdose. Taper benzodiazepines cautiously to prevent seizures in longstanding users.

continued

Chemical/Drug Abuse/Dependence (*continued*)

Drug	Management
Cocaine	Treat cardiac symptoms and seizures, benzodiazepines for agitation, antipsychotics for psychotic symptoms.
Amphetamines	Benzodiazepines for agitation, antipsychotics for psychotic symptoms.
Heroin	For overdose give naloxone. Give methadone for maintenance.

EMOTIONAL DISORDERS

Schizophrenia

Presentation: college age (20s) in males but a bit older (30s) in females; patients tend to be born in winter months with older fathers.

Phase	Presentation	Management
Prodromal phase	Social isolation, may have new interest in religion/philosophy	
Positive symptoms in psychotic phase	Delusion, hallucination, strange behaviors	Respond to most anti-psychotic agents
Negative symptoms in psychotic phase	Flat affect, social withdrawal	Respond a little to atypical drugs
Residual phase	Between psychotic episodes flat affect, taking things personally that have nothing to do with the patient (i.e., TV talks to patient)	

Management:
- Step 3 likely to present a patient in the prodromal phase and ask about the next step in diagnosis or counseling of parents.
  - □ 1% risk in general, 50% for twins, 40% if *both* parents have it, 10% if *one* parent has it.
  - □ Suicide risk is high.
  - □ Disease may stabilize in middle age.
- In acute episode
  - □ First gently try to talk the patient into a calm state.
  - □ Consider chemical sedation.
  - □ Haloperidol is a nice choice for acute psychosis if Step 3 asks you to pick a medication.
- This is a chronic debilitating disease.

- Medically speaking, a lot of what you do as a primary care or emergency physician is to look out for side effects of medications:
  - Excess dopamine may contribute. Haloperidol, chlorpromazine work at this level. Look for "man breasts" and other side effects of increased prolactin.
  - Dopamine and serotonin (the other theory) can be affected by clozapine, but watch for agranulocytosis. Get regular CBCs.
  - Atypical antipsychotics such as risperidone, olanzapine, and quetiapine have the fewest side effects
  - Check electrolytes; hyponatremia is common.
  - Extrapyramidal symptoms include parkinsonlike symptoms, dystonia (young men). Reduce doses and give amantadine, benztropine, diphenhydramine (Benadryl).
  - Watch for tardive dyskinesia, which is characterized by writhing movements of mouth/tongue. Stop the medication and substitute another.
  - Watch for neuroleptic malignant syndrome: rigidity, fever, renal failure. Get creatine phosphokinase (CPK) level. Stop medications, teat with IV fluids and dantrolene.

Paranoid States

Presentation: isolated paranoid delusions with no other features of schizophrenia.

State	Presentation
Paranoid	Distrustful, suspicious; responsibility always belongs to someone else
Schizoid	Voluntary social withdrawal without psychosis. The patient may live alone in a cabin in Montana and is content.
Schizotypal	Magic thinking—odd but not psychotic. Patient likes to walk in the woods and talk to the birds.

Anxiety Disorders

Disorder	Presentation	Management
Panic attacks	Most common in women: tachycardia, shortness of breath, diaphoresis, feeling of dread.	Rule out medical cause such as hyperthyroidism, stimulants/caffeine intake. Start fluoxetine (Prozac) and short-term benzodiazepines for new presentation. Beta blockers are sometimes prescribed. Associated with mitral valve prolapse.
Generalized anxiety disorder	Middle-aged woman with heart palpitations, shortness of breath, stomach pain for at least 6 months.	Start SSRI. Benzodiazepines can be given but may result in dependence.
Adjustment disorders	Anxiety and/or depression to life events that impairs functioning.	Psychotherapy and SSRIs are appropriate.

Post-traumatic Stress Disorder/Acute Stress Disorder

Presentation: symptoms of hyperarousal and withdrawal in survivor of violent crime, terrorist attack

Management:

- Symptoms must last over 1 month for diagnosis of post-traumatic stress disorder; otherwise the diagnosis is acute stress disorder.
- Psychotherapy as soon as possible after traumatic event is first-line therapy.
- SSRIs may be used for depression.
- Beta blockers may be used for autonomic symptoms.

Bereavement

Presentation: loss, actual or symbolic, followed by a period of mourning and grief. On Step 3 look for widow(er).

	Presentation
Normal	Minor weight loss, mild insomnia, guilt about things left undone or unsaid, illusions (briefly seeing the person), sadness. Severe symptoms resolve in 2 months and moderate symptoms within 1 year.
Abnormal	Extreme guilt, hallucinations/delusions, social dropout, suicidal, severe symptoms over 2 months and moderate symptoms over 1 year.

Management:

- Know the stages of loss: denial → anger → bargaining → depression → acceptance.
- Establish that the patient is not suicidal; hospitalize suicidal patients.
- For normal grief give psychological support, benzodiazepines for sleep. SSRIs are not out of the question.
- Abnormal grief: definitely give SSRI, even antipyschotics and electroconvulsive therapy.

Depressive Disorders

Disorder	Presentation
Major depressive episode	Over 2 weeks of depressive symptoms required for this diagnosis, see below
Dysthmia	Chronically depressed mood with occasional episodes of major depression
Seasonal affective	Depressed in winter with reduced daylight
Adjustment disorder	Depression and/anxiety in response to stressor that interferes with function

Presentation: SIGECAPS inventory: **s**leep, **i**nterest, **g**uilt, **e**nergy, **c**oncentration, **a**ppetite, **p**sychomotor status, **s**uicidal ideation. Depressive disorders tend to be more common in women.

Management:

- Establish that the patient is not suicidal.
- Get detailed history; ask patients about:
  - Mood
  - Interest in activities that gave pleasure formerly (e.g., sex, sports)

- Weight loss/gain
- Insomnia/hypersomnia (especially early morning awakening)
- Agitation/slowness
- Fatigue
- Feeling worthless
- Inability to think or concentrate
- Thoughts of death or suicidal ideation
- Especially ask about suicide attempt and specific plan to commit suicide.

- Major depression lasts longer than 2 weeks.
- Give SSRI as front-line drug.
- Wait 2–6 weeks for effect.
- Make certain that the patient is compliant.
- Consider tricyclic antidepressant (TCA) or monoamine oxide inhibitor (MAOI).
- Know the side effects
  - SSRI: GI symptoms, reduced orgasm. Interestingly, in some studies men with premature ejaculation take SSRI to help with this problem.
  - MAO: hypertension, crisis with tyramine foods.
  - TCA: cardiac effects in overdose.
  - Bupropion: seizures.
- Advise physical activity and exercise.
- For patients with seasonal affective disorder (SAD), consider light therapy.

SAMPLE CCS INPUT: Simple Depression

PE complete
CBC, CMP, UA, TSH
Serum ethanol
Urine drug screening
Depression index (this is the actual CCS command)
Sertraline hydrochloride (Zoloft) PO
Refer patient, psychiatry
Suicide contract
Discharge patient to home follow-up 1 month

Bipolar Disorders

Disorder	Presentation
Bipolar I	Mania with major depression
Bipolar II	Hypomania with major depression
Cyclothymia	Hypomania with mild depression

Presentation: the classic presentation is mania with spending spree, hypersexuality, not sleeping. Patients may also be irritable or have psychotic aspects with grandiosity.

Management:

- Take detailed history. Ask about and look for sense of grandiosity/exaggerated self-importance, little need for sleep, excessive or pressured speech, flight of ideas and distractibility, and excessive eating, sleeping, or spending.
- There is a strong genetic component.
- Hospitalize patients who present danger to self or others.
- Lithium is the first-line medication. Check TSH frequently and monitor renal function.
- Carbamazepine is used for "rapid cyclers" (i.e.,quick mood changes). Watch for bone marrow suppression.
- Valproic acid is most effective at stopping manic phase.
- Insight-oriented and cognitive therapy are helpful.

GENERAL ISSUES

Psychological Factors Associated with Other Medical Condition

Presentation	Condition
Depression	Huntington's chorea Pancreatic cancer Multiple sclerosis
Anxiety	Anemia Mitral valve prolapse Cushing's syndrome Pheochromocytoma Pulmonary disease
Mania	Porphyria Multiple sclerosis Systemic lupus erythematosus

Personality Disorders

Disorder	Characteristics	Presentation
Cluster A	Avoids social interaction	Paranoid (blames everyone else for problems) Schizoid (loner) Shizotypal (magic thinking, odd)
Cluster B	Emotional and dramatic	Histrionic (seductive, theatrical) Narcissistic (sense of entitlement) Antisocial (psychotic, no empathy, cruel, criminal) Borderline (impulsive and unstable mood)
Cluster C	Fearful and anxious	Avoidant (sensitive to rejection) Obsessive/compulsive (perfectionistic) Dependent (poor self-confidence; let others make decisions for them)

Management:

- Few treatment options; psychotherapy may have some benefit.
- Step 3 seems to focus on recognition rather than management.

Confusional States

Presentation:

State	Presentation
Delirium	Acute and dramatic onset Frequently caused by illness, toxin Characterized by fluctuating arousal
Dementia	Chronic/insidious Frequently caused by Alzheimer's disease, infarct Usually attention and arousal are normal

Management:

- Get lab tests; check electrolytes, blood counts, and certainly glucose.
- Thiamine, liver function tests, and ammonia levels are not unwarranted.
- Get urine drug screen and alcohol levels in the ED.
- Consider pancultures of blood, urinalysis, chest x-ray.
- Look for neck rigidity, and consider lumbar puncture after CT. Consider empirical treatment for meningitis.
- Ask about exposure to various parasites that can infect the brain.
- Consider CT of the head.
- Consider "banana bag" or rallypack (IV fluids with folic acid, vitamins, electrolytes) for alcoholics to correct thiamine deficiency. Look for ataxia, nystagmus, or Korsakoff memory loss with confabulation.
- Above all, treat the cause of delirium.
- Dementia treatment includes withholding medications that increase dementia.
- See section about about central nervous system for Alzheimer's disease and treatment modalities.

Postconcussion Syndrome

Presentation: depression, anxiety, memory problems, academic difficulties. Athlete suffering from poor performance in school after suffering concussion while playing contact sports

Management:

- This is a controversial topic; be nonjudgmental to patient and family.
- Consider CT/MRI to look for organic defect.
- Prognosis is generally good for patients with symptoms up to 6 months after injury.
- If symptoms persist after 1 year, the patient is not likely to improve.

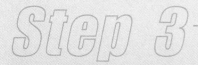

CHAPTER 19

Renal System and Urology

RENAL SYSTEM
- Malignant neoplasm of kidney
- Nephrotic syndrome/nephritis
- Chronic renal failure/insufficiency
- Acute renal failure
- Cystic kidney disease
- Urinary calculus/renal colic/nephrolithiasis

UROLOGY
- Malignant neoplasm of prostate
- Malignant neoplasm of bladder
- Neurogenic bladder
- Urethritis
- Hematuria/urethral stricture
- Enuresis
- Stress incontinence, female
- Symptoms referable to genitourinary system

RENAL SYSTEM

Malignant Neoplasm of Kidney

Presentation: hematuria, flank pain/symptoms of urinary tract infection, mass. Most common form is renal cell carcinoma.

	Etiology
Exposure	Smoking, asbestos, cadmium, trichloroethylene are classic
Hereditary	Von Hippel-Lindau syndrome, in which patient has hemangioblastoma of the eyes and brain/spinal cord, as well as cystic pancreas, pheochromocytoma

Management:
- Hematuria is the first presenting symptom in most cases.
- By the time you have diagnosed it, about 33% of your patients will already have metastases. The lungs are a frequent site of metastasis.
- Watch out for paraneoplastic syndromes manifested by high serum calcium, excess of erythrocytes, and liver dysfunction.

- Get CBC, CMP, liver function tests, erythrocyte sedimentation rate, prothrombin time, partial thromboplastin time, and urinalysis.
- CT with contrast is the test to choose for diagnosis and to look for metastases.
- Consider bone scan to rule out metastases to bone.
- Radical nephrectomy is the standard surgical procedure.
- Follow up with chemotherapy (adjuvant therapy not beneficial for renal cell carcinoma).
- Radiation therapy is palliative in advanced cases.
- Follow up with basic lab tests and CT of the abdomen at regular intervals.

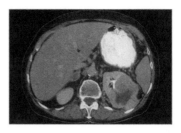

Figure 1. Clear cell renal cell carcinoma. (From Resnick MI, Schaeffer AJ: Urology Pearls. Philadelphia, Hanley & Belfus, 2000, p 80.)

Nephrotic Syndrome/Nephritis

Presentation:

Syndrome	Presentation	Cause
Nephrotic syndrome	Proteinuria, hypoalbuminemia, hyperlipidemia, edema	Numerous causes including diabetes, autoimmune disease, drugs, hepatitis B or C
Nephritis	Hematuria, red blood cell casts, mild proteinuria, hypertension, edema	Poststrepococcal infection is frequent cause.

Management:

- Steroid therapy is the mainstay of treatment.
- Give Lasix for significant edema. Albumin should be considered as well.
- Give statins for hyperlipidemia.
- In all cases restrict protein intake.
- Get international normalized ratio, prothrombin time, and partial thromboplastin time, and be prepared to give anticoagulation for hypercoagulability.
- Specific treatments:

Disease	Presentation	Management
Minimal change disease	Foot process fusion	Prednisone
Membranous nephropathy	IgG/C3 deposits	Prednisone
Membranoproliferative	Hepatitis C	No treatment needed
Idiopathic	RPG postviral	Prednisone
Anti-GBM (including Goodpasture's syndrome)	Glomerulonephritis with rapidly progressive renal failure	Cyclophosphamide and prednisone
Lupus	Azotemia	Prednisone
Wegener's granulomatosis	Upper respiratory symptoms, hemopytsis, ANCA blood tests	Cyclophosphamide and trimethoprim/sulfamethoxazole
Poststreptococcal disease	Strep throat followed by renal failure	No treatment needed

RPG = rapidly progressive glomerulonephritis, GBM = glomerular basement membrane, ANCA = antineutrophilic cytoplasmic antibody.

Chronic Renal Failure/Insufficiency

Presentation:

	Presentation
Chronic renal failure	GFR is under 30 cc/min
Chronic renal insufficiency	GFR is 30-70 cc/min

GFR = glomerular filtration rate.

Management:
- Same factors that cause acute renal failure can lead to chronic renal failure (CRF) or chronic renal insufficiency (CRI). Diabetes and hypertension are the most common causes.
- Early in diabetic CRI you should give maximal dosage of angiotensin-converting enzyme (ACE) inhibitor to protect the kidneys from further damage. Get rid of ACE if the patient has bilateral renal stenosis or single kidney with renal artery stenosis.
- Treat hypertension aggressively.
- Treatment varies, depending on glomerular filtration rate (GFR), but protein, potassium, and magnesium restriction should be considered.
- Treat anemia with erythropoietin. Check CBC and get reticulocyte count to see if erythropoietin is needed.
- In CRF treat hyperkalemia, acidosis, and hypervolemia with regular dialysis.
- Watch for development of secondary hyperparathyroidism due to hypocalcemia.
  - □ Restrict phosphates and give phosphate binder such as calcium acetate (PhosLo).
  - □ Give calcitriol and calcium supplements.
  - □ Remove parathyroids, if needed.
- Consider renal transplant as ultimate treatment.

Acute Renal Failure

Presentation: acute renal failure (ARF) manifests as a rapidly rising creatinine level and a decline in urine output.

Management:
- Hypoperfusion manifests as prerenal azotemia with a blood urea nitrogen (BUN)-to-creatinine (Cr) ratio greater than 15. IV fluids should be given. Give a fluid challenge and follow with Lasix. Sepsis and heart failure can also underperfuse the kidneys.
- If the patient is on an ACE inhibitor, stop it.
- Stop NSAIDs as well.
- Is it obstructive? Insert a Foley catheter in all cases of ARF.
- Does the patient have intrinsic renal failure? Look for history of radiocontrast, aminoglycosides, pigment, penicillin, or sulfa drugs.
- Other causes to consider in renal failure include lupus, Goodpasture's syndrome, Wegener's granulomatosis. Get a urine sample and look for WBCs and RBC casts. Consider tests for antinuclear antibody and antineutrophilic cystoplasmic antibody.
- Patient should be put on low protein and low salt diet immediately.
- Always consider possible dialysis in the presence of severe potassium excess, acidosis, volume overload, hyperuremia.
- Uremia can lead to pericarditis and/or encephalitis.

Cystic Kidney Disease

Presentation:

	Presentation	Management
Autosomal dominant polycystic kidney disease	Adults 30–60 years old Associated with berry aneurysms in the brain Hematuria, dilute urine	Oral water intake, salt restriction Treat hypertension with calcium channel blockers. Get MR angiography to rule out aneurysms in the brain.
Autosomal recessive polycystic kidney disease	High mortality in neonates Older children show growth retardation and liver disease as well.	Treat pulmonary manifestations in the neonate and look for pneumothorax. Consider dialysis.

Management:
- Ultrasound or CT can be used to see cysts.
- Renal carcinoma can also present as cysts.

Urinary Calculus/Renal Colic/Nephrolithiasis

Presentation: extreme flank pain worse than childbirth!

Management:

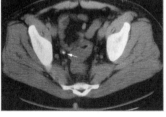

- Get a kidney-ureter-bladder (KUB) study initially and look for stones.
- Spiral CT and intravenous pyelography are considered equivalent for diagnosis of stones that are too small to see on KUB.
- Stones less than 5 mm are likely to pass spontaneously. Patient should attempt to catch the stone (use a coffee filter).
- Stones larger than 5 mm may require percutaneous nephrostomy or stent placement.
- When calculus is in the ureter, cystoscopy can retrieve the calculus, or ultrasonic lithotripsy can be used to break the stone up that the pieces can be easily suctioned out or allowed to come out on their own.

Figure 2. Obstructing right ureteral uric acid calculus. (From Resnick MI, Schaeffer AJ: Urology Pearls. Philadelphia, Hanley & Belfus, 2000, p 71.)

- Patient needs to be hospitalized for severe pain or in the face of associated sepsis/infection.
- Give NSAIDs, acetaminophen (Tylenol), and opioids for pain control.
- Give nifedipine to help relax the ureter, enhancing passage of the stone.
- Give prednisone for swelling in the ureter; prednisone also enhances passage.
- Trimethoprim/sulfamethoxazole or levofloxacin is used to treat infection and prevent possible urosepsis.
- Consider work-up for repeated occurrences. Such stones are usually calcium oxalate, but they may be uric acid, struvite, or cystine and can be detected with 24-hour urine sample for crystals.
- Hydrochlorothiazide can be used to protect against future occurrences of calcium variety.

UROLOGY

Malignant Neoplasm of Prostate

Presentation: often found in elderly men on routine digital rectal exam (DRE).

Management:

- Put on gloves, and insert a finger in the rectum for the DRE. A firm, hard/rocky, asymmetrical prostate definitely should cause concern.
- Get a prostate-specific antigen (PSA) level and correlate with age. PSA rises as the prostate enlarges.
- Look for low level of free PSA in the malignant prostate.
- If the PSA shoots up unexpectedly, even within the age-approprate range, this is also concerning.
- Get a biopsy with use of transrectal ultrasound.
- Get CT of abdomen and pelvis to find metastases.
- Consider bone scan to find metastases.
- If the patient is old, consider watchful waiting without intervention.
- Radical prostatectomy is the most common treatment.
- External radiation therapy or brachytherapy/implants are also used.
- Anti-androgens are implanted commonly.
- Treat impotence, which frequently occurs after surgery.

Malignant Neoplasm of Bladder

Presentation: painless hematuria.

Management:

- Risk factors are smoking, schistosomiasis, dye/rubber/aluminum/leather workers, truck drivers, agricultural/pesticide exposure.
- Urinalysis is the routine first step.
- Intravenous pyelography is also used.
- Cystoscopy with biopsy and cytology gives the most definitive information.
- Chemotherapy is used only if the lesion is superficial to mucosa.
- Transurethral resection of the bladder (TURB) is used if the lesion involves lamina propria only.
- Bladder removal + lymph node dissection + removal of prostate, ovaries, and vaginal wall are used for invasion of muscles and fat.
- Bladder removal with chemotherapy is appropriate if distant metastases are present.
- Recurrence rate is high; cystoscopy and cytology should be done every 4 months.

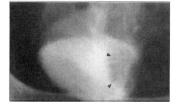

Figure 3. Transitional cell carcinoma of the bladder. (From Resnick MI, Schaeffer AJ: Urology Pearls. Philadelphia, Hanley & Belfus, 2000, p 38.)

Neurogenic Bladder

Presentation: urinary retention or incontinence.

Management:

- Typically caused by CNS tumor, trauma/surgery, Parkinson disease, multiple sclerosis.
- Patients may have detrusor and/or sphincter underactivity or overactivity.
- Get a urinalysis to rule out infection. Look for hematuria. Proceed with cystoscopy and cytology if blood is found in urine. You do not want to miss a malignancy.
- Have the patient keep a voiding diary.

- Voiding cystometrogram is the test to check for obstruction as well as poor contractility of bladder.
- The first step is behavioral changes (i.e., scheduled trips to the bathroom). Restrict fluids after dinner.
- Have patient do Kegel exercises to strengthen the pelvic muscles. This is not the most effective strategy for pure neurogenic bladder and generally is used for stress or mixed incontinence.
- Estrogen increases tone at the urethra and should be considered in some cases.
- Pseudoephedrine tightens the sphincter and may be used for pure sphincter dysfunction.
- Oxybutynin chloride (Ditropan) is used for urge incontinence; it relaxes the bladder.
- Pads may be worn in some cases.
- Catheter options include intra-urethral, "straight" self-catheterization, or suprapubic catheter (more permanent option). In a person with spinal cord injury a suprapubic catheter may be the best option.
- Surgery can be effective in some cases to increase tone or relax bladder.
- Monitor for urinary tract infections.

Urethritis

Presentation: discharge with or without burning.

Management:

- In patients younger than 35 years, assume sexually transmitted disease such as chlamydial infection or gonorrhea.
- In patients over 35, assume *Escherichia coli*, *Klebsiella* sp., or *Ureaplasma urealyticum*.
- Some cases are idiopathic or due to chemical sensitivity.
- Urethritis can progress to cystitis, pyelonephritis, epididymitis, orchitis, or prostatitis.
- Get a triple void urine specimen with initial stream, midstream, and after prostate massage. Expect elevated WBC count in initial stream with gonorrhea.
- Get cultures for gonorrhea and chlamydial organisms.
- Empirical therapy should cover gonorrhea and nongonococcal urethritis without getting these studies if the patient has symptoms—especially if he or she is not likely to return for treatment.
- Ceftriaxone IM and doxycycline PO cover both and can be used empirically. A single dose of azithromycin may be better alternative to 7-day course of doxycycline.

Hematuria/Urethral Stricture

Presentation: trauma in the pelvic area, sexually transmitted diseases, tumors, scar tissue.

Management:

- Did a Foley catheter cause this problem?
- Diagnose by cystoscopy.
- Dilate the stricture if needed.

Enuresis

Presentation: involuntary urination with bedwetting after age 5.

Management:

- Get a history of fluid intake, how often and how much patient voids during the day, how frequently the bedwetting occurs. Suggest that patients keep a diary.
- The patient should void at bedtime every night.
- Make sure that the patient does not have a urinary tract infection or treatable cause.
- Get a urinalysis.
- Get a voiding cystourethrogram if you suspect an anatomic problem.
- Alarm therapy should be tried first.

- Desmopressin can reduce urine production during sleep and is the first pharmacologic agent used.
- Oxybutynin is added for patients with small bladders.
- Add imipramine to treat if desmopressin and oxybutynin fail.
- Be aware that enuresis causes significant psychological stress.

Stress Incontinence, Female

Presention: loss of urine with coughing, sneezing, laughing, or physical activity.

Management:
- In history ask about multiple pregnancies.
- Do a pelvic exam and look for cystocele, rectocele, pelvic prolapses.
- Get a urinalysis to rule out infection. Look for hematuria. Proceed with cystoscopy and cytology if blood is found in urine. You do not want to miss a malignancy.
- Have the patient keep a voiding diary.
- Voiding cystometrogram is the test to order to check for obstruction as well as poor contractility of bladder.
- The first step is to institute behavioral changes, such as scheduled trips to the bathroom and restriction of fluids after dinner.
- Have patients do Kegel exercises to strengthen the pelvic muscles. This technique is most effective for stress or mixed incontinence generally.
- Estrogen increases tone at the urethra and should be considered in some cases.
- Pseudoephedrine tightens the sphincter and may be used for pure sphincter dysfunction.
- Oxybutynin chloride (Ditropan) is used for urge incontinence; it relaxes the bladder.
- Pads may be worn in some cases.
- Catheter options include intra-urethral catheter, "straight" self-catheterization, or suprapubic catheter (more permanent option). In a person with spinal cord injury a catheter may be the best option.
- Surgery can be an effective tool in some cases to increase tone or relax bladder.
- Monitor for urinary tract infections.

Symptoms Referable to Genitourinary System

Presentation	Cause
Obstruction	Benign prostatic hypertrophy
	Tumor
Incontinence	Stress
	Urge
	Overflow
	Functional
Retention	Urinary tract infections
	Medication
	Neurologic
Hematuria	Urinary tract infections
	Urolithiasis
	Renal tumors
	Trauma (Foley catheter is common cause)
	Hemangiomas or AV malformations

continued

Symptoms Referable to Genitourinary System (*continued*)

Presentation	Cause
Hematuria (*continued*)	Glomerulonephritis
	Strictures
	Urethritis
Flank pain	Pyelonephritis
	Nephrolithiasis
	Diverticulitis
	Aortic aneursym
	Appendicitis
	Bile duct stones
	Adnexal masses
Bladder pain	Urinary tract infections
	Interstitial cystitis
	Trauma

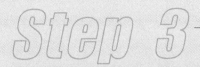

CHAPTER 20

Respiratory System

GENERAL ISSUES

Chronic obstructive pulmonary disease/
    chronic airway obstruction
Asthma
Pneumoconioses
Sarcoidosis
Cystic fibrosis
Pulmonary embolism and infarction
Pulmonary hypertension
Pleurisy without effusion
Spontaneous tension pneumothorax
Mediastinitis
Wegener's granulomatosis
Dyspnea
Cough
Hemoptysis
Stridor
Hoarseness

INFECTIOUS DISEASES

Croup
Acute bronchitis
Acute bronchiolitis
Pneumonia
Pulmonary tuberculosis
Influenza with other respiratory
    manifestations

MALIGNANCY

Malignant neoplasm of bronchus and
    lung, primary and secondary
Small cell or oat cell cancer
Non-small cell cancer

GENERAL ISSUES

Chronic Obstructive Pulmonary Disease/
Chronic Airway Obstruction

	Presentation
Bronchitis	Inflammation of bronchi
Obstructive chronic bronchitis	Cough every day with production of sputum for 3 months and for at least two years
Emphysema	Permanently enlarged air spaces distal to bronchioles that are destroyed but not fibrotic

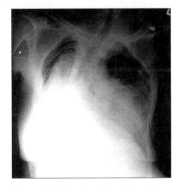

Figure 1. Chronic obstructive pulmonary disease. (From Mazzagatti FA, Lebowitz LC, Schluger NW: Respiratory Care Pearls. Philadelphia, Hanley & Belfus, 1997, p 159.)

Asthma

Presentation: wheezing, shortness of breath, tightness, and cough. Can be exercise-induced. Twice as common in boys before puberty; the incidence equalizes in adolescence; women predominate in adulthood in regard to new cases.

Management:

- Asthma is chronic inflammation of the airway with intermittent obstruction and bronchial hyper-responsiveness.
- In history ask about family history as well as possible triggers such as environmental exposure, medications such as aspirin and beta-blockers, cold dry air with exercise.
- Ask about seasonal occurrence as well as time of day (i.e., early morning and at night). Is anyone in the home a smoker?
- Listen for wheezing on exam. Look for polyps in nose. Allergic rhinitis is associated with asthma. Pulsus paradoxus may be present (systolic blood pressure drops with inspiration). Atopic dermatitis may be present on skin.
- For acute exacerbation that presents in ED, first give supplemental oxygen.
- Next give frequent, inhaled, high-dose beta agonist by nebulizer.
- Then give oral or IV steroids.
- Admit patients who do not respond to ED treatment; certainly admit to MICU if intubation is required.
- Stepwise approach to ongoing treatment:

Intermittent	Brief and less than once a week with nocturnal symptoms fewer than twice per month	1. No daily medication needed 2. Albuterol for exacerbations
Mild persistent	Exceeds once per week but not daily and affects activity/sleep, with nocturnal symptoms exceeding two nights per month	1. Inhaled steroid (Flovent or cromolyn) 2. Albuterol for exacerbations
Moderate persistent	Daily symptoms that affect activity/sleep and nocturnal symptoms exceed once a week	1. Inhaled steroid (Flovent) 2. Salmeterol 3. Theophylline or beta$_2$ agonist tablets 4. Albuterol for exacerbations
Severe persistent	Continuous symptoms with frequent exacerbations and physical activities/sleep limited	1. Inhaled steroid (Flovent) 2. Salmeterol 3. Theophylline or beta$_2$ agonist tablets 4. Prednisone by mouth 5. Albuterol for exacerbations

Pneumoconioses

Presentation:

Course	Presentation
Early	Cough, dyspnea
Late	Cor pulmonale; as lung fibrosis develops, you can see A wave in very advanced disease

Management:

- Good history is the key: look for coal, dust, asbestos exposure, smoking history.
- Pneumoconiosis is non-neoplastic response of lung to inhaled mineral or organic dusts.
- Get pulmonary function tests.
- Recommend cessation of smoking; smoking greatly worsens disease.
- Give oxygen for hypoxemia.
- Give influenza and pneumococcal vaccines.

Pitfall:

- Failure to diagnose tuberculosis superinfection.

Sarcoidosis

Presentation: young blacks (10 times more common in blacks than whites) with noncaseating granulomas in lungs, brain, kidney, eye, and liver.

Management:

- Chest x-ray is key imaging modality.
- Use chloroquine, hydroxycholoroquine, methotrexate for severe mucocutaneous disease.
- Use glucocorticoids for significant extrapulmonary involvement. including heart.
- Get an EKG.
- Order an ophthalmic exam.
- Check serum calcium, 24-hour urinary calcium, and ACE level.
- T cells play a part in the disease process, and tumor necrosis factor is elevated.

Cystic Fibrosis

Presentation: most patients are white with Northern European heritage. Infants may present with meconium ileus at birth. Also be alert to steatorrhea, sterility, chronic cough, and nasal polyps.

Management:

- Order sweat chloride test.
- Cystic fibrosis is caused by CFTR gene defect.
- The inheritance pattern is autosomal recessive.
- Do DNA testing.
- Check for fecal fat.
- Get upper GI and small bowel series.
- Measure pancreatic function.
- Treat pulmonary manifestations in which bronchiectasis progresses to COPD with physiotherapy, bronchodilators, dornase alfa, steroids, oxygen.
- Treat extrapulmonary manifestations such as pancreatic insufficiency, which causes fat malabsorption. with enzymes like pancrelipase (Creon).
- Treat diabetes mellitus.
- When choosing antibiotics, go for antipseudomonal coverage with penicillin + gentamicin, cephalosporins (cefepime/ceftazidime), and inhaled tobramycin.

Pulmonary Embolism and Infarction

Presentation: female, pregnant, smoker, immobile after surgery, estrogen supplements.

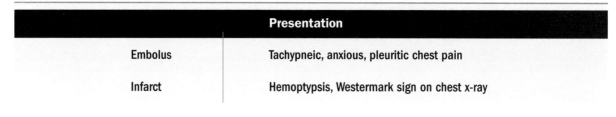

Presentation	
Embolus	Tachypneic, anxious, pleuritic chest pain
Infarct	Hemoptypsis, Westermark sign on chest x-ray

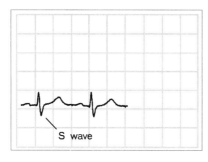 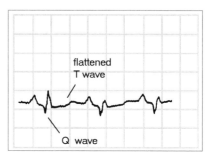

Figure 2A. S1.   Figure 2B. Q3 T3.

(From Jenkins RD, Gerred SJ: ECGs by Example. New York, Churchill Livingstone, 1997, p 157.)

Management:

- D-Dimer, while nonspecific, is a sensitive lab test for pulmonary embolism.
- Arterial blood gas analysis may show large A:A gradient.
- On ECG look for classic S1Q3T3 pattern with prominent S wave in lead I, Q wave and inverted T wave in lead III. Usually you see only sinus tachycardia. Other signs on ECG include T-wave inversion in leads V1–V3, right bundle branch block.
- Get VQ scan or spiral CT.
- Do not forget Doppler ultrasound of the legs to look for deep vein thrombosis.
- Angiography is the gold standard, although hardly ever ordered.
- Give oxygen and heparin bolus + drip.
- Start warfarin with heparin.
- Consider internal vena cava filter.

Pitfalls:

- Failure to diagnose pulmonary embolism in patient after orthopedic surgery patient or in obstetric/gynecologic patients.
- Failure to start treatment with high clinical suspicion before all diagnostic studies are completed.

Pulmonary Hypertension

Presentation: dyspnea, fatigue, and syncope.

Management:

- Pulmonary hypertension can be primary or secondary to COPD, fen-phen.
- Get chest x-ray.
- Order pulmonary function tests, exercise testing.
- Get ECG, VQ, pulmonary artery catheterization.
- Give oxygen + vasodilator + anticoagulation with warfarin.
- Lung transplant is the definitive treatment.

Pitfall:
- Do not forget that oxygen is the only "medication" to reduce vasoconstriction and alter course of disease (i.e., right heart failure).

Pleurisy Without Effusion

Presentation: pleuritic chest pain that resolves with breath-holding. Pain may be referred to shoulder or neck.

Management:
- Listen for pleural friction rub. It is pathognomonic.
- Consider ruptured esophagus, amebic empyema, pancreatitic pleurisy, and neoplastic cells as causes
- Treat the underlying disease.
- Chest wrap is usually helpful.
- Use NSAIDs with or without narcotics for pain control to reduce inflammation of the pleura.
- Urge patient to breathe deeply and cough.
- Consider antibiotics and bronchodilators for bronchitis.

Spontaneous Tension Pneumothorax

Presentation: decreased breath sounds unilaterally, hypotension, jugular venous distention, pulsus paradoxus, chest pain, dyspnea, anxiety, fatigue. In addition, a patient on a ventilator may suddenly require high inspiratory pressures. Often presents in tall thin men with COPD who have a ruptured bleb.

Management:
- Spontaneous tension pneumothorax can be a life-threatening emergency.
- Give oxygen.
- Order arterial blood gas analysis.
- Get chest x-ray. Look for air in pleural cavity with deviation of mediastinum and absent lung markings peripherally.
- Get needle thoracostomy to second intercostal space at midclavicular line on affected side.
- Perform tube thoracostomy: insert chest tube to vacuum with waterseal and watch for bubbles.
- Get another chest x-ray.
- Transfer to MICU (if the patient is in ED or other location).
- After bubbles have ceased for about 24 hours, turn vacuum down.
- Remove chest tube.

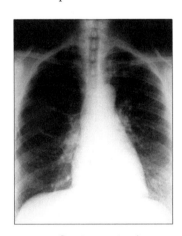

Figure 3. Spontaneous tension pneumothorax. (From Mazzagatti FA, Lebowitz LC, Schluger NW: Respiratory Care Pearls. Philadelphia, Hanley & Belfus, 1997, p 122.)

Pitfalls:
- Bear in mind that the chest x-ray may be misleading with regard to the extent of pneumothorax. A few centimeters of air space can represent a 50% pneumothorax.
- A skin fold can mimic pneumothorax in appearance.
- **Very important:** if pneumothorax is suspected in an unstable patient, defer the chest x-ray and immediately perform the needle thoracostomy and chest tube procedures. **Do not wait for the chest x-ray!**
- **Do not use positive ventilation, which can convert a simple pneumothorax into a tension pneumothorax.** Try this on the Sample Case and see how fast the case ends: intubate and ventilate the patient with pneumothorax.

Mediastinitis

Presentation: fever, chills, pleuritic chest pain, shortness of breath, confusion, sore throat, swelling in the neck, pertussis.

Management:

- Be alert to history of an upper respiratory tract infection, intubation of esophagus with rigid stylet, or recent dental infection.
- Mediastinitis is usually a clinical diagnosis. It is a surgical emergency.
- Get a chest x-ray and look for wide mediastinum.
- Protect airway.
- Patient should be scheduled for emergent surgery.
- Start third-generation cephalosporin + metronidazole or clindamycin.

Wegener's Granulomatosis

Presentation: nose bleeds, frequent sinus infections, fatigue in a middle-aged man.

Management:

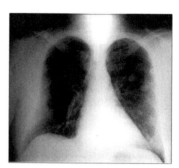

- Wegener's granulomatosis is an autoimmune disorder that classically affects lungs, kidneys, and mucous membranes/sinuses.
- Get chest x-ray. Look for round cavities with a hemorrhage inside; it looks like an abscess.
- CT of the chest is a better diagnostic tool.
- Get cytoplasmic antineutrophilic cytoplasmic antibody (c-ANCA) level.
- Get urinalysis to look for renal involvement.
- Consider biopsy because Wegener's granulomatosis can mimic other lesions in the lung.
- Consider bronchoscopy to look for tracheal involvement; you may need to relieve strictures with tracheostomy.
- Methotrexate and prednisone can be attempted as treatment.
- With cyclophosphamide and corticosteroids, complete remission can be expected in 90% of cases. Old data give mean survival time of 5 months.

Figure 4. Wegener's granulomatosis. (From Mazzagatti FA, Lebowitz LC, Schluger NW: Respiratory Care Pearls. Philadelphia, Hanley & Belfus, 1997, p 117.)

Dyspnea

Presentation: abnormally uncomfortable awareness of breathing—not pain per se. May herald pulmonary edema, pulmonary embolism, pneumothorax, pneumonia, or worsening asthma.

Management:

- Good history and physical exam of pulmonary and cardiovascular systems are crucial. Listen for crackles and S3; look for jugular venous distention.
- Get chest x-ray.
- The rest of the diagnostic regimen should follow the clinical history and severity of presentation.
- Consider arterial blood gases, echocardiograms.

Cough

Presentation: upper respiratory infection, smoking, gastoesophageal reflux disease (GERD), angiotensin-converting enzyme (ACE) inhibitor, tumor, infectious disease.

Management:

- History provides the most valuable information. Is the cough acute or chronic? Is it seasonal? Is it associated with wheezing, postnasal drip, or GERD? Is sputum produced? If so, of what color and consistency? Does the patient smoke? Is the patient immunocompromised? Ask about environmental exposures and ACE inhibitor.
- Stop ACE inhibitor, if any.
- Get chest x-ray; look for infiltrate, hilar adenopathy.

- If chest x-ray is abnomal, get sputum cytology, CT, bronchoscopy, cardiac studies—but use your clinical judgment based on patient history.
- If chest x-ray is normal, try to eliminate any irritants.
- Evaluate for most common causes: postnasal drip, GERD, asthma.
- Still no luck? Proceed to sputum cytology, CT, bronchoscopy, cardiac studies—but use your clinical judgment based on history.
- If you still do not have the answer, consider psychological etiology. This is a diagnosis of exclusion.

Hemoptysis

Presentation: spitting of blood or of blood-stained sputum; a nonspecific symptom that may indicate infection, neoplasm, cardiovascular disease, pulmonary embolism, autoimmune disease, drugs.

Management:
- Get thorough history and physical exam.
- Admit patient if loss of blood is life-threatening.
- Get chest x-ray at the minimum.
- Get sputum cultures.
- Order urinalysis.
- Order bronchoscopy for localizing abnormality on chest x-ray.

Stridor

Presentation: harsh, musical sound produced in obstructed airway.

Management:
- Check oxygen saturation at the minimum, and get arterial blood gas analysis if warranted.
- History and physical exam for acute stridor: ask about recent intubation/trauma; look for possible foreign body, infection.
- History and physical exam for chronic or ongoing stridor: consider congenital anomalies, neoplasms. Laryngomalacia is the most frequent congenital anomaly. It is usually seen at 2 months of age and increases over 6 months. Pediatric patient usually outgrows problem by age 2 years.
- Get x-rays of neck and chest.
- CT can be helpful, of course
- Direct laryngoscopy + bronchoscopy is the gold standard—once you have ruled out acute epiglottitis, of course.

Pitfalls:
- Manipulating acute epiglottis. Symptoms include sore throat, difficulty with breathing, inspiratory stridor, hoarseness, and swallowing trouble.
- Failure to diagnose retropharyngeal/peritonsillar abscess, which requires surgical intervention.

Hoarseness

Presentation: rough quality of voice may be key presenting sign of neoplasm or simple irritation or infection.

Management:
- In history look for clues such as GERD history, smoking, signs and symptoms of infection. Ask about trauma (e.g., surgical trauma) in which recurrent laryngeal nerve may have been sliced.
- Physical exam: do ENT exam using either direct or indirect laryngoscopy.
- Obtain ENT consultation if you have any doubt or if you have difficulty with the exam.

Pifall:
- Failure to diagnose neoplasm.

Infectious Diseases

Croup

Presentation: harsh, barking cough with wheezing, and difficulty in breathing; appears in patients age 3 months to 6 years after upper respiratory infection.

Management:

- Initial treatment: moist air.
- Consider racemic epinephrine.
- Look for steeple sign on neck x-ray showing narrowing of the tracheal air column at the larynx and distention of the hypopharynx.
- Admit patients with respiratory distress or stridor.
- Give steroids.

Pitfall:

- Failure to note aspirated foreign body or other cause.

Acute Bronchitis

Presentation: productive cough, pleuritic pain, or pain with coughing; caused by inflammation of bronchi.

Management:

- Treat the symptoms.
- Albuterol is effective.

Pitfall:

- Do not give antibiotics; they have not been found to be truly useful.

Acute Bronchiolitis

Presentation: respiratory distress in a child less than 18 months old; symptoms include tachypnea, tachycardia, retractions, fine rales, and fine wheezing.

Management:

- Acute respiratory illness due to respiratory syncytial virus (RSV) leads to edema and infiltration of bronchial walls.
- Start oxygen mask or tent.
- Use bronchodilators such as albuterol. Steroids are controversial.
- Nasal washings can diagnose RSV via antigen testing.
- Order chest x-ray, posteroanterior and lateral views. Look for patchy infiltrates, atelectasis, flat diaphragm, increased anteroposterior diameter.
- Chest x-ray may suggest pneumonia or foreign body aspiration.
- Get arterial blood gas analysis, and, if needed, proceed to mechanical ventilation (rarely necessary).

Pneumonia

Type	Presentation	
Lobar	Fever, tachypnea, crackles, consolidation	
Bronchopneumonia (localized to the bronchioles/ surrounding alveoli)	Coughing, chest pains, fever, blood-streaked sputum, chills, and difficulty in breathing. Most common at age extremes: infants and elderly	

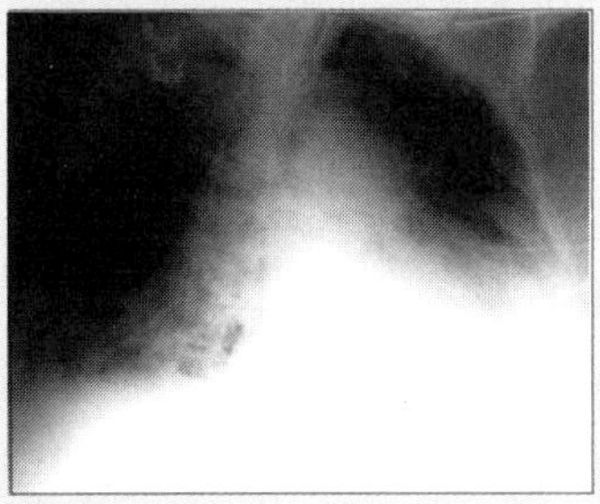

Figure 5. Pneumonia. (From Mazza-gatti FA, Lebowitz LC, Schluger NW: Respiratory Care Pearls. Philadel-phia, Hanley & Belfus, 1997, p 159.)

Management:
- Classic regimens based on setting:

Presentation	Management
For immunocompetent outpatient	Macrolide (e.g., azithromycin or tetracycline)
For outpatients older than 60	Cephalosporin, amoxicillin/clavulanic acid with or without macrolide
For hospitalized patients	Second- or third-generation cephalosporin or betalactam with macrolide
For ICU patients	IV macrolide with an IV cephalosporin (e.g., cefepime) and vancomycin

Pulmonary Tuberculosis

Presentation: fever, cough, hemoptypsis, night sweats, weight loss; may resolve or go dormant.

Management:
- Risk factors are HIV infection or other immunocompromise, low socioeconomic status, alcohol abuse, homelessness, occupational exposure; more likely in prison inmates, immigrants, health care workers.
- Get chest x-ray; look for upper cavitary lesions.
- Give purified protein derivative (PPD) test. If a wheal is raised after 48 hours, the test maybe positive. PPD may not react in immunocompromised patient.
- Get sputum testing with acid-fast bacilli.
- Treatment regimen is summarized by the mnemonic **SPIRE**: **s**treptomycin, **p**yrazinamide, **i**soniazid, **r**ifampin, **e**thambutol.
  - First 2 months: isoniazid, rifampin, and pyrazinamide.
  - Next 4 months: just isoniazid and rifampin.
  - Start ethambutol or streptomycin until susceptibility tests return.
  - For prevention: isoniazid alone for up to 1 year.

Pitfalls:
- Keep in mind that streptomycin is ototoxic.
- With isoniazid always give pyridoxine.
- Do not forget to warn patient that rifampin turns urine orange.
- Do not fail to do ophthalmic exam with ethambutol because of possible optic neuritis.

Influenza with Other Respiratory Manifestations

Presentation:

Stage Presentation Early: respiratory symptoms with influenza are mild at start: sore throat, dry cough, and coryza. Late: progression to lower respiratory symptoms later in course of disease, with a cough that may be productive. Hemorrhagic bronchitis and pneumonia can occur. Secondary bacterial infection usually manifests after about 2 weeks. A gram-positive organism is the most likely culprit; infection manifests as fever and cough. The cough will worsen and become productive or bloody.

Management:

- Give an antiviral such as oseltamivir (Tamiflu).
- Give antibiotics.
- Hospitalize, if needed.

MALIGNANCY

Malignant Neoplasm of Bronchus and Lung, Primary and Secondary

General Presentation: weight loss and respiratory distress, usually late in disease; otherwise an incidental chest x-ray finding.

Small Cell or Oat Cell Cancer

Presentation: many endocrine/paraneoplastic syndromes, weight loss, superior vena cava syndrome, frequent metastases, gynecomastia, hyperpigmentation, and carcinoid syndrome.

Management:

- Small cell or oat cell cancer is associated with cigarette smoking; radiation is synergistic in its development. It is a very aggressive tumor.
- On chest x-ray the tumor is usually centrally located.
- Order CT; remember that the brain is a frequent site of metastatic small cell lung cancer.
- Order CBC, liver function tests, blood urea nitrogen/creatinine.
- Order BMP to rule out paraneoplastic effects such as hypoglycemia and hypocalcemia.
- Consider getting cortisol to look for Cushing syndrome, urine electrolytes to look for SIADH, and parathyroid hormone (PTH) or PTH-related peptide to look for hyperparathyroidism.
- Typical chemotherapy regimen: etoposide + cisplatin + vincristine.
- Also use radiation therapy.

Pitfalls:

- Failure to diagnose neoplasm on chest x-ray.
- Do not recommend surgery; patients with small-cell lung cancer are rarely candidates.
- Failure to treat paraneoplastic syndromes.

Non-small Cell Cancer

Presentation:

	Presentation
Adenocarcinoma	Peripherally located on chest x-ray Can present in nonsmokers Hypercoagulability Clubbing
Squamous cell carcinoma	Centrally located on chest x-ray Hypercalcemia due to PTH-related peptide Obstructive pneumonia Wheezing Hemoptysis
Large cell carcinoma	Peripherally located on chest x-ray Gynecomastia
Bronchoalveolar carcinoma	Enormous amount of watery sputum

Management:
- Non-small cell lung cancer is associated with asbestos, radon, smoking.
- Order chest x-ray.
- Get sputum cytology.
- Order bronchoscopy or CT-guided transthoracic needle biopsy.
- Get CBC, liver function tests, blood urea nitrogen/creatinine.
- Get BMP to rule out paraneoplastic effects.
- CT of chest and abdomen is the **minimal** imaging required for staging.
- Get CT of head in patients with neurologic symptoms.
- If needed, order skeletal survey to rule out metastases to bone. The spine is a common site for metastases.
- Staging of disease guides therapy:
  - Platinum-based chemotherapy
  - Surgical resection
  - Radiation therapy

Pitfalls:
- Failure to diagnose neoplasm on chest x-ray.
- Failure to diagnose spinal cord compression.
- Failure to treat paraneoplastic syndromes.
- Failure to treat side effects of chemotherapy regimens.

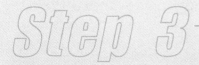

CHAPTER 21

Statistics

FUNDAMENTAL CONCEPTS OF QUANTITATIVE MEASUREMENT
    Mean, median, and mode
    Standard deviation
    Scales of measurement
    Distribution/central tendency
    Variability
    Probability
    Disease incidence and prevalence
    Disease outcomes
    Associations
    Health impact
    Sensitivity, specificity, predictive values

FUNDAMENTAL CONCEPTS OF STUDY DESIGN
    Advantages and disadvantages of different study designs
    Sampling and sample size
    Potential bias in clinical studies
    Outcome assessment

FUNDAMENTAL CONCEPTS OF HYPOTHESIS TESTING AND STATISTICAL INFERENCE
    Confidence interval
    Type I/type II errors
    Clinical importance vs. statistical significance
    Interpreting results of clinical studies/experimental data or biometric studies

FUNDAMENTAL CONCEPTS OF QUANTITATIVE MEASUREMENT

Mean, Median, and Mode

Mean	Sum of data divided by n
Median	Central point of data
Mode	Most frequently observed data value

Standard Deviation (SD)

- "Mean of the mean" used to determine how tightly the data are clustered around the mean in a set of data.

SD	= square root [sum(x – avg x)^2 / (n–1)]
x	= value in set of data
avg x	= mean of all values x
n	= the number of values x

2.5th percentile	2 SD below mean
16th percentile	1 SD below mean
25th percentile	$^2/_3$ SD below mean
50th percentile	mean
75th percentile	$^2/_3$ SD above mean
84th percentile	1 SD above mean
97.5th percentile	2 SD above mean

Scales of Measurement

Nominal: Same Scale Value	Ordinal: Higher Scale Value	Interval: Adjacent Scale Values Equal with Attribute Being Measured	Ratio: Zero Point for Scale
Gender M, F	Pain ratings 1,2,3	Step 3 scores	Time
Step 3 Pass, fail		IQ	

Distribution/Central Tendency

Normal distribution/central tendency	Follows bell curve with scores more concentrated in the middle than in the tails	Mean = median
Positive skew	Lot of high values	Mean > median
Negative skew	Lot of low values	Mean < median

Variability

Variability	Degree to which scores differ from each other

Probability

Simple probability	Number of favorable outcomes divided by total number possible outcomes
Conditional probability	Probability of an event given that another event occurs
Independent	$p(A \text{ and } B) = p(A) \text{ times } p(B)$
Mutually exclusive	$p(A \text{ or } B) = p(A) \text{ plus } p(B)$

Disease Incidence and Prevalence

Incidence	Number of new cases. Probability of disease in whole population any point in time
Prevalence	Total cases, both new and old. Probability that patient without disease will develop disease during time interval

- Remember: if survival time increases, the prevalence increases, but the incidence remains unchanged.
- With short duration of the illness, the incidence exceeds the prevalence.

Disease Outcomes

- Generally given as number per 100,000 population
- Number of fatalities/population = fatality rate

Associations

Correlation	Strength of association between two variables converted to metric units	Height and weight are good examples
Covariance	Similar to a correlation but uses units of original variables	

- Remember: height and weight correlate, but they do not **cause** each other.
- But they can help us predict weight given height.

Health Impact

Risk difference	Difference in event rate between two comparison groups (P1 – P2). Zero indicates no difference. Less than zero = effective in reducing risk of outcome.
Relative risk (RR)—prospective study	Compares risk of disease in exposed group to unexposed control group
Odds ratio (OR)—retrospective study	Odds of exposure in diseased patients vs. those without disease

RR/OR

	Disease	No Disease
Exposure	a	b
No exposure	c	d

RR	a/(a+b) / c/(c+d)
OR	ad/bc

Sensitivity, Specificity, Predictive Values

Sensitivity	Probability that a diseased patient will have a positive test result	Good screening test
Specificity	Probability that a nondiseased patient will have a negative test result	Good confirmatory test
Positive predictive value (PPV)	Probability that a patient with a positive test actually has the disease	
Negative predictive value (NPV)	Probability that a patient with a negative test actually does not have the disease	

	Disease	No Disease
Positive test	a	b
Negative test	c	d

Sensitivity	a/(a+c)
Specificity	d/(b+d)
PPV	a/(a+b)
NPV	d/(c+d)

FUNDAMENTAL CONCEPTS OF STUDY DESIGN

Advantages and Disadvantages of Different Study Designs

Study	Use	Features	Advantages	Disadvantages
Case control	Retrospective: ascertain odds ratio from possible exposures in the past	Cases with and without disease identified	Cheap	Recall bias; survivorship bias
Case series	Very rare diseases	Report on the treatment of individual patients	May help others with rare disease	No statistical validity
Cohort	Prospective	Sample group and control followed to see if disease develops to calculate relative risk	Good for rare exposures	Expensive and time-consuming
Clinical trial	Prospective study in which there are two identical groups and one variable. No one involved knows who is in which group.	Treatment or control randomized and/or double-blinded	Gold standard	Expensive and time-consuming
Cross-sectional survey	Looks for disease prevalence in a population	Population survey at single time period	Calculates prevalence	Cannot establish cause and effect
Meta-analysis		Pooling together a lot of studies, usually from literature	High statistical power	Methodologic/statistical problems when combining studies

Sampling and Sample Size

- Standard deviation does not change with increasing number, but the standard error of measurement does change as sample size increases.
- N = 30 generally is considered the minimal sample size.

Potential Bias in Clinical Studies

Enrollment	Sickest patients may be deliberately enrolled in nonplacebo group, making outcome worse for the nonplacebo group.
Lead-time	Testing can lead to earlier diagnosis and make it seem subjects survived longer.
Length	Screening test can detect slow progressive disease yet miss rapid diseases; makes it seem that the test is more effective than it really is.
Observational	Participant or observer may respond or evaluate differently if aware of placebo vs. intervention.

Recall	Participants may not remember past events or suffer memory lapses that affect results.
Self-selection	Participants may enroll because they do not respond to standard treatments; very sick individuals may make outcome seem worse.

Outcome Assessment

Internal validity	Establishes cause and effect relationship between treatment and observed outcome
External validity	Degree to which conclusions of study would hold true for other persons/places/times

FUNDAMENTAL CONCEPTS OF HYPOTHESIS TESTING AND STATISTICAL INFERENCE

Confidence Interval (CI)

90% CI	10% chance does not contain real mean
95% CI	5% chance does not contain real mean
99% CI	1% chance does not contain real mean

Type I/Type II Errors

- A null hypothesis is the presumption that an event will not occur. Example: a study of whether consumption of red wine can reduce heart attacks.
- Your null hypothesis would be that red wine consumption does **not** reduce heart attacks (the opposite of what you hope to prove). You then calculate a p value. A p value is a measure of whether an event may have occurred randomly.
- $p < 0.05$ is considered statistical significance. This p value tells you that there is less than a 5% chance that an event occurred randomly. When p is statistically significant, you can reject the null hypothesis that the event would not occur—in this case that red wine consumption does **not** reduce heart attacks. You would then accept the alternative hypothesis that red wine consumption **does** reduce heart attacks.
- A type I error is rejection of the null hypothesis when it should not be rejected. You would be saying that red wine does reduce heart attacks when in reality it does not.
- A type II error is acceptance of the null hypothesis when it should be rejected. You would be saying that red wine does not reduce heart attacks when in fact it does.

Clinical Importance vs. Statistical Significance

- A p-value threshold of < 0.05 may be met, but it is outcome that matters.
- Even with statistically significant changes, the outcome may still be trivial when you compare relative risk and absolute risk. For example, coffee exposure may be associated with a 400% increase in the risk of developing malignancy. If 1 in 100,000 people currently develops cancer from imbibing espresso, a 400% increase in risk affects only 4 in 100,000 people.

Interpreting Results of Clinical Studies/Experimental Data or Biometric Studies

Source/where study is reported	Study report should undergo extensive peer-review before publication
Source of funding for study	Follow the dollars to look for conflicts of interest.
Agreement with or contradiction of past research	A single study that appears to have the opposite conclusion of a vast body of evidence should raise some skepticism.
Who was focus of the research	If the study looked at a narrow patient population, it may not be applicable to the population at large.
Type of study	Randomized clinical trials should be given more weight than other studies.
Timing of study	Preliminary report of phase I of an ongoing trial does not have the same weight as a completed phase III study.
Duration of study	The longer the better
Validity	If a test concludes that smoking decreases lung cancer, it is illogical and invalid.
Precision	Is the study reproducible, and does it give consistent results when repeated?
Distribution	Is it bell-shaped or skewed? In a skewed distribution, statistical measures of SD and mean are not as useful.
Power	The larger the sample size, the more likely the study is to reject a null hypothesis when it really is false.

Index

A

Abacavir, 123
ABCDEs for trauma, 38
ABCs
    for burns, 28
    for poisoning, 34
Abdominal aortic aneurysm, 16, 61
Abdominal pain, 61–62
    appendicitis and, 66
    cholecystitis and, 69
    pelvic inflammatory disease and,
        81–82
    peritonitis and, 68
    ulcers and, 65
Abdominal trauma, 40
Abortion, 181
Abruptio placentae, 183
Abscess
    anal, 66
    brain, 161–162
    breast, 79
    intestinal, 68
    pelvic, 187
    peritonsillar, 203, 231
    retropharyngeal, 231
    skin, 116–117
Absolute neutrophil count in
        agranulocytosis, 99
Abuse
    child, 81, 134, 135, 153, 154
    of other person, 207–208
Acanthosis nigricans, 25
Acarbose, 45
Acetaminophen, 34, 36, 70, 101
Acetazolamide, 36, 194
Acetylcysteine, 34
Achalasia, 65
Achondroplasia, 147
Acid burns, ocular, 31
Acid reflux, 62
Acid/base disorders, 51–52

Acidosis
    diabetes-related, 46, 61
    metabolic, 51
    renal failure and, 219
    respiratory, 52
Acne, 20
Acoustic neuroma, 165
Acquired immunodeficiency syndrome.
        See HIV infection/AIDS.
Acromioclavicular arthritis, 144
Acute abdomen, 61
Acute coronary syndrome, 12–13
Acute lymphocytic leukemia (ALL),
        105
Acute myelogenous leukemia (AML),
        105
Acute renal failure (ARF), 219
Acyclovir
    for chickenpox, 121
    for herpes, 81, 125, 131, 161
    for viral conjunctivitis, 120
Addison's disease, 47, 49
Adenocarcinoma
    colorectal, 71
    cutaneous signs of, 24, 25, 26
    esophageal, 72
    pancreatic, 71
    prostatic, 137–138
    pulmonary, 235
Adenoma
    benign intestinal, 72
    microcystic pancreatic, 71
    pituitary, 165
    prostatic, 138
Adenosine, 5, 8
Adenovirus infections, 120, 127
Adjustment disorders, 212, 213
Adolescent pregnancy, 181
Adrenal gland, disorders of, 49
Adrenal hyperplasia, congenital, 49
Adrenal insufficiency, 47, 49

Adrenocorticotropic hormone (ACTH),
        49
Adults
    blood loss in, 41
    fluid bolus for, 38, 40
AEEIOU TIPPS for coma, 169
Agammaglobulinemia, X-linked, 54
Agranulocytosis, 36, 99, 212
AIDS-related complex (ARC), 123. See
        also HIV infection/AIDS.
Airway management
    for anaphylaxis, 175
    for poisoning, 34
    for tetanus, 157
    for trauma, 38
Airway obstruction
    asthma and, 226
    chronic, 225
    stridor in, 231
Albendazole, 146
Albumin, ascites and, 63
Albuterol, 35, 51, 226
Alcohol abuse/alcoholism, 92–93, 210
    ascites and, 62–63
    cardiomyopathy and, 8
    cirrhosis and, 69–70
    delirium and, 216
    hepatomegaly and, 63–64
    neuropathy and, 170
    pancreatitis and, 70
Alcohol poisoning, antidotes for, 35
Alcohol use
    acetaminophen and, 36
    atherosclerosis and, 16
    hypoglycemia and, 47
    metronidazole and, 37
Aldosterone, 49
Alkali burns, ocular, 31
Alkalosis, 52
Allergens, desensitization to, 92, 175
Allergic conjunctivitis, 120

Allergic contact dermatitis, 19
Allergic rhinitis, 203, 226
Allergies/allergic reactions, 175
    drugs associated with, 36, 37
    newborn feeding problems and, 191
    skin tests for, 19, 92
    transfusion-related, 101
    urticaria in, 21
Allopurinol, 53, 144
Alpha-1 blockers, 36
Alpha thalassemia, 98
Alpha-fetoprotein, seminoma and, 138
Alternative therapies, 135
Alzheimer's disease, 162, 216
Amantadine, 212
Amblyopia, 196
Amenorrhea, 74, 77, 78–79
American College of Obstetricians and
    Gynecologists, guidelines of,
    184
Amino acid cream for cervicitis, 81
Aminocaproic acid, 102, 106
Aminoglycosides, 36, 201, 219
Amiodarone, 5, 36, 45, 196
Amitriptyline, 76, 171, 175
Ammonium chloride, 95
Amoxicillin
    for H. pylori, 58, 65
    mononucleosis and, 111, 129
    for otitis media, 113, 200
    for Salmonella, 117
    for strep throat, 202
Amoxicillin/clavulanate, 42, 112, 233
Amphetamines
    abuse of, 95, 211
    for attention deficit/hyperactivity
        disorder, 209
    for narcolepsy, 171
    weight loss and, 177
Amphotericin B, 114, 115, 123
Ampicillin
    for endocarditis, 15
    for meningitis, 160
    for otalgia, 201
    for pneumococcal infection, 113
    for Pseudomonas, 111
    for Shigella, 117
    for staph or strep infections, 112
AMPLE history for trauma, 38–39
Amsler grid, 198
Amylase, pancreatitis and, 70
Amyloidosis, 25, 170, 171
Amyotrophic lateral sclerosis (ALS),
    163
Anabolic steroids, 37, 53
Anal abscess or fissure, 66
Anal hemorrhage, 59, 62
Anaphylaxis, 21, 101, 175
Androgen-secreting tumors, 49

Anemia, 97–98
    macrocytic, neuropathy and, 171
    pregnancy and, 183
    renal failure with, 219
Anesthesia, adverse reactions to, 32
Aneuploidy, 179
Aneurysms
    abdominal aortic, 16, 61
    coronary, 122
    intracranial, 166, 220
    optic, 197
Angelman's syndrome, 177
Angina. See Chest pain.
Angiography
    for intracerebral aneurysm, 166
    for pulmonary embolism/infarct,
        228
Angioplasty, 12
Angiotensin-converting enzyme (ACE)
    inhibitors
    adverse effects of, 36, 230
    for diabetes, 46
    for hypertension, 10
    for myocardial ischemia/infarction,
        12
    for renal insufficiency, 219
Animal bites, 41–42, 159
Anion gap
    in antidepressant overdose, 96
    in diabetic ketoacidosis, 46
Anisocoria, physiologic, 197
Ankle fractures, 154
Ankylosing spondylitis, 155
Anorexia nervosa, 177, 210
Anovulation, 80
Antacids, constipation and, 58
Antenatal screening, 90
Anterior cruciate ligament (ACL) tears,
    143
Anterior drawer sign, 143
Antibiotics. See also specific antibiotic.
    acute bronchitis and, 232
    adverse effects of, 36, 37
    allergic reactions to, 175
    desquamation from, 26
    hemolysis from, 99
Anticholinergics, antidote for, 34
Antidepressants
    abuse/overdose of, 95–96
    adverse effects of, 37, 214
    antidote for, 34
    for neurogenic pain, 46, 131, 171
    weight gain and, 177
Antidotes, 34–35
Antidysrhythmic drugs, antidotes for,
    34
Antiemetics, 60–61
Antifungal drugs, 114, 115, 123
Antihistamines, 34, 175

Antioxidants, atherosclerosis and, 16
Antipsychotic drugs, 169, 211, 212
Antiretroviral drugs, 123
Antisocial personality disorder, 208,
    215
Antithrombin III, 102
Anxiety disorders, 212, 215
Anxiolytic abuse, 94
Aorta, coarctation of, 11, 16
Aortic aneurysm, abdominal, 16, 61
Aortic regurgitation, 14
Aortic rupture, traumatic, 40
Aortic stenosis, 14
Aphasia, 171–172
Apnea, sleep, 171
Appendicitis, 61, 66
Apt test, 183
Arrhythmias, 1–8
Arsenic, antidote for, 35
Arterial embolism/thrombosis, 16
Arteriosclerotic disease/atherosclerosis,
    16, 46
Arteritis, temporal, 142, 146
Arthritis, 149–150
    gouty, 53
    pain in, 151
    rheumatoid, 143
    septic, 113
    of shoulder, 144
Arthropathy, 150, 151
Ascites, 62–63
Ascorbic acid for alkali burns, 31
Asphyxia, cerebral palsy and, 165
Aspiration
    foreign body, 30, 232
    meconium, 188, 190
Aspirin
    adverse effects of, 36
    antidote for, 35
    for arteriosclerosis, 16
    asthma and, 226
    children and, 121
    gout and, 53
    niacin and, 37, 53
    Reye syndrome and, 167
    for transient cerebral ischemia, 166
Associations, statistical, 239
Asthma, 36, 226
Astigmatism, diplopia and, 195
Asystole, 6
Ataxia, 172
Atelectasis, 32
Atenolol, 182
Atlantoaxial instability, 143
Atomoxetine, 209
Atopic dermatitis, asthma with, 226
Atrial fibrillation and flutter, 2, 14
Atrial septal defect (ASD), 15
Atropine, 34, 35

Attention deficit/hyperactivity disorder
  (ADHD), 169–170, 208–209
Audiometry, 201
Autistic disorder, 209
Autoimmune disorders
  cutaneous signs of, 25, 26
  hemolysis in, 99
  joint pain in, 151
Autoimmune thrombocytopenia, 102
Autonomy, patient, 133
Avoidant personality disorder, 215
Avulsions, 41
Azithromycin
  for gonorrhea, 81
  for M. avium complex, 123
  for pneumococcal infections, 113
  for streptococcal infections, 112
  for trachoma, 120
Azotemia, 219

B
Back sprains, 155
Bacteremia, pneumococcal, 113
Bacterial infections. See also specific infection.
  conjunctival, 120
  enteric, 33, 58–59, 117
  general, 110–113
  influenza with, 234
  sepsis/septic shock in, 174–175
Bacterial vaginosis, 81, 116
Balanitis, 140
"Banana bag," for alcoholics, 216
Barbiturates, antidotes for, 34, 210
Barrett's esophagus, 62, 72
Bartonella henselae, 120
Basal cell carcinoma, 23
Battle's sign, 39
B-cell lymphoma, 107
Bedwetting, 222–223
Bee stings, allergic reactions to, 175
Behavioral disorders, 89, 207–210
Behçet's syndrome, 141
Benign neoplasms
  of breast, 85
  gastrointestinal, 71, 72
  ovarian, 84
  uterine, 82–83
Benign prostatic hypertrophy, 135, 138
Benzodiazepines
  abuse of, 210
  as antidote, 34, 35
  antidote for, 34
  for anxiety disorders, 212
  for chorea gravidarum, 169
  for drug abuse/withdrawal, 93, 94,
    95, 96, 210, 211
Benzoyl peroxide, 20
Benztropine, 212
Bereavement, 213

Beta₂ agonists for asthma, 226
Beta blockers
  adverse effects of, 36
  antidote for, 34
  asthma and, 226
  for atrial fibrillation, 2
  for congestive heart failure, 9
  contraindications for, 2, 95
  for hypertension, 10
  for myocardial ischemia/infarction,
    12
  for thyroid hormone excess, 35
Beta thalassemia, 98
Bias in clinical studies, 241–242
Bicarbonate
  for antidepressant overdose, 96
  as antidote, 34, 35
  for diabetic ketoacidosis, 46
  for electrolyte and fluid disorders, 51
  serum, acid/base disorders and,
    51–52
Bile acid sequestrants, 53
Bile duct, stricture of common, 70
Bile reflux, 62
Biliary atresia, 189
Biometric studies, interpreting, 243
Bipolar disorders, 214–215
"Bird beak" achalasia, 65
Birth. See also Delivery.
  prehospital, 187
  respiratory problems after, 189
  trauma during, 188–189
Birth control pills. See Oral contraceptive
    pills (OCPs).
Birth defects. See Congenital anomalies.
Bisphosphonate, 48
Bites, 41–42, 159
Bladder
  malignant neoplasm of, 221
  neurogenic, 221–222
  pain in, 224
Blastomycosis, 115
Bleeding. See also Hemorrhage.
  abnormal uterine, 74–75, 79
  third-trimester, 183
  trauma-related, control of, 38, 40–41
Bleomycin, 36
Blindness
  diabetes and, 46
  herpes zoster and, 130
  sudden bilateral, 196
  trachoma and, 120
Blisters, burn, 28
Blood
  expectoration of, 231
  fecal, 59, 60, 62
Blood loss
  femur fracture and, 154
  trauma-related, 40, 41

Blood pressure
  blood loss and, 41
  elevated, 10 (See also Hypertension)
  hyperthyroidism and, 44
Blood sugar
  diabetes and, 45, 46
  high or low, 47
Blood transfusions. See Transfusions.
Blood urea nitrogen:creatinine ratio in
    renal failure, 219
Bloody show, 183
Body surface area, burn severity and, 28
Boerhaave's syndrome, 68
Bone infection. See Osteomyelitis.
Bone/bone marrow, metastases to, 148,
    176
Borderline personality disorder, 215
Bordetella pertussis, 117
Borrelia burgdorferi, 119
Botulism, 117
Bouchard nodes, 149
Brachial plexus injury, birth-related,
    180, 188
Brain
  abscess of, 161–162
  metastases to, 176
  tumors in, 165
Brain death, 136, 164
Breast milk jaundice, 191
Breastfeeding, 191
  antithyroid drugs and, 44
  oral contraceptives and, 187
  retroviral infections and, 128
Breasts
  examination of, 84, 91
  fibrocystic, 85
  neoplasms of
    cutaneous signs of, 26
    female, 84–85
    male, 137
    metastasis of, 176
  signs and symptoms in, 79
Breathing in trauma management, 38
Broad ligament laceration syndrome,
    77
Broca's aphasia, 172
Bromocriptine, 78, 85, 162
Bronchiolitis, acute, 232
Bronchitis
  acute, 232
  obstructive chronic, 225
Bronchoalveolar carcinoma, 235
Bronchopneumonia, 233
Bronchoscopy
  for oropharyngeal neoplasms, 206
  for stridor, 231
  for tracheal foreign body, 30
Bronchus, malignant neoplasms of,
    234–235

Bruising
systemic disease and, 25
trauma-related, 152
Bruton's disease, 54
Bulimia, 210
Bullae, 26
"Bulls-eye" rash, 25, 119
Bupropion
adverse effects of, 36, 214
for attention deficit/hyperactivity
disorder, 169, 209
for tobacco use disorder, 93,
210
Burkitt lymphoma, 107
Burns, 27–28
ocular, 31
Pseudomonas infection in, 111
Bursa, ganglion and cyst of, 145
Bursitis, 145
"Butt and gutt" for gonorrhea/chlamy-
dial infection, 125, 139
Butterfly rash, 25, 142

C
Café-au-lait macules, 25
CAGE survey for alcohol abuse, 92
Calcific tendinitis of shoulder, 144
Calcitriol, 48
Calcium carbonate, 35
Calcium channel blockers
adverse effects of, 36
antidote for, 34
constipation and, 58
contraindications for, 2, 9
for hypertension, 10
Calcium chloride, 34
Calcium gluconate, 31, 51
Calcium imbalance. *See* Hypercalcemia;
Hypocalcemia.
Calcium oxalate calculi, 220
Calculus
gallbladder, 69
urinary, 111, 220
Campylobacter infection, 59
Cancers, most prevalent, 176. *See also*
Malignancy; Neoplasms; *specific
type.*
Candidiasis, 114
HIV/AIDS and, 123
vaginal/vulvovaginal, 81
"Can't see, can't pee, can't climb a
tree," 150
Capillary refill, blood loss and, 41
Capsaicin, 131, 171
Caput succedaneum, 189
Carbamazepine, 34, 164, 215
Carbon dioxide, acid/base disorders
and, 51–52
Carbon monoxide poisoning, 35

Carcinoma. *See also* Adenocarcinoma;
Squamous cell carcinoma.
basal cell, 23
bladder, 221
bronchial and lung, 235
intraductal, 26
renal cell, 217, 218
thyroid, 43
Carcinoma in situ, vulvar, 84
Cardiac arrest, 6
Cardiac catheterization, 12
Cardiac tamponade, 40
Cardiomegaly, 10
Cardiomyopathy, 8
Cardiotoxicity, tricyclic antidepressants
and, 96
Cardiovascular disease
menopause and, 79
screening for, 91
syncope or ataxia in, 172
Cardiovascular system
arrhythmias of, 1–8
heart failure in, 8–9
hypertension in, 10–11 (*See also*
Hypertension)
ischemia in, 12–13
valvular diseases of, 13–16
vascular diseases of, 16–17
Cardioversion, 2, 5, 8
Caries, 205
Carpal tunnel syndrome, 45, 170
Case control studies, 241
Case series, 241
Case simulations
guidelines for, v–vii
sample input for, vii–x
Casting of fractures, 153
Cataract, 193–194
Catheterization
cardiac, 12
urinary, 39, 111, 222, 223
Cat-scratch disease, 120
Caudal regression syndrome, 180
Cauliflower ear, 155
Caustic ingestions, antidotes for, 35
CD4 count for HIV/AIDS, 123
Cecal volvulus, 58
Cefepime, 110, 111
Cefotaxime, 195
Cefoxitin, 82
Ceftazidime, 200
Ceftriaxone
for conjunctivitis, 120, 194
for general infections, 113
for gonorrhea, 81, 125, 139, 222
for Lyme disease, 120
for meningitis, 160
for osteomyelitis, 110
for otitis media, 199, 200

for pelvic inflammatory disease, 82
for spontaneous bacterial peritonitis,
63
for strep throat, 202
for urinary tract infections, 115, 116
Celecoxib, 149
Celiotomy for abdominal trauma, 40
Cellulitis, 116–117
orbital, 195, 204
pelvic, 81–82
streptococcal infection in, 112
Central nervous system
disorders of, 157–169
surgical complications of, 32
trauma to, 40
Central pontine myelinosis, 48, 52
Central tendency, 238
Cephalexin, 112, 117, 149
Cephalhematoma, 189
Cephalosporin, 111, 160, 202, 233
Cerebral atrophy, 162
Cerebral embolism and thrombosis, 167
Cerebral hemorrhage, 166
Cerebral ischemia, transient, 166, 167
Cerebral palsy (CP), 164–165
Cerebrospinal fluid analysis
for encephalitis, 161
for meningitis, 160
for West Nile virus/fever, 118
Cerebrovascular disease, 167
Cervical radiculopathy, 144
Cervical spine
stabilization of, 38, 40
unstable, rheumatoid arthritis and,
143
Cervicitis, 80–81, 125
Cervix
infertility related to, 80
intrapartum dilation of, 185
malignant neoplasm of, 83
pap smears of
abnormal, 75, 128
routine, 88, 89, 90
Cesarean delivery, 184
follow-up for, 91
indications for, 180, 182, 183, 185,
186
"Chandelier" sign in pelvic infections,
82, 125
Charcoal for poisoning, 34
Charcot's joint, 150
Chemical burns, ocular, 31
Chemical dependence, 210–211
Chemotherapy. *See also* Drugs; *specific drug.*
agranulocytosis and, 99
nausea and vomiting in, 61
prophylactic, 92
for conjunctivitis, 120
for malaria, 119

for migraine, 168
for rabies, 159
Chest pain, 173
myocardial ischemia/infarction with, 12
palpitations with, 8
pleuritic, 229
Chest trauma, 38, 40
Chest tubes for hemo/pneumothorax, 38, 229
Chest x-rays. *See under* X-rays.
Chickenpox (varicella), 92, 121, 130
Child abuse, 207–208
fractures indicating, 153, 154
reporting, 134, 135
sexual, vaginitis and, 81
Children
behavioral disorders in, 89, 208–209
consent for treatment of, 134
developmental disorders in, 89, 174
diarrhea in, 59
fluid bolus for, 38, 40
fractures in, 153, 154
infectious diseases in, 121–122, 232
Reye syndrome in, 167
routine health check for, 88
scoliosis in, 148
strabismus in, 196
stridor in, 231
vaccinations for, 91, 92
CHIMPANZEES for hypercalcemia, 50
Chlamydial infection
cervicitis and, 80, 81
conjunctivitis and, 120, 194
gonorrhea with, 125
orchitis or epididymitis and, 139
pelvic inflammatory disease and, 82
trachoma and, 120
urethritis and, 222
Chloramphenicol, 36, 99, 119, 161
Chloride imbalance, 52
Chlorine gas, antidotes for, 35
Chloroquine, 119
Chlorpromazine, 212
Chocolate cyst, ovarian, 74, 77
Cholangiopancreatography, endoscopic retrograde, 69
Cholangitis, 113
Cholecystitis, 61, 69
Cholera, 117
Cholestasis, pregnancy and, 183
Cholesterol, serum
high total, 53
testing, 89
Cholestyramine, 35, 53
CHOP chemotherapy for Burkitt lymphoma, 107
Chorea/chorea gravidarum, 168–169

Chorioretinitis, 198
Chromium deficiency, 55
Chromosomal anomalies, 179–180
Chronic disease, anemia of, 98
Chronic fatigue syndrome, 129, 174
Chronic lymphocytic leukemia (CLL), 106
Chronic myelogenous leukemia (CML), 105–106
Chronic obstructive pulmonary disease, 225
Chronic renal failure/insufficiency (CRF/CRI), 219
Ciprofloxacin, 110, 111, 125, 139
Circulation in trauma management, 38
Circumferential burns, 28
Cirrhosis of liver, 69–70, 100
Cisplatin, 36
Clarithromycin, 58, 65
Clavicle fracture
birth-related, 188, 189
management of, 153, 154
Cleft lip/palate, 180
Clindamycin, 36, 81, 82, 117
Clinical importance, statistical significance vs., 242
Clinical studies
advantages/disadvantages of, 241
interpreting results of, 243
potential bias in, 241–242
Clofibrate, rhabdomyolysis and, 53, 146
Clomiphene, 75, 80
Clonidine, 94
Clopidogrel, coronary artery bypass and, 33
Closed fractures
of lower extremity, 154
mandibular/facial, 152
of upper extremity, 153
Closed reduction of fractures, 153
Closed-angle glaucoma, 194
Clostridium difficile, 59
Clostridium tetani, 157
Clotrimazole, 123
Clozapine, adverse effects of, 36, 99, 212
Cluster headache, 168
Coagulation disorders
cirrhosis with, 70
hemorrhagic, 101–102
thrombotic, 16, 17, 102
Coarctation of aorta, 11, 16
Cobalamin deficiency, 55, 97, 171
Cocaine abuse, 94–95, 177, 211
Coccidioidomycosis, 115
Cohort studies, 241
"Coining," 135
Colchicine, 53, 144

Cold, common, 127, 130
Colic
neonatal, 191
renal, 220
Colitis
neonatal, 191
pseudomembranous, 36, 117
ulcerative, 26
Collagen synthesis problems, 25
Colles' fracture, 153
Colon, diverticula of/irritable, 67
Colon cancer, 71
metastasis of, 26, 84
rectal bleeding and, 59
Colonoscopy, 67, 89
Colposcopy, 75, 83
Coma, 47, 169
Commitment, guidelines for, 136
Community-related prevention, 87
Compartment syndrome, 152
Competence
Alzheimer's and, 162
definition of, 135
Complement deficiency, 54
Complete blood count (CBC)
for anemias, 97, 98
routine, 88
Computed tomography (CT)
for bronchial or lung neoplasms, 234, 235
for cerebral hemorrhage, 166
for cirrhosis, 70
for coma, 169
contrast
for appendicitis, 66
for brain abscess, 161
for brain tumors, 165
for chronic sinusitis, 204
for kidney neoplasms, 218
for meningitis, 160
for diverticula, 67
for encephalitis, 161
for head trauma, 39, 40
for HIV-related infections, 123
for peritonitis, 68
for peritonsillar abscess, 203
for transient cerebral ischemia, 166
Computer-based case simulations (CSS)
guidelines for, v-vii
sample input for, vii-x
Concussion, 39, 216
Conditional probability, 239
Conduct disturbance, 208
Conduction disorders, cardiac, 1, 2–4
Condylomata acuminata, 128
Cone biopsy, cervical, 75, 83
Confidence interval (CI), 242
Confidentiality of medical records, 134
Confusional states, 216

Congenital adrenal hyperplasia, 49
Congenital anomalies, 180
  cardiac, 15–16
  drugs associated with, 36, 37
  musculoskeletal, 147
  rubella and, 122
  stridor in, 231
  TORCH-related, 116, 190
Congenital infections, 190
Congestive heart failure, 8–9
Conjunctiva, diseases of, 120
Conjunctivitis
  bacterial, 120, 194
  viral, 127, 130
Conn syndrome, 49
Connective tissue diseases, 141–142, 146
Consciousness, loss of
  coma and, 169
  concussion and, 39
  transient, 172
Consent
  informed, 133
  for treatment of minors, 134
Constipation, 58, 187
Contact dermatitis, 19
Contraception. See also Oral contraceptive
    pills (OCPs).
  counseling for, 89
  postpartum, 187
  surveillance and management of, 90
Controlled substances, prescribing, 136
Contusions, 152
Conversion in somatoform disorder, 209
Convulsions, 168. See also Seizures.
Coping strategies, post-crisis, 39
Copper deficiency, 55
Cord compression, 185
Corneal abrasion, 31, 111, 194
Corneal infection, 111
Corneal reflex, brain death and, 136,
    164
Coronary artery bypass graft (CABG),
    12, 33
Correlation, statistical, 239
Corticosteroids. See Steroids.
Cortisol, adrenal disorders and, 49
Cost containment, 134
Costochondritis, 173
Cough, 230–231
  in bronchitis, 225, 232
  in croup, 232
  in influenza, 234
  "whooping," 117
Counseling, 88
  for adolescent pregnancy, 181
  on contraception, 89
  genetic, 90
  postpartum, 91
  on sexual practices, 81, 82, 125

Covariance, statistical, 239
COWS mnemonic for nystagmus, 197
Coxsackievirus infection, 116, 127, 129
Cradle cap, 21
Cranial injuries, 39, 40
Cranial nerves, visual disturbances
    related to, 195
Craniopharyngioma, 165
Craniosynostosis, 147
CREST syndrome, 26, 142
Creutzfeldt-Jakob disease, 159
Cri-du-chat, 180
Crohn's disease, 59
Cross-sectional survey, 241
Croup, 232
Cryptosporidium infection, 123
Cullen's sign, 25
Cultures for strep throat, 111, 202
"Cupping," 135
Cushing syndrome, 11, 49, 234
Cutaneous lupus erythematosus, 25
Cuts, 41
Cyanide poisoning, 35
Cyanoacrylate, 41
Cyanosis, tetralogy of Fallot and, 15
Cyclophosphamide, 142, 218
Cyclothymia, 214
Cystadenoma, ovarian, 84
Cystic fibrosis, 227
Cystic kidney disease, 220
Cystic teratomas, benign ovarian, 84
Cystine calculi, 220
Cystitis, acute, 116
Cystocele, 74, 76
Cystometrogram, voiding, 222, 223
Cystoscopy and cytology for bladder
    neoplasms, 221
Cysts
  ovarian, 74, 76–77, 80, 177
  renal, 220
  sebaceous, 24–25
  of synovium/tendon/bursa, 145
Cytomegalic inclusion disease,
    129–130
Cytomegalovirus infection, 129–130
  chorioretinitis and, 198
  congenital, 190
  HIV/AIDS and, 123
  pregnancy and, 116

D
Danazol, 74, 78, 85
Dantrolene, 35, 36, 212
Dapsone, 115, 124
Dark-field microscopy for syphilis, 124
"Date rape" drug, antidotes for, 34
Death
  brain, 136, 164
  rabies-related, 159

Decelerations, fetal heart, 184,
    185–186
Decubitus ulcer, 20
Deep vein thrombosis (DVT), 17, 102
  cerebral embolism and, 167
  oral contraceptives and, 89
  postoperative, 32
  pregnancy and, 183
  pulmonary embolism and, 228
Deferoxamine, 35
Defibrillation, 5, 6
Deformities. See also Congenital anomalies.
  congenital musculoskeletal, 147
  neonatal head, 189
Delirium, 162, 216
Delivery
  cesarean, 184
  complications of, 184
  post-term, 188
  prehospital, 187
  of twins, 185
  uncomplicated, 185–186
Dementia, 135, 162, 216
Dental problems, 201, 205
Dependence, chemical, 210–211
Dependent personality disorder, 215
Depression, 213–214
  Alzheimer's disease and, 162
  bipolar disorder with, 214
  medical conditions with, 215
  mental retardation and, 169
  multiple sclerosis and, 163
  Parkinson disease and, 162
  postpartum, 187
  terminal illness and, 134, 176
  weight gain or loss and, 177
Dermatitis
  atopic, asthma with, 226
  contact, 19
  exfoliative, 26
  seborrheic, otitis externa vs., 200
Dermatitis herpetiformis, 25
Dermatology
  general issues in, 19–22
  infectious diseases in, 22
  malignancy/tumors in, 23–25
  systemic disease manifestations in,
    25–26
Dermatomyositis, 25, 142, 146
Dermatophytosis, 114
Desensitization to allergens, 92, 175
Desmopressin, 222
Desquamation, 26
Developmental disorders, 89, 174
Dexamethasone, 113, 162, 165, 166
Dexamethasone suppression test, 49
Dextroamphetamine, 209
Dextrose, head trauma and, 40
Diabetes insipidus, 48, 51

Diabetes mellitus, 45–46
    arthropathy in, 150
    fungal infections in, 114, 203, 204
    gangrene in, 46–47
    gestational, 183
    hyperlipidemia in, 53
    hypoglycemia in, 47
    malignant otitis externa in, 200
    maternal, anomalies related to, 180
    myocardial ischemia and, 12
    neuropathy in, 170, 171
    ophthalmologic manifestations of, 197
    renal disorders in, 11, 219
Diabetic ketoacidosis (DKA), 46, 61
Dialysis
    for drug overdose, 34, 35
    for electrolyte and fluid disorders, 51
    for renal failure, 219
    for Reye syndrome, 167
Diaphragmatic hernia, 69, 180
Diarrhea, 58–59
    food poisoning with, 33
    traveler's, 113, 117
    viral infections with, 127, 130
Diastolic blood pressure, hypertension and, 10
Diazepam, 210
Diazoxide, 47
Dicloxacillin, 112, 117, 121, 149
Dideoxyinosine (ddI), 36
Diet
    gout and, 53
    for hyperlipidemia, 53
    for hypertension, 10
    for phenylketonuria, 52
    for renal failure, 219
    surveillance of, 91
Diethylstilbestrol (DES), 83
DiGeorge syndrome, 54, 189
Digibind, 34
Digital rectal exam (DRE), 137, 221
Digoxin, 5, 34, 36, 173
Dilated cardiomyopathy, 8
Dilation and curettage (D&C), 181
Diltiazem, 2
Dimercaprol, 35
Diphenhydramine, 36, 101, 175, 212
Diphtheria, tetanus, pertussis (DTP) vaccine, 92, 117
Diplopia, 195
Disability, trauma survey for, 38
Disc degeneration, 147, 151
Disease, statistical analysis of, 239–240
Dislocations, joint, 154–155
Disseminated intravascular coagulation (DIC), 102, 105, 181
Distribution, statistical, 238, 243

Disulfiram, 210
Diuretics
    adverse effects of, 37
    for ascites, 63
    for congestive heart failure, 173
    for electrolyte and fluid disorders, 51
    for hyperparathyroidism, 48
    for hypertension, 10
    for intracranial pressure reduction, 165, 166, 169
    loop, aminoglycosides and, 36
    for urinary calculus, 220
Diverticulosis/diverticulitis, 59, 61, 67
Dix-Hallpike maneuver, 200
Dobutamine, 9, 175
"Doll's eyes," 174
Donepezil, 162
Dopamine, 175, 212
Dopamine antagonists, 169
Double-blinded clinical trials, 241
Down syndrome, 179
Doxorubicin, 36
Doxycycline
    for cat-scratch disease, 120
    for chlamydial infections, 81, 125, 139, 222
    for *H. influenzae*, 113
    for Lyme disease, 119, 120
    for malaria prophylaxis, 119
    for pelvic inflammatory disease, 82
    for rickettsiosis, 118
Drug abuse. *See* Alcohol abuse/alcoholism; Substance abuse.
Drug "mule," 30
Drugs. *See also* Chemotherapy; *specific drug.*
    adverse effects of, 36–37
        cutaneous signs of, 26
        hemolysis and, 99
        infertility and, 140
        rhabdomyolysis and, 93, 94, 95, 146
        toxic, 34–35
        weight gain or loss and, 177
    prescription practices for, 88, 136
Duodenal atresia, 180
Duodenal ulcer, 65
Duodenitis, 65
Duodenum, benign neoplasm of, 72
Dysfunctional uterine bleeding (DUB), 75
Dysmenorrhea, 78–79
Dyspareunia, 76
Dyspepsia, 57–58
Dysphagia, 64
Dyspnea, 230
Dysthymia, 213
Dystonia, 168–169, 212

E
Ears
    cauliflower, 155
    foreign body in, 29
    issues related to, 199–202
Eating disorders, 177, 210
Echocardiogram
    for atrial fibrillation, 2
    for hypertensive heart disease, 10
Echovirus infections, 130
Eclampsia, 164, 182
Ecstasy, 93, 94, 95
Ectopic pregnancy, 182
    abdominal pain in, 61
    infertility and, 80
    pelvic inflammatory disease and, 82
Eczema herpeticum, 125
Edema
    eclampsia and, 182
    macular, 197
    pulmonary, 9, 166
Edetate (EDTA), 35
Edward syndrome, 179
Ehlers-Danlos syndrome, 25
Elbow
    bursitis of, 145
    dislocation of, 154–155
    fractures of, 153, 154
Elderly
    abuse of, 207
    diphenhydramine and, 36
    pneumonia in, 233
Electrocardiograms
    for antidepressant overdose, 96
    for arrhythmias, 2–7
    for hypertensive heart disease, 10
    for Kawasaki disease, 122
    for myocardial ischemia/infarction, 12
    normal, 1
    for pericarditis, 9
    for pulmonary embolism/infarct, 228
    routine, 91
Electrolyte imbalances, 50–51
    adrenal disorders and, 49
    diabetic ketoacidosis and, 46
    hyperparathyroidism and, 48
    renal failure and, 219
Emancipated minors, 134
Embolism. *See also* Pulmonary embolism (PE).
    arterial, 16
    cerebral, 167
    venous, 17
Emergencies. *See also* Trauma.
    burn/exposure, 27–29
    ear, nose, and throat, 29–30
    ophthalmic, 31–32, 194, 195
    surgical, 32–33
    toxicologic, 33–37

Emotional disorders, 211–215
Emphysema, 225
Encephalitis, 161
    measles and, 121
    viral, 127, 130
Encephalopathy, hepatic, 63, 70
Endocarditis, 14–15, 111, 112
Endocervicitis, 80–81
Endocrine disorders, 43–49
Endometrial biopsy, 75
Endometrial cancer, 82
Endometrial hyperplasia, 73
Endometriomas, 74, 77
Endometriosis, 74, 80
Endometritis, 112, 187
Endoscopic retrograde cholangiopan-
    creatography (ERCP), 69
Endoscopy
    for dyspepsia/indigestion, 58
    for gastrointestinal hemorrhage, 60
    for swallowed foreign body, 30
Enemas, 58
Enoxaparin, 12, 166
Entamoeba histolytica, 68
Enteric infections, 33, 58–59, 117
Enterocele, 74, 76
Enterococcal endocarditis, 15
Enterocolitis, necrotizing, 190
Enterotoxigenic E. coli (ETEC), 117
Enthesopathy, 145, 147
Enuresis, 222–223
Environmental exposure
    frostbite and, 28–29
    heat stroke and, 29
    trauma and, 38, 39
Enzyme-linked immunosorbent assay
    (ELISA), 123
Ephedra, 37
Epididymitis, 125, 139
Epidural hematoma, 166
Epigastric pain, 61
Epiglottitis, 113, 202, 231
Epilepsy. See Seizures.
Epinephrine, 5, 34, 101, 175
Epi-Pen, 175
Epiphysis, slipped capital femoral, 147
Episiotomy, 186
Epistaxis, 30
Epstein-Barr virus infection
    mononucleosis and, 129
    pregnancy and, 116
    splenomegaly in, 64, 100
Erb-Duchenne palsy, neonatal, 188
Erectile dysfunction, 208
Errors
    physician, negligence vs., 135
    statistical, 241, 242
Erysipelas, 110
Erythema, necrolytic migratory, 26

Erythema chronicum migrans, 25
Erythema infectiosum, 122
Erythema multiforme, 26
Erythema nodosum, 26
Erythrasma, 110
Erythroblastosis fetalis, 191
Erythromycin
    for cat-scratch disease, 120
    for conjunctivitis, 120, 194
    for impetigo, 121
    for pertussis, 117
    for strep throat, 111, 202
Erythropoietin, 98, 106, 219
Escherichia coli infections, 59, 113, 117
Esophageal candidiasis, 114
Esophageal varices, 64–65
Esophagitis, 65
Esophagoscopy for neoplasms, 206
Esophagus
    Barrett's, 62, 72
    fistula of, 180
    malignant neoplasm of, 72
    rupture of, 68
Essential hypertension, 10
Estrogen
    amenorrhea and, 78, 79
    exogenous
        adverse effects of, 36
        for dysfunctional uterine bleed-
            ing, 75
        for endometriosis, 74
        lactation and, 187
        for menopausal symptoms, 79
        for neurogenic bladder/inconti-
            nence, 222, 223
        for ovarian failure, 77
        for uterine or vaginal prolapse,
            74, 76
Ethambutol, 36, 196, 233
Ethanol as antidote, 35
Ethics, medical, 133–136
Ethylene glycol, antidotes for, 35
Euthyroid syndrome, 44
Exanthem subitum (roseola), 122
Exercise
    asthma and, 226
    atherosclerosis and, 16
    hyperlipidemia and, 53
    management of, 91
Exfoliative dermatitis, 26
Experimental data, interpreting, 243
Experimental therapies, 135
Exposure, environmental
    frostbite and, 28–29
    heat stroke and, 29
    trauma and, 38, 39
External validity, 242
Extrapyramidal symptoms, 168–169,
    212

Extremities
    fractures of, 153–154
    pain in, 151
Exudative retinal detachment, 197
Exudative ("wet") macular degenera-
    tion, 198
Eye
    anterior disorders of, 193–195
    burns of, 31
    foreign body in, 31
    infections of, 120, 127, 130
    injuries to, 32
    Lisch nodules of, 25
    neurologic disorders of, 195–197
    posterior disorders of, 197–198
Eyelids, disorders of, 194

F
Facial bones, fracture of, 152
Factitious disorder, 209
Failure to thrive, 174
Fallopian tubes
    infertility related to, 80
    torsion of, 77
Fasciitis, necrotizing, 112
Fat, fecal, 62, 227
Fat necrosis of breast, 79
Fatigue, 129, 174
Fatty liver, 63
Feeding problems, newborn, 191
Felty's syndrome, 143
Females
    common cancers in, 176
    gonococcal infections in, 125
    infertility in, 80, 82
    stress incontinence in, 223
Femoral hernias, 68
Femur, fracture of, 154
Fentanyl, 175
Fertilization, in vitro, 80
Fetal demise, 181
Fetal growth retardation, 181, 188
Fetal heart tones, 184, 185–186
Fetal hydrops, 191
Fetus, delivery of, 185–186
    cesarean, 184
    prehospital, 187
Fetuses, multiple, 184–185
Fever
    convulsions with, 168
    postpartum, 187
    transfusion-related, 101
    of unknown origin, 173
Fever blisters, herpes simplex, 131, 205
Fibroadenoma of breast, 85
Fibrocystic breasts, 85
Fibromyalgia, 146, 171
Fibula, fractures of, 154
Fifth disease, 122

Filgrastim, 99, 105, 106
Finasteride, 36, 138
Fingers, dislocation of, 154–155
First-degree burn, 27
First-degree heart block, 2
Fissures, anorectal, 59
Fistulas
    anorectal, 59
    tracheoesophageal, 180
Fitz-Hugh-Curtis syndrome, 82
5 Ps of peripheral vascular disease, 17
Flank pain, 220, 224
Flash burn, ocular, 31
Fluconazole, 114
Fluid balance, disorders of, 51–52
Fluids
    intravenous
        for diabetic ketoacidosis, 46
        for electrolyte and fluid disor-
            ders, 50, 51, 52
        for gastrointestinal hemorrhage,
            60
        for sinus tachycardia, 7
        for transfusion reaction, 101
        for trauma, 38, 40, 41
    oral rehydration, 33, 59, 117
Flumazenil, 34, 35, 94, 210
Fluorescein exam for corneal defects,
    31, 111, 194
Fluorescent treponemal antibody,
    absorbed (FTA-ABS) test, 124
Fluoride poisoning, 35
Fluoroquinolones, 36, 116
Fluoxetine, 78, 212
Flushing, ocular, 31
Folic acid
    deficiency of, 55, 171
    for sickle cell anemia, 98
Folk therapies, 135
Follicle-stimulating hormone (FSH)
    amenorrhea and, 79
    female infertility and, 80
    male infertility and, 140
    ovarian failure and, 77
Follicular carcinoma of thyroid, 43
Folliculitis, 20
Follow-up examinations
    management of, 88
    postpartum, 91
Fomepizole, 35
Food allergies, 21, 175, 191
Food poisoning, 33, 117
Foot and mouth disease, 127, 129
Forceps delivery, 186, 189
Forearm, fractures of, 153, 154
Foreign bodies
    aspirated/tracheal, 30, 232
    in ear, 29
    nasal, 29

    ocular, 31
    swallowed, 30
Foscarnet, 125
4 Fs of cholecystitis, 69
4 Hs and Ts of ventricular fibrillation, 6
Fractures, 152–154
    clavicle, birth-related, 188, 189
    limb, 151, 153–154
    mandibular/facial, 152
    orbital, 32
    pathologic, 148
    rib, 153
    vertebral, 151, 152
Fresh frozen plasma for disseminated
    intravascular coagulation, 102
Friedman rules for labor, 185
Frostbite and frostnip, 28–29
Frozen shoulder, 144
Full-thickness burn, 27, 28
Fundal height, measuring, 186
Funding, study, 243
Fundoplication for acid reflux, 62
Fungal infections, 114–115
    diabetes and, 46
    HIV/AIDS and, 123
    vaginal/vulvovaginal, 81
Fungal sinusitis, 203, 204
Furosemide, 48, 51, 166

G
Gabapentin, 175
Gag reflex, brain death and, 136, 164
Gait, abnormality of, 174
Gallbladder
    calculus of, 69
    pain related to, 61
Gamma benzene hexachloride (lin-
    dane), 22
Gamma-hydroxybutyrate (GHB), anti-
    dotes for, 34
Gammopathies, monoclonal, 105, 171
Ganciclovir, 123, 130
Ganglion of synovium/tendon/bursa,
    145
Gangrene, diabetes-related, 46–47
Garlic, 135
Gastric lavage, 34, 60
Gastric ulcer and gastritis, 65
Gastroenteritis
    E. coli-related, 113
    noninfectious, 67
    staphylococcal, 112
    viral, 117
Gastroesophageal reflux disease
    (GERD), 62, 64
Gastrointestinal hemorrhage, 60
    esophageal varices and, 64–65
    stools in, 62
Gastrointestinal obstruction, 61, 64

Gastrointestinal system
    foreign body in, 30
    general issues for, 57–70
    infections of, 33, 117, 127
    neoplasms of, 24, 26, 71–72
    surgical complications of, 32
Gastroschisis, 180
Gemfibrozil, 53
Generalized anxiety disorder, 212
Genetic counseling, 90
Genital herpes, 125, 131
Genital warts, 22, 128
Genitalia, male, disorders of, 137–140
Genitourinary infections
    postpartum, 187
    prepartum, 116
Genitourinary system, symptoms refer-
    able to, 223
Gentamicin, 15, 82, 111, 120
German measles. *See* Rubella.
Gestational diabetes, 183
Giardiasis, 59
Giemsa stain for malaria, 119
Gingivostomatitis, herpetic, 205
Ginkgo, 135
Glaucoma, 194
Gliomas, intracranial, 165
Glipizide, 45
Glomerular filtration rate, renal fail-
    ure/insufficiency and, 219
Glomerulonephritis, 112, 218
Glucagon, 34, 47
Glucagonoma, 26
Glucose–6-phosphate dehydrogenase
    (G6PD) deficiency, 99, 119
Gluten sensitivity, 25
Glyburide, 45
Glycogen storage disease, 47
GoLytely, 30, 34, 35, 58
Gonococcal infections, 125
    of conjunctiva, 120, 194
    of joint, 149, 150
Gonorrhea, 125
    cervicitis and, 80, 81
    orchitis or epididymitis and, 139
    pelvic inflammatory disease and, 82
    urethritis and, 222
Good Samaritan laws, 135
Goodpasture's syndrome, 218, 219
Gout, 37, 53–54, 144
GP TPAL pregnancy history, 186
Grafts, complications of, 33
Granulomatosis, Wegener's, 142, 218,
    219, 230
Granulomatous disease, chronic, 54
Grave's disease, 44
Grieving, stages of, 213
Growing pains, 151
Growth retardation, fetal, 181, 188

Guardians, obtaining consent from, 134
Gynecologic examination, 90, 91
Gynecology
  general issues in, 73–82
  neoplasms in, 82–85

H
Hairy cell leukemia, 106
Hallucinogen abuse, 93–94
Halogen, 36
Haloperidol
  adverse effects of, 212
  for amphetamine abuse, 95
  for attention deficit/hyperactivity
      disorder, 170
  for chorea gravidarum, 169
  for schizophrenia, 211, 212
Hamartomatous polyps, small bowel, 26
Hand
  fractures of, 153
  joint dislocations in, 154–155
Hand, foot, and mouth disease, 127,
      129
Hashimoto's thyroiditis, 44
HDL cholesterol, low, 53
Head shape, abnormal, 147, 189
Head trauma, 39–40
Headache, 165, 166, 168
Health checks, routine pediatric, 88
Health impact of disease, statistical eval-
      uation of, 239–240
Health maintenance
  general issues in, 87–92
  substance abuse and, 92–96
Hearing loss, 200, 201–202
Heart, congenital anomalies of, 15–16,
      180
Heart and Estrogen/Progestin
      Replacement (HERS) Study
      (1998), 79
Heart block, 2–4
Heart disease, hypertensive, 10
Heart failure, 8–9
Heart rate
  blood loss and, 41
  fetal, 184, 185–186
  tachycardias and, 7
Heart valves
  artificial, complications of, 33
  diseases of, 13–16
Heartburn, 62
Heat stroke, 29
Heavy metals
  antidotes for, 35
  neuropathy related to, 170–171
Heberden's nodes, 149
Helicobacter pylori infection, 58, 62, 65
HELLP syndrome, 182
Hemangiomas, small bowel, 72

Hematochezia, 59, 60, 62
Hematology
  anemia in, 97–98
  general issues in, 99–103
  malignancy in, 104–107
Hematoma
  birth-related, 189
  epidural, 166
  of muscle, 152
Hematuria, 222
  causes of, 223–224
  neoplasms and, 217, 221
  neurogenic bladder and, 221
  stress incontinence and, 223
Hemianopia, homonymous, 196
Hemodialysis. *See* Dialysis.
Hemodilution for cerebral vasospasm,
      166
Hemoglobin, routine tests of, 88
Hemoglobin A1c level in diabetes, 46
Hemolysis, 99, 182
Hemolytic disease of newborn,
      190–191
Hemolytic uremic syndrome (HUS),
      102–103
Hemoperfusion for theophylline over-
      dose, 35
Hemophilia, 101–102
Hemophilus influenzae
  infections caused by, 113, 160
  vaccination for, 92
Hemoptysis, 231
Hemorrhage. *See also* Bleeding.
  anorectal, 59, 62
  cerebral, 166
  coagulation disorders with,
      101–102
  gastrointestinal, 60, 62, 64–65
  neonatal subperiosteal, 189
  optic dot-and-blot, 197
  postpartum, 186
  surgery complicated by, 32–33
Hemorrhoids, 59, 65–66, 187
Hemothorax, 38
Henoch-Schönlein purpura, 26
Heparin
  adverse effects of, 36, 102
  for cerebral embolism/thrombosis,
      167
  for disseminated intravascular coag-
      ulation, 102
  for myocardial ischemia/infarction,
      12
  for pulmonary embolism/infarc-
      tion, 228
  surgical procedures and, 33
  for transient cerebral ischemia, 166
  for venous embolism/thrombosis, 17
Hepatic encephalopathy, 63, 70

Hepatitis, 126
  nephrotic syndrome and, 218
  polyarthritis and, 150
Hepatitis B
  pregnancy and, 116
  vaccination for, 92, 126
Hepatitis C, cirrhosis and, 70
Hepatomegaly, 63–64
Hernias
  abdominal, 68–69
  congenital diaphragmatic, 180
  constipation and, 58
  inguinal, 139
Herniation, uncal
  lumbar puncture and, 160, 162
  pupillary signs of, 169, 197
Heroin abuse, 211
Herpangina, 127, 129
Herpes simplex encephalitis (HSE), 161
Herpes simplex virus infection, 131
  cervicitis from, 80, 81
  congenital, 190
  genital, 125
  herpes zoster with, 131
Herpes virus infection
  conjunctival, 120
  desquamation in, 26
  pregnancy and, 116
Herpes zoster virus infection, 130–131
Herpetic gingivostomatitis, 205
Hip dysplasia, 147
Hirschsprung disease, 189
Histoplasmosis, 115
Histrionic personality disorder, 215
HIV infection/AIDS, 123. *See also*
      Immunocompromised patients.
  candidiasis in, 114
  chorioretinitis in, 198
  congenital, 190
  cytomegalovirus infection in, 130
  herpes zoster and, 130
  intracranial lymphomas and, 165
  Kaposi's sarcoma in, 124
  pneumocystosis in, 123
  retroviruses and, 128
  syphilis and, 124
  toxoplasmosis prevention for, 115
Hoarseness, 231
Hodgkin's disease, 104
Homonymous hemianopia/quadran-
      tanopia, 196
Hordeolum, 194
Hormone replacement therapy (HRT),
      79, 89
Horner syndrome, 197
Human diploid cell vaccine (HDCV), 159
Human papillomavirus (HPV), 128
  cervicitis from, 80, 81
  erythema infectiosum and, 122

Human T-cell lymphotropic virus (HTLV), 128
Humerus, fractures of, 153
Humoral immunodeficiencies, 54
Hydralazine, 182
Hydrocarbon insecticides, antidotes for, 35
Hydroceles, scrotal, 139
Hydrochlorothiazide, 10, 220
Hydrogen sulfide, antidote for, 35
Hydroxymethylglutaryl CoA reductase inhibitors, 12, 16, 36, 53
Hymen, imperforate, 76
Hyperaldosteronism, 11
Hypercalcemia, 48, 50, 235
Hypercholesterolemia, 53
Hypergammablobulinemia, Waldenström's, 104, 105
Hyperglycemia, 47. See also Diabetes mellitus.
Hyperglyceridemia, 53
Hyperhidrosis, 21
Hyper-IgE/IgM syndromes, 54
Hyperinsulinemia, cutaneous signs of, 25
Hyperkalemia, 51, 219
Hyperlipidemia, 26, 53
Hypermagnesemia, 50
Hypernatremia, 51
Hyperparathyroidism, 47–48
    lung cancer and, 234
    renal failure and, 219
Hyperphagia, 177
Hyperphosphatemia, 48, 50
Hypersomnia, 171
Hypertension, 10–11
    diabetes and, 46
    drug-induced, 95
    induced, for cerebral vasospasm, 166
    portal, 63, 64, 70
    pregnancy-related, 182
    pulmonary, 228–229
    renal disease and, 11, 219
Hyperthyroidism, 44
    atrial fibrillation and, 2
    hypoglycemia in, 47
    neuropathy and, 171
Hypertrophic cardiomyopathy, 8
Hypertrophic scar, 22
Hyperventilation for intracranial pressure reduction, 40, 166, 169
Hypervolemia, 51
    induced, for cerebral vasospasm, 166
    renal failure with, 219
Hyphema, 32
Hypocalcemia, 50
    lung cancer and, 234
    neonatal, 189
    parathyroidectomy and, 48
    renal failure with, 219

Hypochloremic alkalosis, 52
Hypochondria, 209
Hypoglycemia, 47
    antidiabetic drugs and, 45, 46
    lung cancer and, 234
    postnatal, 188, 189
    seizures and, 164
Hypogonadism, male, 140
Hypokalemia, 46, 51
Hypomagnesemia, 50
Hypomania, 214
Hyponatremia, 51, 212
Hypophosphatemia, 50
Hypopigmentation, skin, 26
Hypospadias, 140
Hypotension
    drugs causing, 36, 37
    orthostatic, syncope and, 172
Hypothermia, 28
Hypothesis testing, 242–243
Hypothyroidism, 44–45
    abnormal uterine bleeding in, 75
    cutaneous signs of, 26
    female infertility and, 80
    lipid disorders in, 53
    neuropathy and, 170, 171
Hypovolemia, 40–41, 51
Hypoxia, seizures and, 164

I
Idiopathic thrombocytopenic purpura (ITP), 103
Ileum, benign neoplasm of, 72
Ileus
    meconium, 190
    postoperative paralytic, 32
Imatinib, 105
Imipramine, 223
Imiquimod, 22, 81
Immunity deficiency, 54
Immunization. See Vaccination.
Immunocompromised patients. See also HIV infection/AIDS.
    cytomegalovirus infections in, 130
    fungal infections in, 114, 115, 203, 204
    herpes infections in, 131
    influenza vaccination for, 91
    Salk vaccine and, 158
Immunoglobulins
    deficiencies of, 54
    for hepatitis, 126
    herpes zoster virus, 131
    rabies, 159
    tetanus, 158
Impaired physician, recognition of, 136
Imperforate hymen, 76
Impetigo, 112, 121
Impingement, rotator cuff, 144, 149

In loco parentis, 134
In vitro fertilization, 80
Inactivated polio virus, 158
Incidence, disease, 239
Incisions for cesarean delivery, 184
Incontinence, urinary, 221–223
Indigestion, 57–58
Indomethacin, 15, 53, 78
Infants. See also Newborns.
    cradle cap in, 21
    diarrhea in, 130
    "floppy," 170
    infectious diseases in, 121–122
    low-birth-weight, teen pregnancy and, 181
    phenylketonuria in, 52
    respiratory infections in, 232–233
    routine health check for, 88
    stridor in, 231
Infections. See also specific infection.
    arthritis and, 113, 144, 149, 150, 151
    of bursa, 145
    congenital, 190
    of conjunctiva, 120
    diabetes and, 46
    hepatomegaly with, 63
    joint, effusion with, 143
    neuropathy or neuralgia with, 171
    opportunistic, 54, 114, 115, 123–124, 130
    postoperative, 33
    postpartum, 187
    secondary, influenza with, 234
    sepsis/septic shock from, 174–175
    splenomegaly with, 100
    wound, 28, 41, 42, 159
Infectious diseases
    dermatologic, 22
    enteric, 33, 58–59, 117
    general, 110–120
    pediatric, 121–122
    respiratory, 232–234
    sexually transmitted and HIV, 123–126
    viral, 126–131
Inference, statistical, 242–243
Infertility
    female, 74, 80, 82, 125
    male, 139–140
Influenza, 234
Influenza vaccination, 91–92
Informed consent, 133
Inguinal hernias, 68, 139
Inhalation injury, burn-related, 28
Inotropic drugs, 9, 175
Insecticides, antidotes for, 35
Insomnia, 171
Insulin therapy, 46, 51

Insulinoma, 47
Intelligence quotient (IQ)
    cerebral palsy and, 165
    mental retardation and, 170
Intercessory prayer, 135
Interferon alpha–2b, 126
Internal validity, 242
International normalized ratio (INR)
    for anticoagulation with artificial
        heart valve, 33
    minimum preoperative, 33
Intestinal abscess, 68
Intestinal obstruction, 58, 67, 68
Intestines
    disorders of, pain in, 61
    diverticula of, 59, 67
    polyps in, 26, 72
Intracerebral hemorrhage, 166
Intracranial aneurysm, 166, 220
Intracranial neoplasm, 165
Intracranial pressure, elevated
    brain abscess and, 162
    cerebral hemorrhage and, 166
    coma and, 169
    encephalitis and, 161
    head trauma and, 40
    intracranial neoplasms and, 165
    meningitis and, 160
    Reye syndrome and, 167
Intraductal carcinoma, 26
Intrauterine growth retardation, 181, 188
Intravenous fluids. *See under* Fluids.
Intravertebral disc disorders, 147, 151
Intussusception, 58, 189
Involuntary movement, abnormal,
    168–169
Iodine deficiency, 44, 55
Iritis, 197
Iron
    antidote for, 35
    deficiency of, 55
Iron-deficiency anemia, 98
Irritable bowel syndrome, 67
Ischemia
    limb pain and, 151
    mesenteric, 61
    myocardial, 12–13
    transient cerebral, 166, 167
Ischemic cardiomyopathy, 8
Isoniazid, 34, 36, 196, 233
Isoproterenol, 34
Isotretinoin, 20, 36
Itraconazole, 114, 115
Ivermectin, 22

J
Jarisch-Herxheimer reaction, 124
Jaundice
    biliary atresia and, 189

pancreatic cancer and, 71
    perinatal, 191
Jaw, disorders of, 149, 205
Jejunum, benign neoplasm of, 72
Joints
    dislocations/separations of, 154–155
    effusion of, 143
    pain or stiffness in, 53, 143,
        149–150, 151
Juvenile chronic arthritis, 150

K
Kaposi's sarcoma, 124
Kawasaki disease, 122
Kayexalate, 51
Kegel exercises
    for neurogenic bladder/inconti-
        nence, 222, 223
    for uterine or vaginal prolapse, 74, 76
Keloid, 22
Keratoderma, acquired, 24
Keratolytics, 20, 22, 24
Keratoses, seborrheic, 24, 26
Kerr's sign, 61, 64
Ketoacidosis, diabetic, 46, 61
Ketoconazole, 114
Kidney
    cystic disease of, 220
    infections of, 115–116
    malignant neoplasms of, 217–218
Kidney-ureter-bladder (KUB) study for
    calculus, 220
Klinefelter syndrome, 180
Knee
    fractures of, 154
    internal derangement of, 143
    osteoarthritis of, 149
    prepatellar bursitis of, 145
Koplik spots, 121
Krukenberg tumor, 72, 84
Kuru (Creutzfeldt-Jakob disease), 159
Kwashiorkor, 55
Kyphoscoliosis, 148

L
Labetalol, 95, 182
Labor
    complications of, 184
    induction of, 181, 182
    stages and cardinal movements of,
        185
    uncomplicated, 185–186
Laboratory tests
    routine, schedule for, 88–89
    sensitivity and specificity of, 240
Lacerations, 41
Lacrimal system, disorders of, 194
Lamivudine, 123
Laparoscopy for infertility, 80

Laparotomy for silent abdomen, 68
Large cell carcinoma of lung, 235
Laryngomalacia, 231
Laryngoscopy
    for oropharyngeal neoplasms, 206
    for stridor, 231
Larynx, malignant neoplasm of, 205
Lateral collateral ligament (LCL) tears,
    143
Laxatives, 58
LDL cholesterol, high, 53
Lead poisoning
    antidote for, 35
    screening for, 89
Lecithin-sphingomyelin ratio, 189
Left ventricular hypertrophy (LVH), 10
Legal and ethical issues, 133–136
Legg-Calvé-Perthes disease, 147
Leiomyoma
    gastric, 72
    uterine, 75, 82–83
Leiomyosarcoma, gastric, 72
Leser-Trelat sign, 26
Leukemia, 26, 105–106
Levodopa, 162
Levofloxacin, 111, 113, 115, 220
Levothyroxine, 45
Lewy bodies, 162
Lhermitte's sign in multiple sclerosis, 163
Lichen sclerosis, vulvar, 84
Lidocaine, 6, 201
Lidocaine with epinephrine, 41
Lifestyle modifications
    for hyperlipidemia, 53
    for hypertension, 10
Ligaments, sprains or tears of, 143, 152
Limbs
    fractures of, 153–154
    pain in, 151
Lindane, 22
Liothyronine, 45
Lip, malignant neoplasm of, 206
Lipase, pancreatitis and, 70
Lipid metabolism, disorders of, 53
Lipid profile
    for diabetes, 46
    routine, 89, 91
Lipoma
    intestinal, 72
    subcutaneous, 24
Liposarcoma, 24
Lisch nodules of eye, 25
Listeria infection, meningitis from, 160
Lithium, 34, 37, 45, 215
Liver
    cirrhosis of, 69–70
    drugs toxic to, 36, 37
    malignant neoplasm of, 71
    metastases to, 176

Liver disease, splenomegaly and, 100
Liver enzymes, HELLP syndrome and, 182
Liver function tests
    for hepatomegaly, 63
    for Reye syndrome, 167
Lobar pneumonia, 233
Lochia, 187
Loop diuretics, 36, 37
Loperamide, 33
Lopinavir, 123
Lorazepam, 164
Low birth weight, teen pregnancy and, 181
LSD abuse, 93
Lumbar puncture (LP)
    brain abscess and, 162
    cerebral hemorrhage and, 166
    coma and, 169
    for encephalitis, 161
    intracranial neoplasms and, 165
    for meningitis, 160
    for West Nile virus/fever, 118
Lumbosacral sprain, 155
Lump, localized superficial, 21
Lung
    malignant neoplasms of, 234–235
    metastases to/from, 176
Lupus
    cutaneous, 25
    renal failure in, 218, 219
    shoulder problems in, 144
    systemic, 142
    thrombocytopenia in, 102
Luteinizing hormone (LH)
    amenorrhea and, 78–79
    female infertility and, 80
    male infertility and, 140
Lyme disease, 25, 119–120
Lymphocytes, defects in, 54
Lymphocytic leukemias, 105, 106
Lymphoma
    Burkitt, 107
    central nervous system, 165
    cutaneous signs of, 26

M
Macrocytic anemia, 97, 171
Macrolide antibiotics for pneumonia, 233
Macrosomia, 180, 188
Macular degeneration, 198
Macular edema, 197
Magnesium imbalance, 50
Magnesium sulfate, 182
Magnetic resonance imaging (MRI)
    for encephalitis, 161
    for knee injuries, 143
    for visual disturbances, 196

Major depressive episode, 213
Malabsorption, feeding problems and, 191
Malaise, 174
Malar (butterfly) rash, 25, 142
Malaria, 92, 118–119
Males
    breast neoplasms in, 137
    common cancers in, 176
    gonococcal infections in, 125
    reproductive system disorders in, 137–140
Malignancy
    cutaneous signs of, 25, 26
    dermatologic, 23–25
    hematologic, 104–107
    hepatomegaly and, 63
    otolaryngologic, 205–206
Malignant melanoma, 23, 176
Malignant neoplasms
    of bladder, 221
    of breast, 84–85, 137
    bronchial and lung, 234–235
    central nervous system, 165
    gastrointestinal, 71, 72
    gynecologic, 82, 83–84
    laryngeal, 205
    lip, oral, or pharyngeal, 206
    male reproductive, 138
    prostatic, 137–138, 221
    renal, 217–218
    secondary bone/marrow, 148
    of thyroid, 43–44
    unspecified or secondary sites of, 176
Malignant otitis externa, 200
Malingering, 209
Mallory-Weiss tear, 68
Malnutrition, 55
Mammograms, 84, 85, 91
Mandible, closed fracture of, 152
Manganese deficiency, 55
Mania, 214, 215
Mannitol, 165, 166, 169
Mantoux tuberculin test, 92
Maple syrup urine disease, 47
Marasmus, 55
Marijuana abuse, 210
Mass, localized superficial, 21
Mastitis, 79, 187
Mastoiditis, 112, 199
McMurray test for meniscal tears, 143
MDMA abuse, 93, 94, 95
Mean, statistical, 237
    confidence interval and, 242
    score distribution and, 238, 243
    standard deviation from, 238
Measles, 121

Measles, German. *See* Rubella.
Measles, mumps, rubella (MMR) vaccination, 92
Meclizine, 201
Meconium aspiration, 188, 190
Meconium ileus, 190
Medial collateral ligament (MCL) tears, 143
Median, statistical, 237, 238
Mediastinitis, 229–230
Medical care, withholding, 134
Medical conditions
    follow-up for, 88
    laboratory tests for, 89
    psychological factors associated with, 215
Medical examination, general, 88
Medical law and ethics, 133–136
Medical records, confidentiality of, 134
Medications. *See* Chemotherapy; Drugs; *specific drug.*
Medullary carcinoma of thyroid, 43
Mefloquine, 119
Megestrol, 177
Melanoma, malignant, 23, 176
Melena, 59, 60, 62
Membranous nephropathy, 218
Ménière's disease, 197, 200, 201
Meningiomas, 165
Meningitis, 160–161
    bacterial, 111, 113
    delirium and, 216
    viral, 127, 130
Meniscal tear of knee, 143
Menometrorrhagia, 74
Menopause
    premature, 77
    symptoms of, 79
Menorrhagia, 74, 75, 79
Men's health, 137–140. *See also* Males.
Menstrual disorders, 74–75, 78–79
Mental retardation, 169–170
Mental status changes, 216. *See also* Consciousness, loss of; Intracranial pressure, elevated.
    Alzheimer's and, 162
    blood loss and, 41
    postoperative, 32
    thrombocytopenia and, 102
Meperidine, 37, 69
Mercury, antidote for, 35
Mescaline abuse, 93
Mesenteric ischemia, 61
Meta-analysis, 241
Metabolic acidosis, 46, 51
Metabolic alkalosis, 52
Metabolic disorders, 52–54
    hepatomegaly in, 63
    weight gain in, 176

Metastasis, neoplasm, 176
to bone/marrow, 148
to brain, 165
from breast, 137
from kidney, 217, 218
from liver, 71
from lung, 234, 235
to ovary, 84
from prostate, 137, 221
from stomach, 72
to thoracic spine, 151
from thyroid, 43, 44
umbilical, 26
to vagina, 83
Metformin, 45
Methadone, 94, 211
Methanol, antidotes for, 35
Methicillin-resistant S. aureus, brain
abscess from, 162
Methimazole, 44
Methotrexate, 182
Methyldopa, 37, 99
Methylene blue, 35
Methylphenidate, 170, 171, 209
Methylprednisolone, 35
Metoclopramide, 60
Metoprolol, 12
Metronidazole
adverse effects of, 37
for E. coli, 113
for H. pylori, 58, 65
for infectious diarrhea, 59
for orbital cellulitis, 195
for pelvic inflammatory disease, 82
for pseudomembranous colitis, 36,
117
for trichomoniasis, 81, 126
for vaginosis, 116
Metrorrhagia, 74, 75
Microaneurysm, optic, 197
Microcystic adenomas, pancreatic, 71
Microcytic anemia, 98
Migraine, 168
Milk allergy, neonatal, 191
Milwaukee shoulder, 144
Mineral deficiencies, 55
Mineral metabolism, disorders of, 50
Minimal change disease, 218
Minors, treatment of, 134
Minoxidil, 37
Misoprostol, 182
Mitral regurgitation, 14
Mitral stenosis, 14
Mixed connective tissue disease, 142,
146
Mobitz type I/II heart block, 3
Mode, statistical, 237
Molluscum contagiosum, 129
Mongolian spots, 190

Monoamine oxidase inhibitors
(MAOIs), 37, 95, 96, 214
Monoarthritis, 150
Monoclonal gammopathies, 105, 171
Mononucleosis, infectious, 129
distinguishing strep throat from,
111, 202
splenomegaly in, 64, 100
Monosomy X, 179
Morphine, 9, 69
Mosquito-borne illnesses, 118–119
Mourning, 213
Movement, abnormal involuntary,
168–169
MPTP (synthetic heroin), Parkinson dis-
ease and, 162
Mucinous cystadenoma, ovarian, 84
Mucocutaneous lymph node syndrome,
122
Mucus, fecal, 62
Multiple endocrine neoplasia (MEN),
43, 48
Multiple myeloma, 25, 104, 105
Multiple sclerosis (MS), 163, 196
Mumps, 92, 128
Munchausen syndrome, 209
Mupirocin, 121
Murmurs, heart, 13, 14, 15
Murphy's sign, 61, 69
Muscle pain, 146, 151
Muscle trauma, 152
Musculoskeletal system
general issues for, 141–151
trauma to, 39, 40, 152–155
Mushrooms
hallucinogenic, 93
poisonous, antidotes for, 35
Myalgia, 146
Myasthenia gravis (MG), 170
Mycobacterial infections, idiopathic dis-
seminated, 54
Mycobacterium avium complex (MAC), 123
Mycoplasma infection, 26
Mycoses, 115
Myelinosis, central pontine, 48, 52
Myelodysplastic syndrome, 106
Myelogenous leukemias, 105–106
Myocardial infarction (MI), 12–13
arrhythmias associated with, 2, 3, 4
chest pain and, 173
neuropathies and, 171
Myocarditis, viral, 127, 130
Myoclonus, 168–169
Myositis, 146
Myositis ossificans, 146, 152
Myxedema, 45

N

Nafcillin, 110, 112, 162, 195

Nails
infections of, 112, 114
ingrowing, 21
Naloxone, 34, 94, 211
Naltrexone, 94
Narcissistic personality disorder, 215
Narcolepsy, 171
Narcotics
abuse/overdose of, 94, 211
antidote for, 34
constipation and, 58
for pain control, 69, 175
Nasal cavity, diseases of, 204
Nausea and vomiting, 60–61
food poisoning with, 33
postoperative, 32
Necrolytic migratory erythema, 26
Necrotizing enterocolitis, 190
Necrotizing fasciitis, 112
Needle thoracentesis, 38
Needle/tube thoracostomy, 229
Negative predictive value (NPV), 240
Neglect, 207
Negligence, physician error vs., 135
Neisseria meningitidis, 160
Neonates. See Newborns.
Neoplasms
bladder, 221
bronchial and lung, 234–235
central nervous system, 165
gastrointestinal, 71–72
gynecologic, 82–85
hoarseness related to, 231
laryngeal, 205
lip, oral, or pharyngeal, 206
male breast and reproductive,
137–138, 221
renal, 217–218
secondary bone/marrow, 148
thyroid, 43–44
unspecified/secondary sites for, 176
Neostigmine, 170
Neovascularization, optic disc, 197
Nephritis, 218
Nephrolithiasis, 220
Nephropathy, membranous, 218
Nephrotic syndrome, 218
Nerve damage
fracture-related, 153, 154
optic, 32
Nesiritide, 9
Neural tube defects, 180
Neuralgia, 170–171
Neuritis
generalized, 170–171
optic, 163, 196, 233
Neurofibromatosis (NF), 25
Neurogenic bladder, 221–222
Neurogenic pain, 151, 170–171, 175

Neuroleptic agents, 35, 95
Neuroleptic malignant syndrome, 35, 212
Neurologic disorders
  dysphagia in, 64
  ophthalmic, 195–197
  syncope or ataxia in, 172
Neurologic survey
  for coma, 169
  for trauma, 38
Neurology
  central nervous disorders in, 157–169
  general issues in, 169–172
Neuropathic arthropathy, 150
Neuropathy, 170–171
  compressive optic, 196
  diabetic, 46
Neutropenia, 54, 99
Newborns. See also Infants.
  anomalies in, 179–180
  birth trauma in, 188–189
  congenital infections in, 190
  conjunctivitis in, 194
  cystic fibrosis in, 227
  delivery of, 185–186
    cesarean, 184
    prehospital, 187
  feeding problems in, 191
  hemolytic disease of, 190–191
  hypocalcemia in, 189
  jaundice in, 191
  myasthenia gravis in, 170
  perinatal conditions in, 189–190
  phenylketonuria screening for, 52
  post-term, 188
  respiratory problems in, 189
  rubella and, 122
Niacin
  adverse effects of, 37
  deficiency of, 55
  for hypercholesterolemia, 53
Nicotine dependence, 93, 210
Nifedipine, 220
Nissen fundoplication, laparoscopic, 62
Nitrates
  aortic stenosis and, 14
  for congestive heart failure, 173
  sildenafil and, 37
Nitroglycerin, 12, 173
Nitrous dioxide, antidotes for, 35
Nonexudative ("dry") macular degeneration, 198
Nonketotic hyperosmolar hyperglycemic coma (NKHHC), 46
Non-small cell cancer of lung, 235
Nonsteroidal antiinflammatory drugs (NSAIDs)
  for arthritis, 143, 149, 150
  for gout, 53
  renal disease and, 11

Norepinephrine, 175
Norwalk virus infection, 117
Nose
  foreign body in, 29
  issues related to, 202–204
Nosebleed, 30
Null hypothesis, 242, 243
Nutritional disorders, 55
Nystagmus, 197
Nystatin swish-and-swallow, 114, 123

O
O negative blood, 41
Oat cell cancer of lung, 234
Obesity, 177, 210
Observational bias, 241
Obsessive-compulsive disorder, 209, 215
Obstetrics. See also Pregnancy.
  anomalies in, 179–180
  postnatal issues in, 188–191
  pregnancy-related issues in, 181–187
Occult blood, fecal, 62
Octreotide, 65
Ocular injury, 32. See also Eye.
Oculocephalic/oculovestibular reflexes, brain death and, 136, 164
Oculomotor nerve palsy, 197
Odds ratio (OR), 239–240
Olanzapine, 212
Olecranon bursitis, 145
Oligohydramnios, 188
Oligomenorrhea, 74
Omeprazole, 58, 65
Omphalocele, 180
Oncology. See Malignancy; Neoplasms.
Ondansetron, 61
Open dislocations, 155
Open fractures of lower extremity, 154
Open reduction with internal fixation (ORIF), 153, 154
Open-angle glaucoma, 194
Ophthalmicus, herpes zoster, 130
Ophthalmology, disorders in
  anterior, 193–195
  neurologic, 195–197
  posterior, 197–198
Opioids
  abuse/overdose of, 94
  for chronic pain, 175
  constipation and, 58
  withdrawal from, 94
Opportunistic infections
  cytomegaloviral, 130
  fungal, 114, 115
  HIV/AIDS and, 123–124
  immunodeficiency and, 54
Optic nerve
  damage to, 32
  diseases of, 196

Optic neuritis, 163, 196, 233
Oral cavity
  issues related to, 205
  malignant neoplasm of, 206
Oral contraceptive pills (OCPs)
  for acne, 20
  counseling and examination for, 89
  for dysfunctional uterine bleeding, 75
  for dysmenorrhea/premenstrual tension, 78
  for endometriosis, 74
  lactation and, 187
  side effects of, 90, 177
Oral hypoglycemic drugs, 45, 46, 183
Oral polio vaccine, 92
Oral rehydration therapy (ORT), 33, 59, 117
Orbital blow-out, 32
Orbital cellulitis, 195, 204
Orchitis, 139
Organophosphates, antidotes for, 35
Organs, transplant
  allocation priorities for, 134
  harvesting, 136, 164
Orgasmic disorder, 208
Orthostatic hypotension, 172
Oseltamivir, 234
Osgood-Schlatter disease, 147
Osler-Weber-Rendu syndrome, 26
Osteoarthritis, 149, 150, 151
Osteogenesis imperfecta (OI), 146
Osteomyelitis, 110, 111
Osteoporosis, 79, 148
Otalgia, 200, 201
Otitis externa, 111, 200
Otitis media, 113, 199, 200
Otolaryngology
  ear issues in, 199–202
  malignancy in, 205–206
  nose, sinus, and throat issues in, 202–204
  oral cavity issues in, 205
Ototoxicity, drugs causing, 36, 37, 233
Outcome assessment of study, 242, 243
Outcomes, disease, 239
Ovarian cysts, 76–77
  endometriosis and, 74
  infertility and, 80
  obesity and, 177
Ovarian failure, 77, 79
Ovarian torsion, 61, 77
Ovary, neoplasms of, 84
Overnutrition, 55
Ovulation, checking for, 80
"Owl's eye" cells, 104
Oxacillin, 160
Oxybutynin, 222, 223
Oxycodone, 175

Oxygen therapy
  for carbon monoxide poisoning, 35
  for neonatal respiratory distress,
    189, 190
  for pulmonary hypertension, 228, 229
  for trauma, 38
Oxytocin, 37, 181, 182, 186

P
P value, 242
Packed red blood cells for disseminated
    intravascular coagulation, 102
Paget's disease, 26
Pain. *See also* Abdominal pain.
  chest, 8, 12, 173, 229
  chronic, 175
  ear, 200, 201
  genitourinary, 220, 224
  on intercourse, 76
  joint, 53, 143, 149–150, 151
  limb, 151
  menstrual, 78
  muscle, 146
  in myocardial ischemia/infarction, 12
  neurogenic, 170–171, 175
  psychogenic, 172
  shoulder, 144, 145
  thoracic spinal, 151
Pain control
  for burns or frostbite, 28
  for cholecystitis, 69
  for corneal abrasion, 194
  for dislocations, 155
  for fractures, 153, 154
  for herpes zoster, 131
  for pleurisy, 229
  for terminal illness, 176
  for urinary calculus, 220
Palliative care, 176
Palpitations, 8
Pancreas, neoplasms of, 71
Pancreatic insufficiency, 70, 227
Pancreatitis, 70
  abdominal pain in, 61
  cholecystitis and, 69
  cutaneous signs of, 25, 26
Panic attacks, 212
Pap smears
  abnormal, 75, 128
  routine, 88, 89, 90
Papillary carcinoma of thyroid, 43
Papillomavirus, human. *See* Human
    papillomavirus (HPV).
Paracentesis for ascites, 63
Parametritis, acute, 81–82
Paramyxovirus, 128
Paranoid states, 212, 215
Parental consent for treatment of
    minors, 134

Parkinson disease (PD), 162
Paronychia, 110, 112
Partial-thickness burn, 27, 28
Parvovirus, human, 116
Patau syndrome, 180
Patella, fractures of, 154
Patent ductus arteriosus (PDA), 15
Patient autonomy, 133
PCP abuse, 93
Pediatric patients. *See* Children; Infants;
    Newborns.
Pelvic cellulitis, 81–82
Pelvic examination
  for contraceptive use, 89
  elements in, 90
  routine, 88
  third-trimester bleeding and, 183
Pelvic infections
  gonococcal, 125
  postpartum, 187
Pelvic inflammatory disease (PID), 80,
    81–82
Pelvis
  cancer in, umbilical metastasis and,
    26
  internal injuries of, 40
Pemphigus vulgaris, 26
Penicillins
  adverse effects of, 37
  allergies to, 175
  for brain abscess, 161
  for *H. influenzae* or pneumococcal
    infections, 113
  for impetigo, 121
  for meningitis, 160
  for mushroom poisoning, 35
  renal failure and, 219
  for streptococcal infections, 111,
    112, 202
  for syphilis, 124
  for tetanus, 157
Penis, anomalies of, 140
Pentamidine, 123, 124
Peptic ulcer, 65
Percutaneous transluminal coronary
    angioplasty (PTCA), 12
Pergolide, 162
Pericardectomy, 9
Pericarditis, 9, 130
Perimenopause, 79
Perinatal period, conditions specific to,
    189–191
Peripheral vascular disease, 17
Peritoneal lavage, diagnostic, 40
Peritonitis, 61, 63, 68
Peritonsillar abscess, 203, 231
Permethrin, 22
Pernicious anemia, 97
Personality disorders, 212, 215–216

Pertussis, 92, 117
Pessaries, vaginal, 74, 76
Pesticides, antidotes for, 35
Peutz-Jeghers syndrome, 26
Peyote, 93
Peyronie's disease, 140
pH
  fetal scalp, 185, 186
  serum, acid/base disorders and,
    51–52
  24-hour, for acid reflux, 62
  vaginal, vaginitis and, 81
Phantom limb pain, 151
Pharynx, malignant neoplasm of, 206
Phenazopyridine, 116
Phenobarbital, 35
Phenylketonuria (PKU), 52
Phenytoin, 37, 164
Pheochromocytoma, 11, 49
Phimosis, 140
Phlebitis, 17
Phobic disorders, 209
Phosphenytoin, 164
Phosphorus imbalance, 48, 50
Photosensitivity, 26, 37
Physical abuse, 207, 208
Physician-patient relationship, guide-
    lines for, 134
Physicians
  impaired, recognition of, 136
  negligence vs. errors by, 135
Physiological development, lack of
    normal, 174
Physostigmine, 34
Pica, 98
Pilocarpine, 194
"Pink eye," 120
Pinna, trauma to, 155
Piperacillin, 200
Piperacillin/tazobactam, 111
Pituitary tumors, 165, 196
Placenta, delivery of, 185
Placenta previa, 183
Plasmapheresis for thrombocytopenia, 102
Plasmodium spp., 118, 119
Platelets
  HELLP syndrome and, 182
  transfusion of, 102, 103
Pleurisy without effusion, 229
Pleurodynia, 127
Pneumococcal infection, 113
Pneumococcal vaccination, 92
Pneumoconioses, 226–227
Pneumocystis carinii pneumonia (PCP), 123
Pneumocystosis, 123–124
Pneumonia, 233
  bacterial infections causing, 111,
    112, 113
  P. carinii, 123

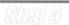

postoperative, 32, 33
rib fractures and, 153
Pneumothorax, 38, 229
Podagra, 53
Podophyllum, 22
Poisoning
by drugs and medicinal substances, 34–35
food, 33, 117
by swallowed foreign body, 30
Polio vaccination, 92
Poliomyelitis, acute, 158
Polyarteritis nodosa, 142
Polyarthritis, 150
Polychondritis, relapsing, 146–147
Polycystic kidney disease, 220
Polycystic ovarian syndrome (PCOS), 76–77, 80, 177
Polycythemia/polycythemia vera, 100
Polyhydramnios, 69
Polymenorrhea, 74
Polymyalgia rheumatica, 142, 146
Polymyositis, 142, 146
Polymyxin B/trimethoprim, 120, 194
Polyps, intestinal, 26, 72
Porphyria, 26, 171
Porphyria cutanea tarda, 26
Portal hypertension, 63, 64, 70
Positive predictive value (PPV), 240
Positive-pressure ventilation, 38, 229
Postconcussion syndrome, 216
Postdate delivery, 184
Posterior cruciate ligament (PCL) tears, 143
Posterior drawer sign, 143
Postnatal issues, 188–191
Postoperative infections, 33
Postpartum care, 91, 186–187
Postpartum hemorrhage, 186
Post-traumatic stress disorder, 213
Potassium chloride, 51
Potassium hydroxide (KOH) prep
for cervicitis, 81
for fungal infections, 114
for trichomoniasis, 126
Potassium imbalance, 46, 51, 219
Prader-Willi syndrome, 177
Prayer, intercessory, 135
Precision, study, 243
Predictive value of test, 240
Prednisone
for asthma, 226
for nephrotic syndrome/nephritis, 218
for nitrous dioxide poisoning, 35
for transfusion reaction, 101
for urinary calculus, 220
weight gain and, 177
Preeclampsia, 182

Pregnancy
adolescent, 181
chorea gravidarum in, 169
complications of, 181–183
coxsackievirus and, 127
cytomegalovirus and, 130
diaphragmatic hernia in, 69
eclampsia-related seizures in, 164
ectopic, 61, 80, 82, 182
finasteride and, 36
genital herpes and, 125
genitourinary infections in, 116
heparin and, 17
hepatitis E and, 126
HIV transmission prevention in, 123
hyperthyroidism and, 44
normal, supervision of, 186–187
pediatric infections and, 121, 122
phenytoin and, 37
podophyllum and, 22
toxoplasmosis in, 115
trauma during, 41
warfarin and, 37
Pregnancy testing
for abdominal pain, 61, 82
for abnormal uterine bleeding, 74
for amenorrhea, 78
Premature ejaculation, 208
Premature rupture of membranes (PROM), 184
Premature ventricular contractions (PVCs), 6
Premenstrual tension, 78
Prenatal care, 186
Prepatellar bursitis, 145
Prepuce, redundant, 140
Prescription practices, appropriate, 136
Presentation, fetal, 185
Pressor agents, 34, 175
Preterm delivery, 181, 184
Prevalence, disease, 239, 241
Priapism, 37, 98
Primaquine, 119
Primary trauma survey, 38
Probability, statistical, 239
Procainamide, 5, 37
Prochlorperazine, 33
Progesterone, 37, 74, 75
Progesterone challenge, 75, 78–79
Progestin, 73, 79, 187
Progressive systemic sclerosis, 26
Prolactinoma, 75, 80
Promethazine, 60
Prophylactic chemotherapy. *See under* Chemotherapy.
Propranolol, 44, 63, 65
Propylthiouracil, 35, 44, 99
Prospective studies, 239, 241

Prostaglandins
for ductus arteriosus patency, 15
for labor induction, 181, 182, 186
Prostate
disorders of, 138
malignant neoplasm of, 137–138, 221
screening for, 89
Prostate-specific antigen (PSA), 89, 137, 221
Prostatic hypertrophy, benign, 135, 138
Prostatitis, 125, 138
Protease inhibitors, 123
Proteinuria, 182, 218
Proteus infection, 111
Prussian blue, 35
Pseudoephedrine
adverse effects of, 37
for neurogenic bladder/incontinence, 222, 223
for priapism, 98
weight loss and, 177
Pseudogout, 53, 144
Pseudomembranous colitis, 36, 117
Pseudomenopause, induced, 74
Pseudomonas infections, 110, 111–112, 200
Pseudopregnancy, induced, 74
Psilocybin mushrooms, 93
Psoriasis, 20, 24
Psoriatic arthritis, 150
Psychalgia, 172
Psychiatric disorders, syncope or ataxia in, 172
Psychiatry
behavioral disorders and substance abuse in, 207–211
emotional disorders in, 211–215
general issues in, 215–216
Psychosis, 211
Pterygium, 193
Pulmonary edema, 9, 166
Pulmonary embolism (PE), 102, 228
cerebral embolism/thrombosis and, 167
chest pain in, 173
deep vein thrombosis and, 17
postoperative, 32
Pulmonary hypertension, 228–229
Pulmonary infarction, 228
Pulmonary tuberculosis, 233
Pulse, blood loss and, 41
Pulsus paradoxus in asthma, 226
Pupils
anomalies in function of, 197
brain death and, 136, 164
coma and, 169
Purified protein derivative (PPD) test, 233

Purpura
palpable, 26
thrombocytopenic, 102–103
Pus, fecal, 62
Pyelonephritis, 115, 183
Pyoderma gangrenosum, 26
Pyrazinamide, 233
Pyridostigmine, 170
Pyridoxine
as antidote, 34, 35
deficiency of, 55
isoniazid and, 36, 233
Pyrimethamine, 115, 123

Q
Quadrantanopia, homonymous, 196
Quality-of-life decisions, 134
Quantitative measurement, 237–240
Quetiapine, 212
Quinsy, 203

R
Rabies, 159–160
Radial nerve injury, 153
Radiculopathy, cervical, 144
Radiocontrast media, renal failure and, 219
Radioiodine scanning and ablation for
thyroid disorders, 43, 44
Radius, fractures of, 153
Rally pack for alcoholics, 216
Randomized clinical trials, 241, 243
Ranitidine, 35, 175
Ranson criteria for pancreatitis mortal-
ity, 70
Rape/crisis adjustment, 39
Rapid plasma reagin (RPR) test for
syphilis, 124
Rashes
amoxicillin, mononucleosis and,
111, 129
"bulls-eye," 119
malar, 142
pediatric infections with, 121–122
staphylococcal/streptococcal, 112
systemic disease-related, 25
Raynaud's symptoms, 104
Recall bias, 241, 242
Rectal prolapse, 59, 66
Rectocele, 74, 76
Rectosigmoid junction, malignant neoplasm of, 71
Rectum
gonococcal infection of, 125
hemorrhage of, 59, 62
neoplasms of, 71, 72
Reduction
of dislocations, 155
of fractures, 153
of hernia, 68

Reed-Steinberg cells, 104
Reflexes, brain death and, 136, 164
Reiter's syndrome, 150
Relative risk (RR), 239–240
Renal artery stenosis, 11
Renal calculi, 111, 120
Renal cell carcinoma, 217, 218
Renal colic, 220
Renal disease, hypertensive, 11
Renal failure
acute and chronic, 219
digoxin and, 36
thrombocytopenia and, 102, 103
Renal insufficiency, chronic, 219
Renal system, disorders of, 217–220
Reporting, guidelines for, 134, 135
Reproductive disorders, male, 137–140
Resource allocation, 134
Respirations, blood loss and, 41
Respiratory acidosis and alkalosis, 52
Respiratory distress syndrome, neona-
tal, 189, 190
Respiratory infections
acute upper, 202
candidal, 114
H. influenzae-related, 113
viral, 127, 128, 130
Respiratory problems, postnatal, 189
Respiratory syncytial virus infection,
128, 232
Respiratory system
general issues for, 225–231
infectious diseases of, 232–234
malignancy of, 234–235
surgical complications of, 32
Restrictive cardiomyopathy, 8
Retinal defects and disorders, 198
Retinal detachment, 32, 197–198
Retinitis, 115, 123, 130
Retinitis pigmentosa, 198
Retropharyngeal abscess, 231
Retrospective studies, 239, 241
Retrovirus infection, 128. *See also* HIV
infection/AIDS.
Rett syndrome, 209
Rewarming for frostbite, 28
Reye syndrome, 167
Rh IgG (RhoGAM), 182, 187, 190
Rh isoimmunization, hemolytic disease
and, 190–191
Rhabdomyolysis
drug-induced, 53, 93, 94, 95, 146
trauma-related, 152
Rhegmatogenous retinal detachment,
197
Rheumatic fever, 112, 150, 202
Rheumatic heart disease, 14
Rheumatoid arthritis, 143, 144
Rhinitis, 203, 226

Rhinovirus infection, 127
Ribavirin, 128
Riboflavin deficiency, 55
Ribs, fracture of, 153
Rickettsiosis, 118
Rifampin, 233
Rinne test, 201
Risk difference, 239
Risperidone, 170, 212
Ritonavir, 123
Rocky Mountain spotted fever, 119
Rofecoxib, 149
Romberg sign, 200
Roseola, 122
Rotator cuff disorders, 144, 149
Rotavirus infection, 59, 117
"Rouleaux" in Waldenström's hyper-
gammaglobulinemia, 104
Rubella, 121–122
congenital, 15, 190
pregnancy and, 116
vaccination for, 92, 187
Rubeola (measles), 121
Rupture of membranes, premature, 184

S
Sacral agenesis, 180
Sacroiliac sprain, 155
Salicylates, antidote for, 35. *See also*
Aspirin.
Salk vaccine, 158
Salmonella infection
diarrhea in, 59
food-borne, 33, 117
osteomyelitis and, 110
Sampling and sample size, 241, 243
Sanity, definition of, 135
Sarcoid, 26
Sarcoidosis, 196, 227
Sarcoma, Kaposi's, 124
Saw palmetto, 135, 138
Scabies, 22
Scalded skin syndrome, staphylococcal,
112
Scales of measurement, statistical, 238
Scalp wounds, 40, 41
Scar, hypertrophic, 22
Scarlet fever, 112
Schizoid/schizotypal personality disor-
ders, 212, 215
Schizophrenia, 211–212
Sciatica, 171
Scleroderma, 26, 142
Sclerotherapy, 17, 65
Scoliosis, 148
Scrapie (Creutzfeldt-Jakob disease), 159
Screening
antenatal, 90
breast cancer, 91

cardiovascular risk, 91
laboratory, 88–89
phenylketonuria, 52
prenatal, 186
routine child/infant, 88
Scrotal disorders, 139
Seasonal affective disorder, 213, 214
Sebaceous cyst, 24–25
Seborrhea, 21
Seborrheic dermatitis, 200
Seborrheic keratoses, 24, 26
Secondary malignant neoplasms. *See* Metastasis, neoplasm.
Secondary trauma survey, 38–39
Second-degree burn, 27, 28
Second-degree heart block, 3
Sedative/hypnotics, 35, 94
Seizures, 164
autistic disorder and, 209
cerebral palsy and, 165
drugs associated with, 36, 37
eclampsia with, 182
febrile, 168
intracranial neoplasms and, 165
Reye syndrome and, 167
Selective serotonin reuptake inhibitors (SSRIs), 37, 78, 212, 214
Selegiline, 162
Selenium deficiency, 55
Self-selection bias, 242
Semen analysis, 140
Seminoma, 138
Sensitivity, test, 240
Separations, joint, 154–155
Sepsis, 174–175
cutaneous signs of, 26
maternal, fetal demise and, 181
neonatal, 190
pneumococcal, 113
Pseudomonas, 111, 112
Septal defects, cardiac, 15
Septic abortion, 181
Septic (infective) arthritis, 149
H. influenzae-related, 113
pain in, 151
of shoulder, 144
Septic shock, 174–175
Septicemia, 99
Serotonin, antipsychotic drugs and, 212
Serous cystadenoma, ovarian, 84
Serum protein electrophoresis (SPEP) for immunodeficiencies, 54
Severe combined immunodeficiency, 54
Sexual abuse, 81, 207, 208
Sexual assault, 39
Sexual dysfunction, 208
Sexual practices, counseling about, 81, 82, 125

Sexually transmitted diseases (STDs), 123–126
cervicitis and, 80–81
orchitis or epididymitis and, 139
pelvic inflammatory disease and, 82
urethritis and, 222
Sézary cutaneous T-cell lymphoma, 26
Shampoos for seborrhea, 20
Shigella infection, 33, 59, 117
Shock
septic, 174–175
traumatic, 40–41
Shoulder
dislocation of, 154–155
disorders of, 144–145
Shoulder dystocia, 180, 188
Sickle cell anemia/disease, 98
erythema infectiosum and, 122
osteomyelitis in, 110
splenomegaly in, 64
SIGECAPS inventory for depression, 177, 213
Sigmoid volvulus, 58
Sildenafil, 37
Silver sulfadiazine, 28, 111
Simvastatin, rhabdomyolysis and, 146
Sinus tachycardia, 7
Sinuses, issues related to, 202–204
Sinusitis, 113, 203, 204
Sister Mary Joseph nodule, 26
SITS muscles of shoulder, 149
Sjögren's syndrome, 142
Skin
general disorders of, 19–22
infectious diseases of, 22
malignancy/tumors of, 23–25
systemic disease signs in, 25–26
Skin infections
bacterial, 111, 112
cellulitis or abscess in, 116–117
fungal, 114
local, 110
Skin sensitization tests, 19, 92
Skin tags, 26
Skull, trauma to, 39, 40
Sleep disturbances, 171
Slings for fractures, 153
Slipped capital femoral epiphysis, 147
Small cell cancer of lung, 234
Small intestine
diverticula of, 67
hamartomatous polyps in, 26
Smoking
lung neoplasms related to, 234, 235
management of, 93, 210
Snoring, 171
Sodium bicarbonate. *See* Bicarbonate.
Sodium imbalance, 51, 212
Sodium nitrite, 35

Somatization, 209
Somatoform disorders, 172, 209–210
"Spatula test" for tetanus, 157
Specificity, test, 240
Sperm analysis, 140
Spermatoceles, 139
Spherocytosis, 99
Spinal enthesopathy, 147
Spinal stenosis, 148
Spine
disorders of, 147–148
pain in, 151
trauma to, 40, 152
Spiral fractures, 154
SPIRE treatment for tuberculosis, 233
Spironolactone, 20, 78
Spleen, ruptured, 61, 100–101
Splenic sequestration crisis, 64
Splenomegaly, 64, 100, 129
Spondylosis, 147
Spontaneous bacterial peritonitis (SBP), 63, 68
Sprains, 152, 155
Sputum, blood-stained, 231
Sputum evaluation
for cough, 230, 231
for tuberculosis, 233
Squamous cell carcinoma
cervical, 75
cutaneous, 23
esophageal, 72
keratoacanthoma vs., 24
lip, oral, or pharyngeal, 206
lung, 235
vulvar, 83, 84
Squamous hyperplasia, vulvar, 84
St. Anthony's fire, 110
St. John's wort, 135
Standard deviation (SD), 238, 241, 243
Staphylococcal infections, 112
arthritis and, 149, 150
endocarditis and, 15
enteric, 117
impetigo and, 121
meningitis and, 160
methicillin-resistant, brain abscess and, 162
Statins, 12, 16, 36, 53
Statistical significance, clinical importance vs., 242
Statistics
hypothesis testing and inference in, 242–243
quantitative measurement in, 237–240
study design and, 241–242
Status epilepticus, 164
Steatorrhea, 62, 227

Steeple sign in croup, 232

Stents, complications of, 33

Sterilization, female, 89

Steroids

    for adrenal disorders, 49

    anabolic, adverse effects of, 37

    for asthma, 226

    for central nervous system trauma, 40

    for connective tissue diseases, 141, 142

    fungal infections and, 114

    hyperlipidemia and, 53

    for intracranial pressure reduction, 169

    for myalgia/myositis, 146

    for nephrotic syndrome/nephritis, 218

    for poisoning, 35

    for shoulder disorders, 144

Stevens-Johnson syndrome, 26

Stiffness, joint, 151

Still's disease, 150

Stomach

    neoplasms of, 72, 84

    ulcers of, 65

Stool

    abnormal contents of, 62, 227

    blood in, 59, 60

Strabismus, 196

Strains, 152

Strangulated hernias, 68

Streptococcal infections, 112

    arthritis and, 149

    endocarditis and, 15

    impetigo and, 121

    meningitis and, 160

    nephritis following, 218

    rheumatic fever and, 150

Streptococcal sore throat, 111, 112, 202

Streptomycin, 233

Stress

    acute, 213

    chorea gravidarum and, 169

    herpes simplex and, 205

    irritable colon and, 67

Stress incontinence, 222, 223

Stress test, 12, 91

Stridor, 231

Stroke, 167

    heat, 29

    transient cerebral ischemia vs., 166

    visual field defects in, 196

Struma ovarii, 44

Struvite renal calculi, 111, 220

Study designs, 241–242

Stye, 194

Subarachnoid hemorrhage (SAH), 166

Subdeltoid bursitis, 145

Subperiosteal hemorrhage, 189

Substance abuse, 92–96, 210–211

    male infertility and, 140

    weight loss and, 177

Sucralfate swish-and-spit, 129

Suicide, risk of

    bereavement and, 213

    depression and, 213, 214

    schizophrenia and, 211

Sulfa drugs, adverse effects of, 37, 99, 219

Sulfacetamide, 120

Sulfonylureas, 45

Superficial burn, 27

Supraventricular tachycardia (SVT), 7–8

Surfactant, 189, 190

Surgery

    cataract, 194

    complications of, 32–33

    for congenital anomalies, 180

    for ectopic pregnancy, 182

    outpatient, follow-up for, 88

    for pharyngeal neoplasms, 206

    for retinal detachment, 197

Sutures, 41, 42

Swallowing, impaired, 64

Sweet's syndrome, 26

Swelling, localized superficial, 21

Syncope, 172

Syndrome of inappropriate antidiuretic hormone (SIADH), 48, 52

    cerebral hemorrhage and, 166

    encephalitis and, 161

    intracranial neoplasms and, 165

    lung cancer and, 234

Synovitis, 145

Synovium, ganglion and cyst of, 145

Syphilis, 116, 124, 190

Systemic disease, manifestations of, 25–26

Systemic inflammatory response syndrome, 174–175

Systemic lupus erythematosus, 142. *See also* Lupus.

Systolic blood pressure

    blood loss and, 41

    hypertension and, 10

T

Tachycardia, 5, 7–8

Tacrine, 162

Tardive dyskinesia, 169, 212

Teeth, disorders of, 201, 205

Telangiectasias, 26

Temporal arteritis, 142, 146

Temporomandibular joint disorders, 149, 205

Tendinitis, shoulder, 144

Tendons

    ganglion and cyst of, 145

    strains of, 152

Tenosynovitis, 145

Tension headache, 168

Tension pneumothorax, spontaneous, 229

Terazosin, 10, 36

Terbinafine, 114

Terminal illness

    degree of disclosure for, 135

    palliative care for, 176

    quality-of-life decisions for, 134

Testes

    disorders affecting, 139–140

    torsion of, 61, 138

    tumors of, 138

Testosterone, 37, 140

Tetanus, 92, 157–158

Tetanus/diphtheria toxoid, 157–158

Tetracycline, 37, 117, 119

Tetralogy of Fallot, 15

Thalassemias, 98

Thalidomide, herpes and, 131

Thallium, antidote for, 35

Theophylline, antidote for, 35

Thiamine

    deficiency of, 55, 216

    for status epilepticus, 164

Thiazide diuretics, 10, 37, 220

Third-degree burn, 27, 28

Third-degree heart block, 4

Third-trimester bleeding, 183

Thoracentesis, needle, 38

Thoracic outlet syndrome, 144

Thoracic spine, pain in, 151

Thoracic trauma, 38, 40

Thoracostomy, needle/tube, 229

Throat

    emergencies related to, 30

    gonococcal infection of, 125

    issues related to, 202–204

    streptococcal infection of, 111, 112, 202

Thrombocytopenia, 102

Thrombocytopenic purpuras, 102–103

Thrombolytic therapy, 12

Thrombophlebitis, 17, 187

Thrombosis. *See also* Deep vein thrombosis (DVT).

    arterial, 16

    atrial fibrillation and, 2

    cerebral, 167

    coagulation disorders with, 102

    venous, 17

Thrombotic thrombocytopenic purpura (TTP), 102–103

Thrush, 114, 123

Thymus tumor, myasthenia gravis and, 170

Thyroid gland

    functional disorders of, 44–45

    malignant neoplasm of, 43–44

Thyroid hormone excess, antidotes for, 35

Thyroidectomy, 44
Thyroiditis, Hashimoto's or subacute, 44
Thyroid-stimulating hormone (TSH), 44, 45
Thyroxine (T$_4$), 44, 45
Tibia, fractures of, 154
Tick-borne illnesses, 118, 119–120
Ticlopidine, 166
Tics, 168–169
Timolol, 194
Tinea infections, 114
Tobacco use disorder, 93, 210
Tonic-clonic seizures, 164
Tonsillitis, 203
Tophi, 53
TORCH infections, 116, 190
Tourette syndrome, 209
Toxic shock syndrome, 112
Toxicology, 33–37
Toxoplasmosis, 115
    congenital, 190
    HIV/AIDS and, 123
    pregnancy and, 116
Trachea, foreign body in, 30
Tracheoesophageal fistula (TEF), 180
Trachoma, 120
Traction for fractures, 153
Tractional retinal detachment, 197, 198
Transfusions
    adverse reactions to, 101
    for anemias and thalassemias, 98
    for disseminated intravascular coagulation, 102
    for gastrointestinal hemorrhage, 60
    for idiopathic thrombocytopenic purpura, 103
    for Reye syndrome, 167
    for trauma, 40–41
    twin-twin, 184
Transient cerebral ischemia, 166, 167
Transjugular intrahepatic portacaval shunt (TIPS), 63, 65
Transplant organs
    allocation priorities for, 134
    harvesting, 136, 164
Transurethral resection of bladder/prostate (TURB/TURP), 138
Trauma, 38–42
    birth, 188–189
    hemolysis in, 99
    musculoskeletal, 152–155
    ocular, 32
    splenic, 100–101
Trauma center, transfer to, 38, 39
Traumatic shock, 40–41
Traveler's diarrhea, 59, 113, 117
Trazodone, 37
Tremor, 168–169
Treponema pallidum, 124

Tretinoin, 20
Trichinosis, 146
Trichomonal infections, 80, 81, 126
Tricyclic antidepressants (TCAs)
    abuse/overdose of, 95, 96
    adverse effects of, 214
    antidote for, 34
    for neurogenic pain, 46, 131, 171
Trigeminal neuralgia, 171
Triglycerides, high, 53
Triiodothyronine (T$_3$), 44, 45
Trimethoprim/sulfamethoxazole (TMP-SMX)
    for cat-scratch disease, 120
    for enteric infections, 33, 59, 117
    for general infections, 111, 113
    for *P. carinii* pneumonia, 123, 124
    for urinary tract infections, 116, 220
Triple H therapy for cerebral vasospasm, 166
Triple-void urine specimen for urethritis, 222
Trismus, 157
Trisomy, 179–180
Troglitazone, 45
Troponin I, 12
Tuberculin tests, 89, 92, 233
Tuberculosis
    chorioretinitis and, 198
    HIV/AIDS and, 123
    pulmonary, 233
    screening for, 92
Tumor lysis, prevention of, 107
Tumors. *See also* Malignancy; Neoplasms.
    androgen-secreting, 49
    dysphagia related to, 64
    skin, 23–25
    thymus, myasthenia gravis and, 170
    visual defects related to, 196
Turner syndrome, 180
Turner's sign, 26
Twins, management of, 184–185
Tympanic membrane, disorders of, 200
Type I/type II statistical errors, 242
Typhoid fever, 33, 59

U
Ulcerative colitis, 26
Ulcers
    decubitus, 20
    gastrointestinal, 61, 65
Ulnar nerve injury, 153
Ultrasound
    for abdominal pain, 62
    for ascites, 63
    for cholecystitis, 69
    fetal measurement via, 188
    for thyroid neoplasms, 44
Ultraviolet light for psoriasis, 20

Uncal herniation
    lumbar puncture and, 160, 162
    pupillary signs of, 169, 197
Undernutrition, 55
Unorthodox therapies, 135
Uremia, 171, 219
Ureter, calculus in, 220
Urethral stricture, 222
Urethritis, 125, 150, 222
Urge incontinence, 222, 223
Uric acid, gout and, 53
Uric acid calculi, 220
Urinalysis
    routine, 88
    for urethritis, 222
    for urinary tract infections, 115, 116
Urinary calculus, 111, 220
Urinary catheterization
    infection and, 111
    for neurogenic bladder, 222
    for stress incontinence, 223
    trauma and, 39
Urinary incontinence, 221–223
Urinary obstruction, 223
Urinary retention, 221–222, 223
Urinary tract infection (UTI), 115–116
    calculus-related, 220
    E. coli-related, 113
    postoperative, 33
    postpartum, 187
    pregnancy and, 183, 186
    Proteus or *Pseudomonas*, 111
Urine discoloration
    phenazopyridine and, 116
    rifampin and, 233
Urine output, blood loss and, 41
Urology, 221–224
Urosepsis, 115, 220
Urticaria, 21
Uterine bleeding, abnormal, 74–75, 79
Uterine contractions in labor, 185
Uteroplacental insufficiency, 186, 188
Uterus
    endometrial hyperplasia of, 73
    endometriosis of, 74
    gravid, measurement of, 186
    infertility related to, 80
    leiomyoma of, 82–83
    malignant neoplasms of, 82
    prolapse of, 74
Uveitis, Reiter's syndrome and, 150

V
Vaccination, 91–92
    chickenpox, 121
    hepatitis, 126
    measles, 121
    mumps, 128
    polio, 158

pre-splenectomy, 64, 100
rabies, 159
rubella, postpartum, 187
tetanus/diphtheria, 157–158
Vacuum-assisted delivery, 186
Vagal maneuvers for supraventricular tachycardia, 8
Vagina, malignant neoplasm of, 83
Vaginal birth
   multiple fetuses and, 185
   prehospital, 187
   trauma related to, 189
Vaginal birth after C-section (VBAC), 184
Vaginal walls, prolapse of, 76
Vaginismus, 76
Vaginitis, 81, 114
Vaginosis, bacterial, 81, 116
Valacyclovir, 125
Validity, study, 242, 243
Valproate/valproic acid, 35, 215
Valvular heart disease, 13–16
Vancomycin
   adverse effects of, 37
   for brain abscess, 162
   for *C. difficile*, 59
   for endocarditis, 15
   for meningitis, 160
   for pneumococcal infection, 113
   for pneumonia, 233
   for pseudomembranous colitis, 36, 117
   for staphylococcal infection, 112
Variability, statistical, 238
Variables, association between, 239
Varicella (chickenpox), 92, 121, 130
Varicella zoster, 116, 161, 190
Varicoceles, 139, 140
Varicose veins, 17
Vasa previa, 183
Vascular diseases
   types of, 16–17
   visual field defects and, 196
Vasculitis, 142
Vasopressin, 48, 51
Vasospasm, cerebral, 166
Venereal Disease Research Laboratory (VDRL) test, 124
Venous embolism/thrombosis, 17
Ventilation, positive-pressure, 38, 229
Ventral hernia, 68
Ventricular fibrillation, 5–6
Ventricular septal defect (VSD), 15
Ventricular tachycardia, 5, 8
Verapamil, 58
Vertebral fractures, 151, 152
Vertebroplasty, percutaneous, 152
Vertiginous syndromes, 200–201
Villonodular synovitis, pigmented, 145

Villous adenoma, rectal, 72
Viral infections, 126–131. *See also specific infection.*
   conjunctival, 120
   enteric, 117
   polyarthritis in, 150
   splenomegaly in, 64
Viral warts, 22, 128
Viremia, 101
Visual disturbances, 165, 195–196
Visual field defects, 196
Vital signs, blood loss and, 41
Vitamin B_1. *See* Thiamine.
Vitamin B_3. *See* Niacin.
Vitamin B_6. *See* Pyridoxine.
Vitamin B_{12} deficiency, 55, 97, 171
Vitamin deficiencies, 55
Vitamin E, atherosclerosis and, 16
Vitamin K
   for coagulopathies, 33, 70
   deficiency of, 55
   for warfarin overdose, 35
Vitiligo, 26
Voiding cystometrogram, 222, 223
Volvulus, constipation and, 58
Vomiting, induction of, 34. *See also* Nausea and vomiting.
Von Hippel-Lindau syndrome, 217
von Willebrand disease, 101–102
Vulva, malignant neoplasm of, 83–84
Vulvodynia, 76
Vulvovaginitis, 81

W

Waldenström's hypergammaglobuline-mia, 104, 105
Warfarin
   adverse effects of, 37
   antidote for, 35
   aspirin and, 36
   for atrial fibrillation, 2
   for cerebral embolism/thrombosis, 167
   pregnancy and, 183
   for pulmonary embolism/infarc-tion, 228
   for pulmonary hypertension, 228
   for thrombotic disorders, 102
   for transient cerebral ischemia, 166
   for venous embolism/thrombosis, 17
Warts, 22, 128
Water deprivation test for diabetes insipidus, 48
Water restriction
   for hypervolemic hyponatremia, 51
   for syndrome of inappropriate antidiuretic hormone, 48, 52
Weber test, 201

Wegener's granulomatosis, 142, 218, 219, 230
Weight gain
   abnormal, 176–177, 210
   pregnancy and, 186
Weight loss
   abnormal, 177, 210
   postnatal, 191
Weight training, 91
Wenckebach-type heart block, 3
Wernicke's aphasia, 172
West Nile virus/fever, 118
Western blot for HIV infection, 123
White blood cell count
   leukemia and, 105, 106
   sepsis/septic shock and, 174
Whitlow, herpetic, 125
"Whooping" cough, 117
Wilson disease, 162
Wiskott-Aldrich syndrome, 54, 200
Withdrawal, drug or alcohol, 94, 210
Wolff-Parkinson-White syndrome, 4–5
Women's Health Initiative study, 89
Wounds, 41–42
   bite, rabies and, 159
   burn, 28
   infections of
      postoperative, 33
      postpartum, 187
      Pseudomonas, 111

X

Xanthomas, 26
X-rays
   for abdominal pain, 62
   for bone/marrow neoplasms, 148
   chest
      for bronchial or lung cancer, 234, 235
      for bronchiolitis, 232
      for chest pain, 173
      for cough, 230–231
      for hypertension, 10
      for mediastinitis, 230
      for tension pneumothorax, 229
      for tuberculosis, 233
      for Wegener's granulomatosis, 230
   for croup, 232
   for dislocations/separations, 155
   for fractures, 148, 152, 153, 154
   for shoulder disorders, 144
   for trauma evaluation, 39, 40

Y

Yogurt, candidiasis and, 114

Z

Zidovudine, 123
Zinc deficiency, 55

NOTES